Atlas of Feline Anatomy
FOR VETERINARIANS

SECOND EDITION

LOLA C. HUDSON, DVM, PhD
Professor of Anatomy
North Carolina State University
College of Veterinary Medicine
Department of Molecular and Biomedical Sciences
North Carolina State University
Raleigh, North Carolina

WILLIAM P. HAMILTON, B.A., CMI
Fellow, Association of Medical Illustrators
Marquette, MI

T0273831

TETON NEWMEDIA
INNOVATIVE PUBLISHING OF VETERINARY & HUMAN MEDICINE
www.tetonnm.com

Executive Editor: Carroll C. Cann
Design and Production: www.fiftysixforty.com

Teton NewMedia
P.O. Box 4833
Jackson, WY 83001
1-888-770-3165
www.tetonnm.com

PRINTED IN THE UNITED STATES OF AMERICA

ISBN # 1-59161-044-3

Print number 5 4 3 2 1

Library of Congress Cataloging-in-Publication Data on file.

Contributors

Jill A. Barnes, DVM, PhD
Associate Professor of Anatomy
Department of Molecular Biomedical Sciences
College of Veterinary Medicine
North Carolina State University
Raleigh, North Carolina, 27606

William P. Hamilton, BA, CMI
Medical Illustrator
Fellow, Association of Medical Illustrators
Marquette, Michigan, 49855

Kristina E. Howard, DVM, PhD
Research Assistant Professor
Department of Molecular Biomedical Sciences
College of Veterinary Medicine
North Carolina State University
Raleigh, North Carolina, 27606

Lola C. Hudson, DVM, PhD
Professor of Anatomy
Department of Molecular Biomedical Sciences
College of Veterinary Medicine
North Carolina State University
Raleigh, North Carolina, 27606

Antonella Borgatti Jeffreys, DVM
Assistant Professor
Veterinary Clinical Sciences Department
College of Veterinary Medicine
University of Minnesota
St, Paul, MN 55108

Bonnie J. Smith, DVM, PhD
Associate Professor of Anatomy
Department of Biomedical Sciences and Pathobiology
Virginia-Maryland Regional College of Veterinary Medicine
Virginia Tech
Blacksburg, Virginia, 24061

Mary B. Tompkins, DVM, PhD
Professor of Immunology
Department of Population Health and Pathobiology
College of Veterinary Medicine
North Carolina State University
Raleigh, North Carolina, 27606

Cherie M. Pucheu-Haston, DVM, DACVD, PhD
Postdoctoral Research Associate
Curriculum in Toxicology
University of North Carolina - Chapel Hill CB #7270
Chapel Hill, NC 27599

David J. Waters, DVM, PhD, DACVS
Professor and Associate Director
Center on Aging and the Life Course
Director, Gerald P Murphy Cancer Foundation
Purdue University
West Lafayette, Indiana, 47907

Preface to the First Edition

"The cat is not a small dog" - unknown

This quotation succinctly states why we felt this book was needed. Although cats and dogs share many similarities as carnivores, they each have many unique characteristics. This uniqueness is important to veterinarians if we are to provide the best treatment to the animals in our care. The popularity of cats as pets has rapidly increased, but the pool of readily available information on veterinary medicine specific to cats has lagged behind. This is also true of scientific information on the anatomy of cats that is pertinent to clinical veterinary medicine. Certainly, anatomical information on felines is available if you know where to look. However, all too often, much of it uses archaic nomenclature, is inaccurate, or is tacked on as a paragraph at the end of a chapter or monograph on dogs. Even texts that state that they cover both dogs and cats do not consistently provide information on cats, so the reader is left wondering whether the material for the cat is the same as that for the dog, is unknown, or was just not included. Our frustration at not being able to find information or illustrations on cats led us to produce this atlas.

Most chapters in this text are not highly detailed; for example, the origin and insertion of every muscle in the feline body is not stated. We tried to place emphasis on those areas of anatomy that are frequently encountered in clinical medicine. Therefore, veterinary students may find this text more useful as an additional small animal anatomy text. Practitioners will find the illustrations useful in client education.

Readers will notice that the chapter on special senses is more detailed than other chapters. Because this information is quite difficult to find elsewhere in the literature, this greatly enhances the usefulness of this chapter.

The illustrations have been taken from original dissections, photographs, radiographs and are based on palpation by the authors or editors. We believe that they are accurate. However, should the reader find any inaccuracies in the illustrations or the text, we would appreciate notification for correction in future editions.

The nomenclature used is from *Nomina Anatomica Veterinaria* (with some rare exceptions) in order to bring feline anatomy in line with the terminology of current veterinary texts of other common domestic mammals.

This atlas, which was conceived of and proposed by William Hamilton and developed jointly with Lola Hudson, is a unique collaboration between medical illustrator and veterinary anatomist.

Lola C. Hudson
William P. Hamilton

Abbreviations

Throughout the text and figure legends, certain words are consistently abbreviated. In general, a single letter is used and denotes the singular form. Plurals are indicated by double letters. Other abbreviations or acronyms are defined with the first use in a chapter.

a., aa. artery, arteries

v., vv. vein, veins

n., nn. nerve, nerves

m., mm. muscle, muscles

ln., lln. lymph node, lymph nodes

Contents

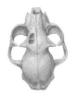

Chapter 1

General Information and Physical Examination

■ Lola C. Hudson

Modified from the original chapter by Jacqueline Bird and Lola Hudson

General Information

The "house" cat was fully domesticated at least by 1600 BC, after domestication of the dog. While a cat skeleton from some 9500 years ago was discovered in Cyprus, this was believed to be during the period of domestication. Most authorities cite Egypt as a location for domestication but a more exact place is not known. It is believed that domestication coincided with the invention of grain silos, and that the human need for rodent control and the cat's need for a ready food source resulted in a mutually beneficial, but still aloof, relationship.

The cat was deified in ancient Egypt, being worshipped as Bastet, the goddess of fertility - both human and agricultural. This special esteem of cats resulted in attempts to prevent their export from Egypt, but eventually domestic cats appeared in other areas of the Mediterranean. The domesticated cat is now found throughout the populated world and over 35 breeds have been developed, although not all breeds are recognized by all groups. The Cat Fanciers Association currently recognizes 37 breeds. An abbreviated list of breeds (Table 1-1) is included in this chapter.

The domestic cat has the scientific name of *Felis catus* (*F. cattus*), but has also been identified under the name *Felis domesticus* (*F. domestica*), as the taxonomy underwent changes in 1996. Cats belong to the family Felidae, which includes the "big cats," to the order Carnivora, and to the class Mammalia. Overall, the cat shows less variation in body size and skull shape than is seen among dogs, which suggests that there is a more uniform genetic makeup in cats. Nevertheless, relatively long-faced cats (Siamese), short-faced cats (Persian) and medium-faced cats (domestic short hair) are found among the various recognized breeds.

TABLE 1-1
Abbreviated List of Recognized Feline Breeds in the United States

Abyssinian*	Cornish Rex*	Oriental*
American Shorthair*	Devon Rex*	Persian†
American Wirehair*	Egyptian Mau*	Ragdoll†
Balinese†	Exotic*	Russian Blue*
Birman†	Havana Brown*	Scottish Fold*
Bombay*	Japanese Bobtail*	Siamese*
British Shorthair*	Korat*	Somali†
Burmese*	Maine Coon†	Sphynx (hairless)
Charteux*	Manx*	Tonkinese*
Colorpoint Shorthair*	Ocicat*	Turkish Angora†

*= shorthair breed, †= longhair breed

The pet cat population in the United States has steadily increased over the last decade. The American Veterinary Medical Association reports that there are more cats than dogs in USA households as the companion animal. Such numbers have influenced the interest of the veterinary profession as seen by the increase in numbers of feline-related seminars at various local, regional, and national professional meetings. This interest has also lead to a boom in textbooks and monographs on feline medicine and surgery for the veterinary profession or inclusion of more feline-related material in "small animal" textbooks.

Physical Examination

A good, thorough physical examination takes only a few minutes to perform but reveals a wealth of information to the veterinarian. In order to be efficient, the routine examination is performed systematically, concentrating on the same things in the same order. The precise order is not important as long as it is done the same way each time. The procedure then becomes second nature and the likelihood of overlooking something is minimized. As many of the examination procedures are irritating to many cats, becoming practiced at a technique is important. A large portion of a physical examination is based on palpation. Which structures are palpable in a normal cat is dependent upon the body condition of the cat and the skill and experience of the veterinarian. The following is one method of performing the physical examination.

First, the cat is removed from its carrier. If it can move about without escaping, the cat is observed walking, noting the mentation, posture and gait for balance and control, as well as its general attitude. Once the cat is placed on an examination table, the hair coat is checked for indications of self-grooming, for areas of alopecia and for ectoparasites.

Next, the head becomes the focus. The dorsum of the skull is palpated while noting the health of the hair and skin. Both eyes are examined for size, shape, and position. The upper eyelid can be retracted to observe the sclera and conjunctiva for color. The presence of a normal tear film is noted by the glistening appearance of the cornea. Using the upper eyelid for protection, each orb is gently pressed to roughly compare intraocular pressure. (This step can be substituted with the use of ocular pressure measuring devices such as a Tonopen®.) During this procedure, the third eyelid may move into clear view and be assessed. The corneas, irides, and pupils are checked for smoothness, clarity, and symmetry. With a strong light source such as a transilluminator, the pupillary light reflex of each eye is assessed. The clarity and uniformity of the lens is evaluated. The fundus is examined taking care to visualize the retinal blood vessels, tapetum lucidum, non-tapetal areas and the optic disc. Both lateral and medial commissures are gently touched to observe the palpebral (blink) reflex, assessing cranial nerve V (sensory) and cranial nerve VII (motor) function. Care is taken not to stimulate the tactile hairs or induce a visual menace response instead of a palpebral reflex by using the tips of closed forceps brought over the head, caudal to rostral. A menace response is elicited by a small, quick hand movement toward each eye or an up and down motion in front of the eye while blocking the view of the other eye. Care is taken not to stimulate any tactile hairs with either the hand or by air movement.

The ears are assessed for normal upright position. The pinnae are examined on the concave and convex surfaces, and the canals are checked for abnormalities. An otoscopic examination of the external auditory canal and tympanic membrane is performed. The hairs inside the pinna are gently touched to elicit a twitch assessing cranial nerve VII motor function to auricular muscles.

The skin and hair coat of the nose are examined. The paranasal sinuses and recesses of the skull are assessed for sensitivity by pressing firmly dorsal to each eye, ventral to each eye, and on each side of the nose. Both nares are examined for symmetry and discharge. Gently touching just inside the nares with closed, blunt hemostats elicits a strong aversive reaction, assessing cranial nerve V sensory function.

The hair and skin of the lips are checked as well as the tactile hairs. The symmetry of the lips is noted. Lifting the lips allows examination of the gums, including color, and teeth. Capillary refill time can be ascertained by pressing the gum with a fingertip to blanch out the blood and observing how quickly the area turns pink again. Gently opening the mouth affords a quick assessment of the teeth, tongue, tonsils, palate, and of jaw tone (cranial nerve V). While the mouth is open, pressure on the intermandibular area will elevate the tongue for a better view of the sublingual region, which should be checked for foreign bodies (especially string). The breath of the cat is smelled for a foul odor indicating infection or a sour odor indicating uremia or ketoacidosis. Careful palpation of the intermandibular space under the jaw and the region ventral to the opening of the external auditory canal allows assessment of the salivary glands and lymph nodes. Generally, these structures are not identified as separate entities, but the abnormal enlargement of any of them may be obvious on palpation.

The hair and skin of the throat area is examined next. The trachea is palpated along its full length, and then firmly rubbed to test for an abnormal cough response. At the dorsolateral junction of larynx and trachea, the thyroid glands should be palpated. Lateral to the trachea, palpation is performed the length of each jugular furrow checking for lumps or signs of discomfort. Next the wings of the atlas are palpated along with the rest of the cervical vertebrae. The muscles of the neck are massaged. The head is moved dorsally, ventrally and to each side to check range of motion in the neck and the oculovestibular responses. The thoracic inlet is palpated for lumps or sensitivity.

The hair and skin of the thoracic region is assessed. The muscular and the bony prominences of the forelimbs are palpated. Continuing down the thoracic limbs, each joint is moved through its full range of motion. Each paw is placed on its dorsum for the cat to replace properly (proprioceptive positioning). The pads and claws of each paw are checked.

The ribs are palpated and the rib cage is pressed to assess compressibility. The pattern and rate of respiration are noted. The location of superficial cervical lymph nodes and axillary lymph nodes are checked, although again, only abnormally large lymph nodes may actually be readily palpated.

Auscultation of the heart is performed on both sides just caudal to the thoracic limb (see Chapter 4 also). The normal heart rate is 118 ± 11 beats per minute for a resting, relaxed cat. In a hospital environment where they are likely to be more anxious and stressed, cats may have a mean heart rate of 182 ± 20 beats per minute.

Each lung field is auscultated in the triangular area of the lateral thorax caudal to the forelimb (see Chapter 7 also) and in the axilla region cranial to the heart. The entire lung field is not completely accessible due to overlying limb and epaxial musculature. The trachea is also directly auscultated in the ventral neck.

The respiratory rate is about 26 breaths per minute. Purring, which is unique to cats, occurs on both inspiration and expiration and can complicate pulmonary auscultation. (Sometimes, it can be very difficult to stop the cat's purring. Techniques that may stop purring include blowing on the cat's nose, gently tapping the cat's nose, and running water in a sink in the same room in which the cat is located.)

The hair and skin of the abdominal region is examined next. A flea comb is drawn through the hair coat, especially over the dorsal rump area checking for fleas, flea eggs, and flea dirt (feces).

In the abdomen, both kidneys are generally readily palpated caudal to the costal arch just ventral to the vertebrae, the right kidney being more cranial than the left. Usually, only the caudal pole of the right kidney can be palpated. The edge of the liver is normally detectable at the caudoventral limit of the costal arch. The full stomach is in the left cranial quadrant of the abdomen. The spleen may be palpable in the left, ventral abdomen cranial to the level of the umbilicus. The intestinal tract is palpated for smoothness, slipperiness, and size as loops of bowel pass between the fingers squeezing from dorsal to ventral abdomen. Frequently, feces can be detected in the descending colon. Abdominal masses in any location should be noted. The bladder is assessed in the caudal abdomen, checking for distention, wall thickness, and the presence of calculi. Palpation of the pregnant uterus is easiest at 21-25 days post breeding. The anus and external genitalia are examined for abnormalities.

Each hindlimb is palpated, as with the forelimb, moving all joints through full range, and assessing femoral pulses for rate and quality. The popliteal lymph nodes, located caudal to the stifle, are palpated for size and excess heat. Each paw is placed on its dorsum and the cat is allowed to replace it (proprioceptive positioning). The pads and claws of each paw are checked.

The vertebral column is palpated, pressing firmly between each dorsal spine. The tail should be stroked to detect abnormalities such as kinks. The ventral surface of the thorax and abdomen of the cat is felt giving particular attention to the sternum and xiphoid cartilage, mammary glands, and the superficial inguinal lymph nodes.

The cat's temperature should be taken. Normal body temperature in a healthy, relaxed cat is $38.5 \pm 0.5°C$ ($101.5 \pm 1°F$). Extreme agitation or excitement in a clinical setting may raise the temperature.

Sexual maturity of the female cat occurs in the first year, often at 6-7 months-of-age, in conjunction with the photoperiod. This relatively young age at puberty is a fact that surprises many neophyte cat owners. Queens are seasonally polyestrous from late winter to early autumn. The entire cycle is about 2 weeks long and the actual estrus (heat) lasts for an average of 7days. Coitus generally must occur for the queen to ovulate (induced ovulation) and pregnancy lasts for an average of 65 days. Abdominal palpation of pregnancy for number of kittens is best accomplished at 17-25 days of gestation and age of fetuses can be determined via serial plasma progesterone. Ultrasound after day 14 of gestation can also reliably determine pregnancy but numbers may

Plate 1-1

Major palpable structures of the normal cat, lateral view. In certain animals other structures such as individual muscles may also be identifiable. Some of labeled structures may not be identifiable in obese animals.

1   Thyroid gland
2   Frontal bone and its zygomatic process
3   Zygomatic arch
4   Maxilla
5   Mandible
6   Masseter m.
7   Larynx and trachea
8   External jugular v.
9   Cervical vertebrae
10 Superficial cervical l.n.
11 Dorsal border of scapula
12 Spine of scapula
13 Suprahamate process
14 Hamate process
15 Clavicle
16 Greater tubercle of humerus and its crest
17 Humeral condyle and lateral epicondyle
18 Proximal radius
19 Medial border of radius
20 Olecranon
21 Caudal border of ulna
22 Tendon of m. Flexor carpi ulnaris
23 Accessory carpal bone
24 Proximal and distal rows of carpal bones

25 Metacarpal bones II-V
26 Proximal, middle, and distal phalanges of digits II-V
27 Carpal pad
28 Metacarpal pad
29 Digital pads
30 Cephalic v.
31 Dorsal spines of thoracic vertebrae
32 Manubrium sterni
33 Sternum and xiphoid process
34 Ribs
35 Costal cartilages
36 Costal arch
37 Apex of heart (not palpable)
38 Auscultation triangle
39 Dorsal spines of lumbar vertebrae
40 Lateral epaxial muscles and transverse processes of lumbar vertebrae
41 Kidneys
42 Caudal border of liver
43 Stomach, when full
44 Loops of small intestine
45 Urinary bladder
46 Descending colon
47 Median crest of sacrum
48 Caudal vertebrae
49 Testis
50 Penis

51 Crest of ilium
52 Ischiatic tuberosity
53 Greater trochanter of femur
54 Lateral epicondyle of femur
55 Lateral collateral ligament of stifle joint
56 Fibula
57 Patella
58 Patellar ligament
59 Tibial tuberosity and crest
60 Cranial border of tibia
61 Lateral malleolus
62 Medial malleolus
63 Common calcanean tendon
64 Tuber calcanei
65 Tarsal bones
66 Metatarsal bones II-V
67 Femoral a. (On medial thigh)
68 Popliteal l.n.
69 medial saphenous v.

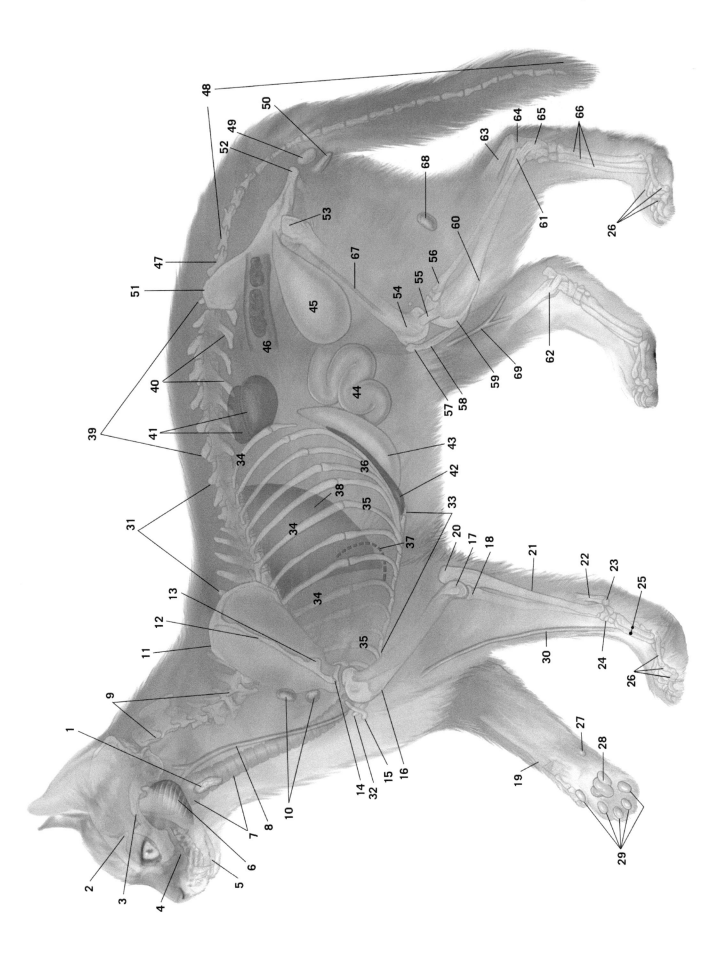

not be accurate. Radiography of the abdomen after day 45 can elicit more accurate numbers of kittens.

The male cat should have testicles descending at the perinatal period and be palpable at 6-8 weeks of age. By 6 months of age, if both testes are not located within the scrotum at all times, the cat should be considered a cryptorchid. Generally, toms will also reach sexual maturity during the second half of their first year.

Kittens are born with hair but with eyes and ears still closed. These structures open and are functional at 3-15 days. Forced weaning can be safely done at 7 weeks-of-age, if the kittens can eat and drink from a dish. If the dam is allowed to wean the kittens, she may allow nursing for several months.

The life span of cats has increased with improvements in veterinary care and nutrition. It is no longer unusual to have feline patients that are in their late teens and even into the early twenties.

Table 1-2 shows the complete blood count (CBC) and common electrolyte and enzyme values for the cat as determined by Clinical Pathology Laboratory of the North Carolina State University Veterinary Teaching Hospital (used with permission).

TABLE 1-2
Feline Hematology and Clinical Chemistry Reference Ranges

Tests		Units	Feline	Tests		Units	Feline
A/G	A/G Ratio		0.6-1.5	pO_2V	PO_2, Venous	mm/hg	30-73
AGAP	Anion Gap		15-32	SDH	Sorbitol Dehydrogenase	IU/L	1.3-8.7
ALB	Albumin	g/dl	3.0-4.2	TCO_2V	TCO_2, Venous		16.3-23.3
ALP	Alkaline Phophatase	IU/L	14-50	TP	Total Protein	g/dl	5.8-8.2
ALT	Alanine Aminotransferase	IU/L	28-88	TRIG	Triglyceride	mg/dl	24-206
AMM	Ammonia	μmol/l	8-52	ALY	Atypical Lymph., Absolute	$10^3/\mu$l	0-0
AMY	Amylase	IU/L	580-1520	ALY%	Atypical Lymph %	%	0-0
AST	Aspartate Aminotransferase	IU/L	16-42	APTT	Activated Partail Thrombo	secs.	10.9-18.1
BAP	Bile Acids	μmol/l	5-18	BAND	Band, Absolute	$10^3/\mu$l	0-0.1
BAP2	Bile Acids, Post 2 Hour	μmol/l		BAND%	Band %	%	0-1.0
BEA	Base Excess, Arterial		-2.0-2.0	BASO	Basophil, Absolute	$10^3/\mu$l	0-0.3
BEV	Base Excess, Venous		-3.9-5.1	BASO%	Basophil %	%	0-3
BILIT	Bilirubin, Total	mg/dl	0.1-0.3	EOS	Eosinophil, Absolute	$10^3/\mu$l	0.1-2.3
BUN	Blood Urea Nitrogen	mg/dl	15-41	EOS%	Eosinophil %	%	1.0-22.0
CA	Calcium	mg/dl	9.3-11.5	FIB	Fibrinogen	mg/dl	50-300
CL	Chloride	mmol/l	113-122	HCT	Hematocrit		32.8-49.8
CHOL	Cholesterol	mg/dl	93-304	HGB	Hemoglobin		10.9-16
CK	Creatine Kinase	IU/L	72-481	LY	Lymphocyte, Absolute	$10^3/\mu$l	1.000-7.400
CREAT	Creatinine	mg/dl	1.0-2.1	LY%	Lymphocyte %		7.0-54
GLOB	Globulin	g/dl	2.4-4.9	MCH	Mean Corpuscular Hemoglobin	pg	13.0-17.7
GLU	Glucose	mg/dl	71-182	MCHC	Mean Corp. Hemo. Concentration	g/dl	31.1-34.0
HCO_3	HCO_3	mmol/l	14-23	MCV	Mean Corpuscular Volume	fl	40.7-53.8
K	Potassium	mmol/l	3.5-5.1	MON%	Monocyte %	%	0-5
LD	Lactate Dehydrogenase	IU/L	49-274	MONO	Monocyte, Absolute	$10^3/\mu$l	0-0.7
LI	Lipase	IU/L	10-64	MPV	Mean Platelet Volume	fl	8.8-21.3
MG	Magnesium	mg/dl	1.8-2.6	PCV	Packed Cell Volume	%	28-45
NA	Sodium	mmol/l	150-159	PLT	Platelet	$10^3/\mu$l	198-434
Na/K	Sodium / Potassium Ratio		30-43	PLTM	Platelet, Manual	$10^3/\mu$l	198-434
C-OSM	Osmolality, Calculated		305-322	PP	Plasma Protein	g/dl	6.5-8.4
pCO_2A	pCO_2, Arterial	mm/hg	23-36	PT	Prothrombin Time	secs.	11.2-15.3
pCO_2V	pCO_2, Venous	mm/hg	25-38	RBC	Red Blood Cell Count	$10^6/\mu$l	6.91-10.49
pHA	pH, Arterial		7.26-7.46	RLY	Reactive Lymph Absolute	$10^3/\mu$l	0-0.2
pHI	pH, Ionized		7.340-7.540	RLY%	Reactive Lymph %		0-2
PHV	pH, Venous		7.26-7.44	SEG	Segmented Neutrophil, ABS.	$10^3/\mu$l	1.6-15.6
PHOS	Phosphorus	mg/dl	2.5-5.5	SEG%	Segmented Neutrophil %		37-83
pO_2A	PO_2, Arterial	mm/hg	78-100	WBC	White Blood Cell Count	$10^3/\mu$l	4.25-14.3

Courtesy of the Clinical Pathology Laboratory at the North Carolina State University Veterinary Teaching Hosptial.

Selected References

1. Beadle M. *The Cat.* New York, Simon and Schuster, 1977; 61-74.

2. Jones D. In: Birchard SJ and Sherding CG (Eds). *Saunders Manual of Small Animal Practice,* 3rd Ed. St Louis, Saunders Elsevier, 2006; 1.

3. Case, LP. *The Cat. Its behavior, nutrition and health.* Ames, Iowa, Iowa State Press, 2003; 1-11.

4. Feldman, EC and Nelson, RW. Canine and Feline Endocrinology and Reproduction, 3rd Ed. St Louis, Saunders Elsevier, 2004; 1016-1029, 1043-1044.

5. Kahn CM (Ed). *Merck Veterinary Manual,* 9th Ed. Whitehouse Station, NJ, Merck & Co., Inc. 2005; 2582-2583.

6. Hamlin R. Heart rate in the cat. *J Am An Hosp Assoc* 1989; 25: 284-286.

7. Hoskins JD. *Veterinary Pediatrics,* 3rd Ed. Philadelphia, WB Saunders, 2001; 1-7

8. Johnston SD, Root Kustritz MV, Olson, PNS. Canine and Feline Theriogenology. Philadelphia, WB Saunders, 2001; 396-405, 503-505.

9. Cat Fanciers' Association. <www.cfainc.org>

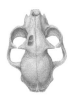

Chapter 2

Integumentary System

■ Cherie M. Pucheu-Haston

Modified from the original chapter by Diane Bevier

The integument (skin) of the cat has unique properties with regards to coat color, skin pigmentation, inflammatory response, and specialized integumentary structures. As is the case for many other species, skin and haircoat condition is often an indicator of general health or internal disease. However, research specifically focusing on the feline integument is less extensive than for some other domestic species.

The skin functions as an enclosing barrier, preventing the loss of such substances as water, electrolytes, and macromolecules. In addition, it prevents entry of exogenous matter, including potentially injurious chemicals, foreign material, and microbiologic agents. The flexibility and elasticity of the skin allow free motion while still maintaining this protective barrier. This protection and immunoregulation are provided in the main by the keratinocytes (epitheliocytes), intraepidermal dendritic cells (Langerhans' cells), dermal dendritic cells and cutaneous lymphocytes. The skin also produces its own antimicrobial coating (which is transported to the surface in sebum and sweat) and even uses the normal surface bacterial and fungal flora to protect against invading pathogens.

The skin is the source of both hair and claws, which provide protection against ultraviolet light, thermal extremes and predators. These structures also facilitate hunting by allowing the cat to blend in with its environment and efficiently capture prey.

The skin also plays an important role in endogenous temperature regulation, as its extensive vasculature facilitates the conservation or dissipation of heat. It functions as a reservoir for electrolytes, water, vitamins, fat, carbohydrates, proteins, and other materials. The skin is a primary sense organ for touch, pressure, pain, itch, heat, and cold. Lastly, the skin can function as an excretory organ to rid the body of unwanted or excessive substances.

Hair Coat
Coat Types

The short-haired cat is the fundamental "wild" type and this coat type is dominant. The longest primary hairs of a long-haired cat may be three times as long as those of a short-haired cat. Three types of hairs have been described in the cat based on gross appearance: (1) primary or guard hairs (thickest, straight, taper evenly to fine tip) (2) awn secondary hairs (thinner, possess subapical swelling below hair tip) and (3) down secondary hairs (thinnest, evenly crimped or undulated). Primary and secondary or undercoat hairs are medullated in the cat. The adult cat does not possess "lanugo" (nonmedullated) hair. In the classic coat types, secondary hairs are more numerous than primary hairs (10:1 dorsally, 24:1 ventrally). The guard hairs of normal cats may vary as much as four to five times in diameter at a given location.

Both primary and most secondary hairs are relatively straight and fine in cats. However, several atypical hair coat types (such as the curly coat in the Devon Rex and Cornish Rex, and the wire-hair coat seen in the American Wirehair breed) have been perpetuated as breed characteristics.

Rex cat breeds are the result of several distinct mutations with a similar phenotype. The two best known Rex breeds are the Cornish

Rex and the Devon Rex. Both have very short, wavy fur. The Cornish Rex appears to lack guard hairs completely, and has a very tight "wave" to the fur. In contrast, the Devon Rex has stunted guard hairs and less wavy fur. Despite their similar appearance the Cornish and Devon Rex breeds arise from two separate autosomal recessive mutations (Rex gene 1 and Rex gene 2, respectively). Even excellent specimens of both breeds tend to be very thinly furred on the head, ventral neck and chest, giving the appearance of pattern alopecia. Other Rex breeds include the Selkirk (plush curly hair, autosomal dominant mutation) and the LaPerm (long or short curly fur, autosomal dominant mutation). Closely related to the Rexes are the American Wirehair breed ("Wh" gene, autosomal dominant with incomplete penetrance) and the Sphynx breed ("hr" gene, recessive), which loses almost all of its fur by maturity.

Coat Distribution

Compared to most other domestic animal species, the cat's skin surface is almost completely covered in fur. The normal cat is thickly furred on all areas of the trunk, legs, neck and tail. Short but dense fur is present between the toes (both ventrally and dorsally), in the axillae, in the inguinal region, and throughout the perineal area (including the scrotum). Most of the head and face is also thickly furred, with the exception of the pinnae and the preauricular skin. These areas may be very thinly furred in even a long-coated cat, with skin easily visible through the sparse hairs.

Coat Growth

The hairs of the coat grow from follicles associated with the dermis. Hairs do not grow continuously, but rather in cycles. Each cycle consists of a growing phase (anagen) during which the follicle is actively producing hair, and a resting period (telogen) when the hair is retained in the follicle as a dead, or "club" hair that is subsequently lost. There is also a transitional period (catagen) between these two stages. Hair replacement in cats is asynchronously mosaic in pattern and predominantly responsive to photoperiod (although ambient temperature may play a contributory role). Cats in colder climates that spend significant periods outdoors will shed noticeably twice a year in the spring and fall. Normal indoor cats will shed all year long.

Hair follicle activity is maximal in the summer and minimal in the winter. In the summer, average hair growth is 289 μg/cm^2 skin/day (with approximately 70% of follicles in anagen at any time), while winter hair growth averages 62 μg/cm^2 skin/day. However, the average fur length is longer in the winter (30 mm for guard hairs and 15 mm for secondary hairs) compared to the summer (25 mm for guard hairs and 12 mm for secondary hairs). The average fur weight of a short haired cat is 19.9 g/kg, while the total yearly hair growth averages 32.7 g/kg.

Coat Colors

The heritability and variety of cat fur colors have long been a subject of fascination for cat fanciers and more recently, for geneticists as well. Careful breeding and observation have combined with modern genetic techniques to provide a detailed picture of the genetic landscape of feline coat color.

With few exceptions, the appearance of any given color and pattern is not a matter of simple "yes or no" genetic inheritance, but rather is the result of the interactions of multiple genes located on several different chromosomes. One of these exceptions is the completely white cat. The solid white ("W") phenotype is dominant over the phenotypes encoded by all other cat color genes. It is uncertain whether the W phenotype is the result of a separate gene, or if it is simply one allele of the gene that governs the presence of white spotting ("S"). Solid white cats with blue eyes are frequently deaf or hear poorly due to a variety of forms of cochlear degeneration.

The tabby gene ("T", chromosome B1) is associated with three striping patterns. The dominant Abyssinian allele ("Ta") codes for minimal striping, with darkly pigmented (eumelanin) hairs striping only the extremities, head and tail. The co-dominant Mackerel allele ("Tm") codes for the "typical" tabby striping pattern, with linear stripes of dark fur on the thorax as well as the head, tail and extremities. The recessive Blotched allele ("tb") codes for linear striping on the extremities, head and tail, but rounded, "blotchy" stripes on the thorax.

All cats carry one or more of the Tabby alleles, but expression of the striped tabby phenotype is dependent upon co-expression of dominant allele of the Agouti ("A") gene. This gene codes for agouti patterned fur-dark eumelanin bands at the base and tip of the hair, with a lighter pheomelanin band in the center. This light-colored pheomelanin banding is not seen if the cat is a homozygote for the recessive allele (the result of a two base-pair deletion of the ASIP gene), and thus the dark tabby stripes are not readily apparent.

Currently, the only known sex-linked cat color gene is the eumelanin-inactivating X-linked Orange ("O") gene. Female cats homozygous for the dominant O allele are orange in color, as are male cats carrying a copy of the dominant allele. Female heterozygotes (Oo) have areas of skin both with and without eumelanin inactivation and are tortoiseshell in appearance. They may be calico if one of the spotting gene alleles is also present.

TYR, the gene for tyrosinase, is located on chromosome D1. The dominant allele ("C") is seen in normally colored cats. Two sub-dominant alleles ("Cb" and "Cs") are associated with two distinct temperature sensitive mutations in the activity of tyrosinase and result in the Burmese and Siamese phenotypes, respectively. Cats homozygous for the third, recessive allele ("c" or "cc") are albino.

TYRP1, the gene for tyrosinase-related protein 1, is located on chromosome D4. This gene controls the "density" or darkness of eumelanin pigment. Cats carrying the dominant allele ("B") are black or have black stripes (if tabby). Cats carrying the sub-dominant allele ("b") are a chocolate brown, while cats carrying the recessive allele ("b1") are a cinnamon red.

Several other genes act as modifiers to the genes listed above. The dominant inhibitor of melanin gene ("I") inhibits pheomelanin, producing white hairs with eumelanin bands at the tips ("smoke" colored cats). The recessive allele of the melanophilin gene ("d")

produces a diluted phenotype (black to blue-grey; orange to cream) by causing clumping of melanin within the hairs ("maltese dilution"). Finally, the spotted gene ("S") can produce a mostly white cat (homozygous dominant; "SS"), a cat with a white belly and/or mittens (heterozygous; "Ss"), or a cat with no white spots at all (homozygous recessive; "ss").

Tactile Hairs (whiskers)

Tactile hairs (vibrissae) are substantially thicker and longer than normal guard hairs. The tactile hair follicle is surrounded by a fibrous capsule and is richly supplied with a venous (blood) sinus. In the walls of the venous sinus are nerve endings responsive to movement of the tactile hair, which is amplified by wave action of the surrounding blood (tactile bodies). Most tactile hairs are found on the face, principally on the upper lip and around the eyes, though others are scattered on the lower lip, chin, and elsewhere on the head and carpus. They are named according to location, e.g., pili tactiles labiales maxillares. The tactile hairs of the carpal region are found on the caudal antebrachium and carpus.

The slightest movement of tactile hairs, even by air currents, stimulates the nerve endings and provides information on the cat's immediate surroundings. The attached arrector pili muscles move the tactile hairs and the hair can be "put on the alert" when required.

Skin

Skin includes the epidermis, dermis, subcutis or hypodermis, the appendageal structures, vascular and nervous supply, and specialized glandular structures.

Pigmentation

In the cat, haired skin is only sparsely populated with melanocytes and melanin. Melanin is found mainly in the epidermis of the lip, pads, planum nasale, prepuce, scrotum, dorsal tail, pinnae, circumanal area, umbilical skin of the fetus and in the hair follicle bulbs. Dermal pigment and melanophages are rarely observed in normal cat skin, except for the scrotum.

Two body regions may develop pigmentation as they age. One is the sparsely haired preauricular/pinnal area. The other is the mucous membranes of the head. This pigmentation occurs most frequently in orange cats with the development of lentigo simplex. The condition often begins development at less than 1 year of age and progresses over time. Affected cats develop asymptomatic macular melanosis typically affecting the lips, gums, eyelids, and nose. Affected cats are at no apparent risk to develop other diseases, including melanoma.

Thickness and Surface of the Skin

The skin of the cat is quite pliable, especially over the neck and trunk. Skin over the dorsal neck and lumbar areas is normally slow to return to its original position when stretched and lifted. This must be kept in mind when attempting to assess hydration by skin tone.

The thickness of normal feline skin varies and decreases from dorsal to ventral regions on the trunk, and from proximal to distal regions on the limbs. The skin is thickest on the dorsal cervical, dorsal lumbar, and dorsal sacral regions; and thinnest on the scrotum and the lateral surfaces of the distal hindlimb, thigh, and distal forelimb. Maximal thickness (on the dorsal neck) has been recorded as 1.9-2 mm, while skin from the lateral thigh may be only 0.36-0.4 mm.

Microscopic, hairless, knob-like enlargements termed integumentary papillae or tylotrich pads are present in the haired skin of cats. These slow adapting mechanoreceptors are comprised of both epidermal and dermal components and are frequently closely associated with one or more hair follicles.

It has been suggested that the skin surface lipids of cats are mainly of epidermal origin (arising from the maturing corneocytes themselves) rather than of sebaceous gland origin. Feline skin surface lipids have been compared to human skin surface lipids. It was found that feline lipids are composed of more sterol esters, cholesterol, cholesterol esters and diester waxes and fewer triglycerides, monoglycerides, free fatty acids, monoester waxes and squaline than those of humans.

The pH of normal feline skin ranges from 5.6 to 7.4 (average about 6.5), which is somewhat less acidic than that of humans.

Microscopic Anatomy and Physiology
Embryology
Initially, the embryonic skin consists of a single layer of ectodermal cells over loosely arranged mesenchymal cells. In the 38-day-old fetus, the epidermis is about five cell layers thick without a stratum corneum and with a very cellular dermis. Aggregations of epidermal cells (the hair germs) project into the dermis at various intervals. These hair germs will form primary hair follicles. Sebaceous glands form as buds from the upper one-third of the developing hair follicle. Below this is another bulge that is the site for arrector pili muscle attachment. At 55 days gestation, the primary hair follicles contain well developed hairs, but secondary follicles may not have external hair shafts until after full term.

At the time of birth, the epidermis of the cat is about two cell layers thick and the dermis is packed with well developed primary hair follicles in anagen. A few days after birth the simple hair follicles are arranged in triads of a large central primary follicle bordered by two or three smaller follicles, which are producing secondary follicles. Subsequently, compound follicles are formed by buds produced from secondary follicles just below the level of the sebaceous glands.

Epidermis
The feline epidermis consists of four distinct layers in the areas of haired skin: the stratum corneum, stratum granulosum, stratum spinosum, and stratum basale. A fifth layer, the stratum lucidum, located between the stratum corneum and stratum granulosum, is present in the nonhaired areas of the pads and planum nasale. In general, the epidermis is thin consisting of two to three nucleated cell layers (about 12-45 μm). The thickest epidermis of the body is found on the pads and planum nasale (about 900 μm).

The epidermis of feline pads has a smooth surface, in contrast to the rough, papillated appearance of canine footpads. The pads and the planum nasale have prominent rete ridges (pegs). These rete ridges are not found in haired areas of normal feline skin.

The stratum corneum (horny layer) has a loose "basket weave" appearance on histopathological sections. This appearance is an artifact of fixation. The cells of this layer are flattened, anucleated, and eosinophilic when stained with hematoxylin and eosin. The thickness of this layer varies in areas of haired skin (3-20 μm), and the thickest layers are seen on the pads and planum nasale (15-35 μm).

Disease processes involving the stratum corneum usually cause increases in the thickness due to increased layers of keratinocytes. This increased thickness is termed hyperkeratosis, which may be subdivided into hyperkeratotic hyperkeratosis (in which keratinocyte nuclei are not retained) and parakeratotic hyperkeratosis (in which keratinocyte nuclei are retained, giving the hyperkeratotic layers a "stippled", somewhat basophilic appearance). The most common clinical syndromes causing hyperkeratosis include the scaling seen with dermatophyte invasion, infestation with surface feeding *Cheyletiella* sp. mites, and xerosis (dryness) of the skin (frequently seen in cats in the wintertime due to low-humidity indoor heating).

The stratum lucidum (clear layer) can be found in the pads and planum nasale, but not in haired skin. It consists of anuclear, homogeneous, hyaline-like material containing refractile droplets (eleidin). There are several layers of these translucent, poorly staining cells. Keratohyaline granules are not visible in these cells.

The stratum granulosum (granular layer) consists of flattened, basophilic, elliptical, or spindle shaped cells with shrunken nuclei and basophilic keratohyalin granules in the cytoplasm. This layer is usually one to two cells thick in haired skin areas except around hair follicle openings where it is often two to four cells thick. It is best developed in the pads and the planum nasale, where it may be 4 to 8 cells thick.

The stratum spinosum (prickle cell layer; spinous cell layer) consists of the daughter cells of the stratum basale. These are nucleated, lightly basophilic, and polyhedral to flattened cuboidal shaped cells. In haired skin this layer is one to two cells thick. The stratum spinosum becomes much thicker at the pads, planum nasale and at mucocutaneous junctions. The keratinocytes of the stratum spinosum are connected by intercellular bridges (desmosomes) that are more prominently visible in nonhaired skin. Ultrastructurally, keratinocytes are characterized by tonofilaments (keratin filaments) and desmosomes.

The stratum basale (basal layer) is a single row of columnar to cuboidal cells resting on the basement membrane zone that separates the epidermis from the dermis. There are three major cell types in this layer: the basal epitheliocytes, melanocytes and intraepithelial macrophages.

The basal epitheliocytes are actively reproducing, and their progeny push upward to replenish the more superficial layers of epidermal cells. The basal cells are nucleated and basophilic and range in shape from slightly flattened to cuboidal or columnar. Mitotic figures (representing actively dividing cells) may be present.

Melanocytes, which are rare in feline haired skin, are derived from neural crest. Melanocytes do not stain readily with hematoxylin and eosin and undergo artefactual cytoplasmic shrinkage during tissue processing. Therefore, they appear as "clear cells" in the stratum basale. Special staining procedures demonstrate their long cytoplasmic extensions (dendrites) that weave among the epitheliocytes. Where melanocytes are present, there is generally one melanocyte for every 10-20 basal cells. Melanocytes are responsible for production and transfer of melanin to a number of epitheliocytes, which together comprise the "epidermal melanin unit."

Intraepidermal macrophages (Langerhans cells) have a round cytoplasm with long dendrites extending between keratinocytes. Like melanocytes, these cells do not stain well with hematoxylin and eosin, and may appear as intercellular vacuoles or "clear cells". These cells are important antigen-capturing and –presenting cells, and increase in number in the face of active allergic inflammation. Immunohistochemical staining has demonstrated that these cells are recognized by antibodies specific for CD18, major histocompatibility class II (MHC II) molecules, CD4 and CD1a. Feline intraepithelial macrophages also possess intracellular structures analogous to human Birbeck's granules, in contrast to similar cells in the dog.

The basement membrane zone is the physiochemical interface between the epidermis and dermis. The basement membrane zone is thin and indistinct on stained sections in areas of haired skin. The zone is important not only in anchoring the epidermis and the dermis, but also plays important roles with regards to barrier function, epidermal nutrition, wound healing and maintaining tissue architecture. This layer is primarily of epidermal origin.

Dermis (Corium)

Because the cat has no rete ridges and dermal papillae in areas of haired skin, there is no clear division between the more superficial (papillary) and deep (reticular) dermis. The dermis is composed of collagen, elastic and reticular fibers, interstitial ground substance, nervous tissue, blood vessels, lymphatics, arrector pili muscles, and various cellular elements.

The superficial dermis is composed of fine, eosinophilic collagen fibers that are mostly parallel to the epidermis and interlace near the dermo-epidermal junction, as well as a network of fine elastic fibers. The collagen fibers have great tensile strength, and are larger than the elastic fibers. They account for the majority of dermal fibers and comprise most of the dermal extracellular matrix. Elastic fibers are composed of fine branches and single fibers that possess great elasticity and account for only a small portion of the dermal extracellular matrix.

The deep dermis consists of dense, irregularly arranged collagen fibers that are about three times larger than those of the super-

ficial dermis. These fibers parallel the skin surface and also encircle hair follicles. Elastic fibers of the deep dermis are thicker and less numerous than those of the superficial dermis. In general, collagenous bundles are smaller and more loosely arranged in areas of skin with particularly high flexibility (such as the interscapular region).

The normal feline dermis contains fibroblasts, mast cells, occasional mononuclear leukocytes (including CD4+ T cells) and, rarely, neutrophils or eosinophils. Cats with dermatitis may have increased numbers of intraepithelial macrophages / dendritic cells, mast cells and eosinophils (as well as CD4+ and CD8+ T cells) in the dermis, and often in the epidermis as well.

The ground (interstitial) substance of the dermis is a mucoid gel-sol of fibroblast origin composed of proteoglycans, dermatan sulfate, and chondroitin sulfates. This provides support and nutrients for the dermal appendageal structures including the hair follicles, sebaceous glands, apocrine, and eccrine sweat glands, arrector pili muscles and the dermal vasculature and nerves. Small amounts of mucin (a granular to stringy appearing substance which stains blue with hematoxylin and eosin) are often seen in normal feline skin, especially around appendages and blood vessels.

Subcutis

The subcutis (hypodermis) is composed of thick bands of collagen fibers and abundant, smaller elastic fibers that interweave and enclose fatty adipose tissue. Inflammation of the subcutaneous fat can occur in cats on diets of red tuna fish, other fish diets, various canned foods and excessive amounts of cod liver oil. The etiology of this syndrome involves deficiency of vitamin E and its antioxidant property. This disorder is termed pansteatitis or yellow fat disease and causes painful subcutaneous nodules. Other causes of subcuticular inflammation (panniculitis) include infections with bacteria, actinomycetes, fungi or mycobacteria, injection of foreign substances, trauma, pancreatitis and vascular inflammation.

Hair Follicles

A hair follicle is the hair and the immediate surrounding structures. There are five major portions to the feline hair follicle: the dermal hair papilla, the hair matrix, the hair, the inner epithelial root sheath and the outer epithelial root sheath, which is an extension of the epidermis. The cells of the hair matrix give rise to the hair shaft and the inner root sheath.

The hair follicle generates a cone-shaped epidermal hair bulb that defines the limit of the dermal papilla. The dermal papilla may induce growth and regulate differentiation within the hair matrix.

The hair shaft is divided into medulla, cortex, and cuticle. The medulla is the innermost region of the hair and is composed of a cord of longitudinal rows of cuboidal cells, or cells flattened from proximal to distal regions. The cells are solid near the hair root, but the rest of the medulla contains air and glycogen vacuoles. The cortex is the middle layer of the hair. It consists of completely cornified, spindle-shaped cells, whose long axis is parallel to the hair shaft. These cells contain the pigment that gives the hair its color. The cuticle, the outermost layer of the hair, is formed by flat, cornified, anuclear cells, arranged like slate tiles on a roof, the free edge of each cell facing the free end of the hair. In the cat, the profile of the hair shaft is distinctly serrated. Secondary hairs have a narrower medulla and a more prominent cuticle than do primary hairs.

Secondary hairs are arranged in clusters of two, three, four, and five groups around a large, central, primary hair. Each peripheral group of hairs usually contains three smaller primary hairs, surrounded by 6 to 12 secondary hairs. Twelve to 20 hairs may emerge from a common opening. Central primary hairs may have their own sebaceous glands, apocrine sweat glands, and arrector pili muscles, while smaller primary hairs and secondary hairs usually share common glands and arrector pili muscles.

Sebaceous Glands

Sebaceous glands are holocrine glands producing sebum and show a characteristic simple alveolar structure. Two or three glandular units empty via ducts into the upper portion of the hair follicle around which they are clustered. Sebaceous lobules are bordered by a basement membrane zone, upon which sits a single layer of deeply basophilic basal cells ("reserve" cells). These cells become progressively more lipidized and eventually disintegrate to form sebum toward the center of the lobule. Sebaceous glands in most haired skin average 20-75 μm in diameter, but glands as large as 700 μm may be seen on the lips and the dorsal surface of the tail.

Sebum is an oily secretion that keeps the skin soft and pliable and gives the hair shafts their glossy sheen. During periods of illness or malnutrition, the haircoat may become dull and dry as a result of inadequate sebaceous secretions. In contrast, hyperactivity of these glands or abnormal secretions may result in or complicate the pathologic conditions of feline acne and stud tail.

The sebaceous glands of the lips and face are numerous and larger than in other regions. Other areas of increased numbers of these glands in feline skin include the chin, which has oval clusters of glands (submental organ), dorsal aspect of the tail (supracaudal organ, preen gland), and the scrotum. Sebaceous glands are not found in pads or the planum nasale.

Apocrine Sweat Glands

Apocrine sweat glands are coiled or saccular, and are distributed throughout all haired skin. These glands range from 15-35 μm in diameter and consist of a single row of flattened to columnar epithelial (secretory) cells and a layer of fusiform myoepithelial cells. The glands are located deep to the sebaceous glands but open through a duct into the canal of the hair follicle superficial to the sebaceous duct opening. Apocrine glands are not present in pads or planum nasale. They are largest and most numerous near mucocutaneous junctions, in interdigital spaces, and over the dorsal neck, and rump. Large (45-110 μm) saccular apocrine glands may be found on the dorsal tail in the supracaudal organ. Hyperfunction of these glands and the associated large sebaceous glands may result in the buildup of waxy, greasy debris ("stud tail").

Eccrine Sweat Glands

Eccrine sweat glands are small, tightly coiled merocrine glands which found only in the pads. They consist of a layer of cuboidal to columnar epithelial cells and a layer of fusiform myoepithelial cells. The excretory duct opens directly to the pad surface. These glands have both adrenergic and cholinergic innervation. They may secrete when the cat is hot or frightened, and may play a role in scent marking.

Feline eccrine sweat is hypertonic, alkaline in pH, and contains high concentrations of sodium, potassium and chloride.

Arrector Pili Muscles

Arrector pili muscles are smooth muscle, and contain intracellular and extracellular vacuoles. Each originates in the superficial dermis and inserts on a bulge of the central, primary hair follicle. These muscles are smaller in diameter than the central primary hair follicle with which they are associated. They are present in all haired skin areas, being most highly developed in the dorsal lumbar, sacral and tail regions. Contraction of this muscle is involuntary and may be stimulated by a low ambient temperature. This results in erection of the hair from its normally oblique posture; when this happens to hairs en masse, the thickened pile traps more air and improves the insulation of the body. A similar effect occurs in the "flight or fight" reaction mediated by the sympathetic nervous system; the pronounced response by the hairs of the neck and back raises the "hackles" that give an animal a threatening appearance. Contraction of these muscles also helps express the sebaceous glands.

Senile changes of the Feline Integument

Certain histologic changes are often encountered in the skin of normal cats that have reached approximately nine or ten years of age. Variable degrees of hyperkeratosis and follicular keratosis are common. Granular, fragmented collagen fibers may be seen. Follicles and sebaceous glands may become atrophic. Sebaceous glands may look vacuolated. Occasional arrector pili muscles may appear fragmented, more vacuolated, and eosinophilic than normal.

Blood Vessels

Blood vessels to the dermis are arranged in three distinct intercommunicating plexi of arteries and veins: the deep (subcutaneous), middle (cutaneous) and superficial (subpapillary) plexi. Simple cutaneous arteries emerge from the fascial planes between underlying muscle masses to supply the deep plexus primarily. Mixed cutaneous arteries supply the muscle mass and eventually terminate in the deep plexus.

The deep plexus is found at the interface of the dermis and subcutis. Branches from this plexus descend into the subcutis, and ascend to supply the lower portion of the hair follicle and the apocrine sweat glands. These vessels continue their ascent to feed the middle plexus that lies at the level of the sebaceous glands. Branches from the middle plexus supply the arrector pili muscles, the middle portions of the hair follicles, sebaceous glands and

supply ascending branches to feed the superficial plexus. Capillary loops emanate from the superficial plexus and are arranged parallel to the skin surface. These vessels supply the epidermis and superficial portions of the hair follicles.

Lymphatic Vessels

Lymphatic vessels are infrequently seen in routine histologic preparations of normal cat skin. They arise from capillary networks, which lie in the superficial dermis and surround the adnexae. These vessels drain into a subcutaneous lymphatic plexus. In edematous or inflamed skin, lymphatic vessels may occasionally be seen as distended, thin walled vessels which are usually lined by a single row of elongated cells.

Nerves

The nerves to the skin are a mixture of motor and sensory nerve fibers. In addition to the important function of sensory perception (touch, heat, cold, pressure, pain and itch), the dermal nerves promote survival and proper functioning of the epidermis ("trophic influences"). Postganglionic neurons of the sympathetic nervous system innervate the smooth muscle walls of the cutaneous blood vessels, the arrector pili muscles, and the myoepithelial cells associated with the sweat glands. The majority of the nerves to the epidermis and dermis are sensory neurons. On the basis of the properties of afferent units, sensory activity in skin can be subdivided into mechanoreceptors, thermoreceptors, and nocioceptors.

Mechanoreceptors in feline hairy skin have been classified as: (1) "rapidly adapting mechanoreceptors" (Pacinian corpuscle, hair follicle receptors), (2) "slowly adapting mechanoreceptors" (tylotrich pad, Ruffini endings), (3) tactile hairs, and (4) nonmyelinated mechanoreceptors.

Nocioceptors are involved in itch and pain perception. Nocioceptors are supplied by A δ fibers (myelinated) and C fibers (nonmyelinated). Proteolytic enzymes, substance P, and vasoactive intestinal peptide have all been demonstrated in the skin of the cat. All are known to be mediators of pruritus in other species.

Plate 2-1

Figure A   Particolored cat showing several coat types and coat colors
Figure B   Schematic illustrations of histological layers of integument
Figure C   Schematic illustration of tactile hair.

1-3 Coat Types
    1   Short hair coat
    2   Rex (curly) coat
    3   Long hair coat

4-6 Coat Color Pattern
    4   Mackerel (tabby)
    5   Abyssinian
    6   Self colored

  a   Epidermis
  b   Dermis
  c   Subcutis
  7   Primary hair
  8   Secondary hairs
  9   Area of sebaceous gland
10   Apocrine sweat gland

11   M. Arrector pili
12   Nerve fiber
13   Cutaneous vessels
14   Tactile hair
15   Fibrous capsule
16   Venous sinus
17   Sensory nerve fibers
18   External root sheath
19   Hair papilla

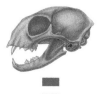

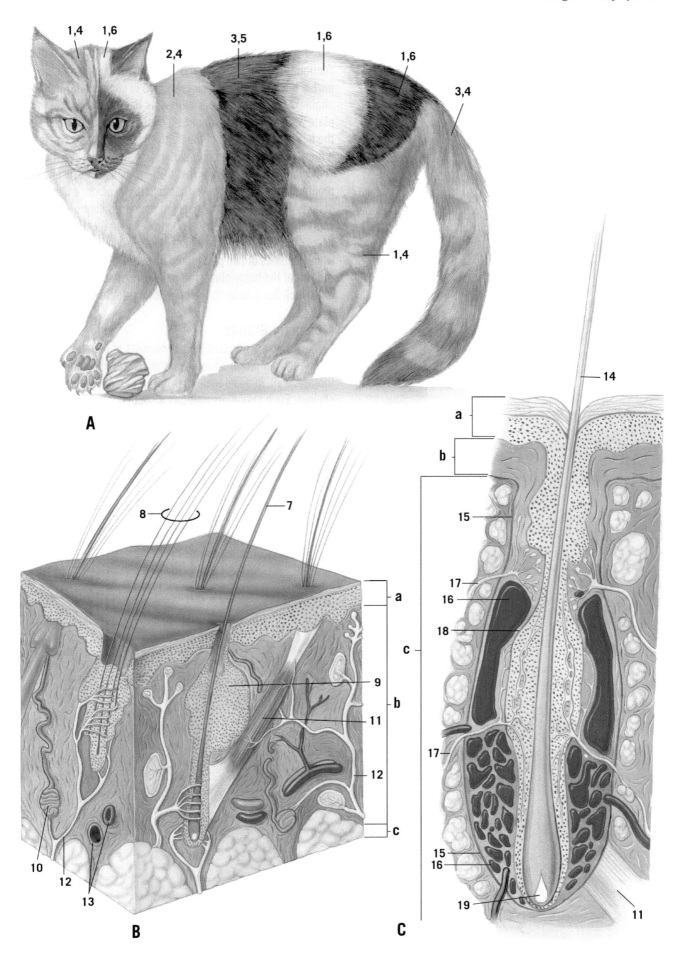

A

B

C

Specialized Integumentary Structures
Pads

The pads (tori) of cats are highly cornified, thickened, highly pigmented, hairless portions of the skin on which cats walk. In the cat digital, metacarpal, and metatarsal pads make ground contact. There is also a carpal pad (which does not normally contact the ground) but no corresponding tarsal pad. The epidermis of pads is the thickest of the body and consists of all five epidermal layers. The surface of the stratum corneum of the pads is smooth in the cat. The dermis of the pad shows prominent dermal papillae interdigitating with epidermal pegs. Very pronounced cushions of adipose tissue are present in the pads and sole that serve as shock absorbers. Sweat glands (eccrine glands) are present.

Planum Nasale

The planum nasale (see Chapter 7 also) is composed of a thickened and highly cornified epidermis devoid of sebaceous and tubular glands. Dermal papillae and rete ridges are found here, as are all five layers of epidermis.

Claw

The claw is a specialized cutaneous structure that is a direct continuation of the dermis and epidermis. The most prominent part is the horny nail, which is shaped to complement the distal phalanx. The epidermis is modified as the hard, resistant horn plate while the corium supplies a connective tissue support for the horn plate. The bed of the horny plate consists of two parts, a proximal coronary bed and a distal, more extensive plate bed. The coronary bed compromises the germinative matrix and it has proliferative epidermal cells that constantly produce new growth of horn. The plate bed is an area of increased dermo-epidermal contact which strengthens the bond between the nail and the deeper tissues. There is a fold of skin surrounding the claw cone which consists of two parts. Dorsally is the claw fold which covers the root of the horny plate. The palmar or plantar part is the digital pad which lies caudal to the horny sole (see Chapter 3 also).

Mammary Glands

The mammary gland of the cat consists of paired mammae (generally four pairs) situated on the ventral abdominal and thoracic wall. In some male cats only a pair of inguinal teats are obvious. Each mammary unit has a small conical teat, which has a moderate epidermal thickness, with dermal papillae and rete pegs. The dermis possesses abundant collagen and elastin fibers intertwined with smooth muscle fibers.

The skin of the teats is covered by fine hairs and has large sebaceous and sweat glands. Four to seven teat canals can be identified on each teat. These openings continue inside the teat as the teat sinuses, which run obliquely towards the center of the teats. The lactiferous ducts run in parallel from the sinuses and arborize into interglandular ducts, which are lined by a double stratified layer of cuboidal to columnar cells overlying a myoepithelial cell layer. These interglandular ducts then enter the glandular parenchyma (secretory lobules). The secretory lobules are formed by tubuloacinar glands and intraglandular ducts. Both structures are lined by cuboidal epithelium on the luminal surface, and flattened myoepithelial cells basally.

Vascularization of the feline mammary gland is from the branches of the cranial superficial epigastric and caudal superficial epigastric arteries and veins and the lateral thoracic arteries and veins. Innervation is derived from the genitofemoral and intercostal nerves. The caudal and cranial mammae are drained by the superficial inguinal and accessory axillary lymph nodes, respectively. However, drainage to the sternal cranial lymph nodes has also been described.

Mastitis in the queen is usually associated with parturition and lactation although occasionally it may be secondary to juvenile mammary gland fibroadenomatous hyperplasia. The most common bacteria causing acute mastitis in queens are staphylococci, streptococci, and coliforms. The organisms are usually introduced through teat fissures rather than by hematogenous or lymphatic routes.

Although mammary tumors are more common in the dog, approximately 80-96% of feline mammary tumors are classified as malignant. These tumors show profoundly aggressive behavior.

Anal Sacs

The anal sacs (sinus paranalis) of the cat are spherical or ovoid structures located in lateral position between the internal and external anal sphincters.

Anal sacs are lined by a smooth, keratinized, stratified squamous epithelium that is perforated by the efferent ducts of sebaceous and apocrine tubular glands. The efferent ducts of the anal sacs are narrow and terminate at the transition between the anus and skin. The anal sacs are surrounded by both smooth and striated muscles which expel the sero-fatty, unpleasant smelling secretion. The scent is utilized for scent marking and individual recognition. Anal sacs rarely cause clinical disease in the cat.

Plate 2-2

Figure A   Mammary gland of non-lactating (top) and lactating (bottom) queen with magnification of papilla (nipple) and sagittal section of papilla

Figure B   Schematic illustration of cutaneous vessels

Figure C   Tori (pads) of thoracic limb (left) and pelvic limb with schematic illustration of histological layers

Figure D   Location of anal sacs in relation to anus, caudal view

1	Caudal thoracic mamma	b	Dermis
2	Cranial abdominal mamma	c	Subcutis
3	Caudal abdominal mamma	11	Dermal papilla
4	Inguinal mamma	12	Superficial plexus
5	Papilla	13	Middle plexus
6	Ostium papillare	14	Deep plexus
7	Papillary duct	15	Carpal pad
8	Caudal superficial epigastric a., v.	**16**	Metacarpal pad
9	Cranial superficial epigastric a., v.	**16'**	Metatarsal pad
10	Lateral thoracic a., v.	17	Digital pads
a	Epidermis	18	Eccrine sweat gland
a'	Stratum basale	19	Anus
a"	Stratum lucidum	20	Paranal sinus (anal sac)
a'''	Stratum corneum	**20'**	Its duct

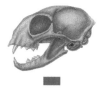

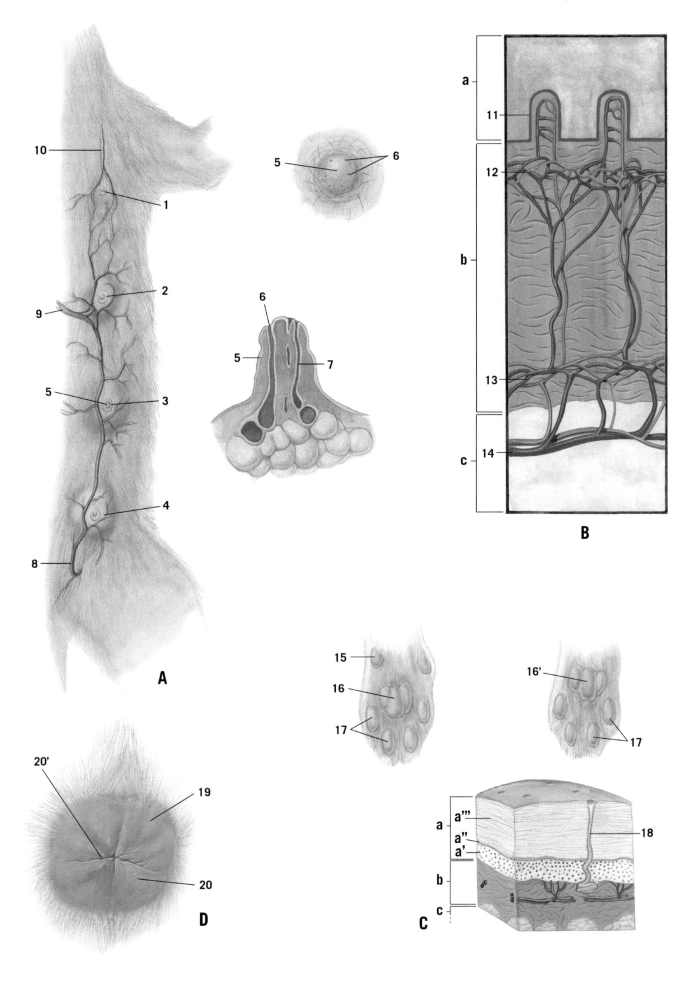

Selected References

1. Al-Bagdadi FK. The integument. In: Evans, HE (Ed). *Miller's Anatomy of the Dog.* 3rd Ed. Philadelphia, WB Saunders, 1993: 98.

2. Banks WJ. Integumentary system. *Applied Veterinary Histology.* 3rd Ed. St Louis; Mosby Year Book, 1993: 298.

3. Cooper MP, et al. White spotting in the domestic cat (Felis catus) maps near KIT on feline chromosome B1. Anim Genet 2006: 37; 163.

4. Grahn RA, et al. Localizing the X-linked orange colour phenotype using feline resource families. Anim Genet 2005: 36; 67.

5. Helgren JA. *Rex cats: everything about purchase, care, nutrition, behavior and housing.* Hauppauge, NY, Barron's Educational Series, 2001.

6. Hendriks WH, Tarttelin MF and Moughan PJ. Seasonal hair growth in the adult domestic cat (Felis catus). *Comparative Biochemistry and Physiology.* 1997: 116; 29.

7. Ishida Y, et al. A homozygous single-base deletion in MLPH causes the dilute coat color phenotype in the domestic cat. *Genomics* 2006:

8. Lemarie SL. Mycobacterial dermatitis. *Vet Clin N Amer Small Anim* 1999: 29; 1291.

9. Lomax TD, Robinson R. Tabby pattern alleles of the domestic cat. *J Hered* 1988: 79; 21.

10. Lyons LA, et al. Tyrosinase mutations associated with Siamese and Burmese patterns in the domestic cat (Felis catus). *Anim Genet* 2005: 36; 119.

11. Lyons LA, et al. Chocolate coated cats: TYRP1 mutations for brown color in domestic cats. *Mamm Genome* 2005: 16; 356.

12. Lyons LA, et al. The Tabby cat locus maps to feline chromosome B1. *Anim Genet* 2006: 37; 383.

13. Prieur DJ, Collier LL. Maltese dilution of domestic cats. A generalized cutaneous albinism lacking ocular involvement. *J Hered* 1984: 75; 41

14. Raharison F, Sautet J. Lymph drainage of the mammary glands in female cats. *J Morphol* 2006: 267; 292.

15. Roosje PJ, et al. Feline atopic dermatitis. A model for Langerhans cell participation in disease pathogenesis. *Am J Pathol* 1997: 151; 927.

16. Roosje PJ, et al. Increased numbers of CD4+ and CD8+ T cells in lesional skin of cats with allergic dermatitis. *Vet Pathol* 1998: 35; 268.

17. Roosje PJ, et al. Mast cells and eosinophils in feline allergic dermatitis: a qualitative and quantitative analysis. *J Comp Pathol* 2004: 131; 61.

18. Schmidt-Kuntzel A, et al. Tyrosinase and tyrosinase related protein 1 alleles specify domestic cat coat color phenotypes of the albino and brown loci. *J Hered* 2005: 96; 289.

19. Scott DW. Feline Dermatology 1900-1978: a monograph. *J Amer Anim Hosp Assn* 1980: 16: 331.

20. Scott DW. Feline Dermatology 1983-1985: "The secret sits". *J Amer Anim Hosp Assn* 1984: 20; 537.

21. Scott DW, Miller WH, Jr., Griffin CE (Eds). *Muller and Kirk's Small Animal Dermatology.* 6th Ed. Philadelphia, WB Saunders, 2001.

22. Strickland JH, Calhoun ML. The Integumentary System of the Cat. *Am J Vet Res* 1963: 24; 1018.

23. Vella CM, et al. In: Vella CM, Robinson R (Eds). *Robinson's genetics for cat breeders and veterinarians* 4th Ed. Oxford, Butterworth Heinemann, 1999.

24. Zappulli V, et al. Feline mammary tumours in comparative oncology. *J Dairy Res* 2005: 72 Spec No; 98.

Chapter 3

Musculoskeletal System

Lola C. Hudson and William P. Hamilton

The skeleton of all mammals, including the cat, has the functions of supporting the body in a semirigid position, and of protecting some deeper soft tissue structures. The support function provides a scaffold for muscle position and allows normal movement only at specialized areas, particularly the synovial joints. Good examples of the protective function are the shielding of the brain by the skull, and sheltering of the heart and lungs within the ribs. However, the bones of mammals also function in producing red blood cells and some white blood cells in the marrow spaces of adult cats, the storage of some minerals, most notably calcium and phosphorous, and the storage of fat. The skeletal muscles function primarily in locomotion with contraction of muscles causing changes in the angulation between bones on opposite sides of an articulation. Most commonly, articulations are viewed as allowing movement but there are situations in the body where articulations restrict or prevent movement such as the sutures of the skull.

Axial Skeleton

The skeleton is often divided into axial and appendicular parts. The axial skeleton corresponds to the part associated with the midline or longitudinal axis of the animal and includes the skull, vertebrae, ribs, and sternum.

Skull

The skull, while often thought of as one structure, is actually a conglomerate of 29 bones (more or less, depending on exactly how a "separate" bone is defined). Most of the bones are found as bilateral pairs; those that are not paired are located on the median plane. Most bones of the skull are joined by suture type articulations. The major exceptions to this are the temporomandibular (jaw) joint, which is a synovial joint and contains an articular disc, and the mandibular symphysis, which is a fibrocartilaginous joint.

In the cat, the skull has a short facial and palatal region as compared to other common domestic mammals. Although selective breeding by humans has not resulted in nearly as much modification of the facial area as in dogs, brachycephalic cats, such as Persians, do exist. This facial bone defect is associated with the process of endochrondral ossification. Also in the facial region are the frontal sinuses and sphenoid sinuses located within the bones of the same name. There is a small maxillary recess located on the medial surface of the maxillae. The sinuses and recesses communicate with the nasal cavity. A median section of the skull often exposes the frontal and sphenoid sinuses to view. The turbinates and conchae that fill much of the nasal cavity also may be seen on this perspective.

The short orbital ligament is found on the lateral portion of the orbit, joining the zygomatic process of the frontal bone, and the frontal process of the zygomatic bone, enclosing the orbit with a connective tissue ring.

The various teeth of the superior arcade are associated with the incisive bones and maxillae (see Chapter 8 also).

The cranium of the skull is proportionally equal in size to other species. This part of the skull houses the brain and has many foramina to allow entry and exit of blood vessels and cranial nerves. The foramina are clustered on the ventrolateral and caudal surface of the skull and are similar to other carnivores. However, the cat does not have an alar canal and, therefore, no rostral or caudal alar foramina. Instead, at the analogous location, the round foramen can be seen on the external surface of the feline skull.

Dorsally, the junction of the left and right frontal and parietal bones (bregma) may be incompletely ossified at the perinatal period resulting in a fontanelle. Kittens with hydrocephalus may fail to close this fontanelle. On the caudodorsal midline of the skull is a sagittal ridge meeting the nuchal crest. The junction of ridge and crest marks the external occipital protuberance.

The rounded tympanic bullae found near the caudoventral surface of the skull contain an incomplete bony septum that divides the middle ear cavity into tympanic and endotympanic parts. This septum bullae can be easily seen on certain radiographic views of the head such as the "open-mouth" view (see Chapter 11 also).

Within the cranial cavity, the large bony tentorium cerebelli that separates the middle and caudal cranial fossae can be seen. This structure is positioned in the deep transverse fissure between the cerebrum and the cerebellum and continues ventrally to surround the brain stem. In a necropsy, this bony partition may need to be removed if the brain is to be collected in one piece. Only a shallow ridge separates the small rostral cranial fossa and middle cranial fossa.

The mandible is not remarkably different from other carnivores and contains the teeth of the lower arcade (see Chapter 8 also). The mandibular symphysis joins the left and right halves.

The very small ear ossicles, malleus, incus, and stapes, are present but are not well appreciated radiographically or clinically (see Chapter 11 also).

The hyoid apparatus articulates with the caudoventral skull dorsally and the thyroid cartilage of the larynx caudally. Only the basihyoid bone crosses the midline as a single bone in the cranioventral neck, the other elements of the hyoid are paired. The hyoid apparatus is associated with respiratory and swallowing functions (see Chapter 7 also).

Plate 3-1

Skeleton, Lateral view

Axial skeleton
a Skull

b Mandible

c Cervical vertebra
1 1st Cervical vertebra = C_1 = atlas
2 2nd Cervical vertebra = C_2 = axis
3 7th Cervical vertebra = C_7

d Thoracic vertebra
4 1st Thoracic vertebra = T_1
5 7th Thoracic vertebra = T_7
6 13th Thoracic vertebra = T_{13}

e Lumbar vertebra
7 1st Lumbar vertebra = L_1
8 7th Lumbar vertebra = L_7

f Sacrum (sacral vertebra)
9 1st Sacral vertebra = S_1
10 3rd Sacral vertebra = S_3

g Caudal vertebra
11 1st caudal vertebra = Cd_1

h Costal arch
12 3rd Rib
13 8th Rib
14 13th Rib

15 Costochondral junction of 12th rib
16 Costal cartilage of 11th rib

i Sternum
17 1st Sternebra = Manubrium sterni
18 8th Sternebra = Xiphoid process
19 Xiphoid cartilage

Appendicular skeleton
Thoracic limb
20 Clavicle
21 Scapula

j Brachium
22 Humerus

k Antebrachium
23 Radius
24 Ulna

l Manus (hand)

m Carpus
25 Carpal bones

n Metacarpus
26 5th Metacarpal bone

o Digits
27 Proximal phalanx of 5th digit

28 Middle phalanx of 5th digit
29 Distal phalanx of 5th digit

Pelvic limb
p Pelvis
30-32 Os coxae (1/2 bony pelvis)
30 Ilium
31 Ischium
32 Pubis

q Thigh
33 Femur
34 Patella

r Crus
35 Tibia
36 Fibula

s Pes (foot)

t Tarsus
37 Tarsal bones

u Metatarsus
38 5th Metatarsal bone

v Digits
39 Proximal phalanx of 5th digit
40 Middle phalanx of 5th digit
41 Distal phalanx of 5th digit

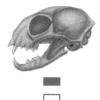

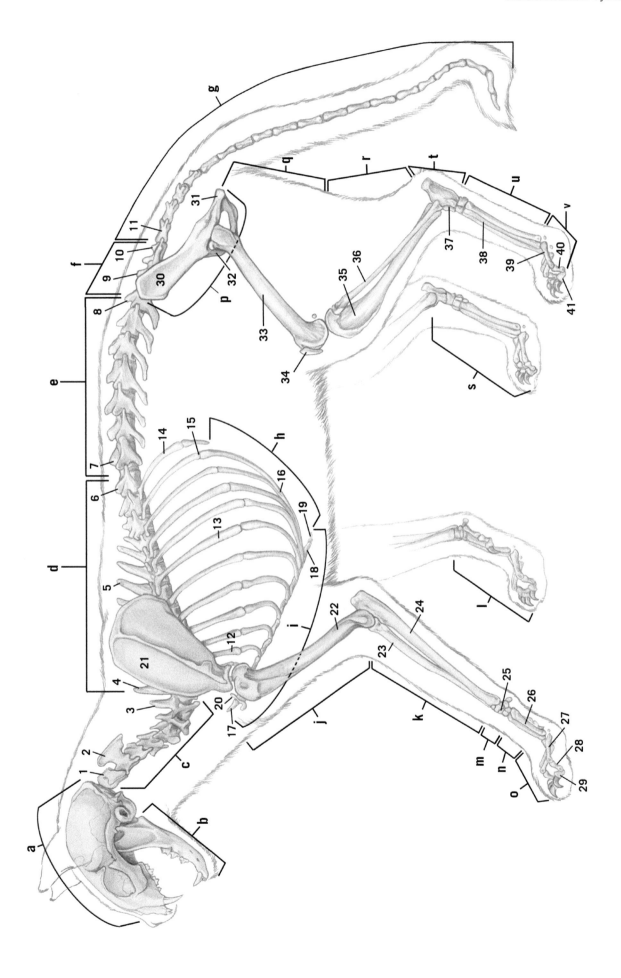

Plate 3-2

Figure A　Skull, dorsal view

Figure B　Skull with mandible, left lateral view

Figure C　Skull with mandible, medial (mid sagittal view)

Figure D　Skull (left), ventral view, and skull with cranial vault opened (right), dorsal view

Figure E　Illustration of positioning (left) to produce radiograph (right) of the head isolating the tympanic bullae, open mouth view. Radiograph provided courtesy of Diagnostic Imaging (Radiology) Service, Veterinary Teaching Hospital, North Carolina State University College of Veterinary Medicine

a　Bones of the face
   1　Incisive bone
   2　Nasal bone
   3　Maxilla
   4　Lacrimal bone
   5　Zygomatic bone
   　5'　Its frontal process
   6　Infraorbital foramen
   7　Maxillary foramen
   8　Dorsal nasal concha
   9　Middle nasal concha
   10　Ventral nasal concha
   11　Hard palate
   12　Choanae
   13　Palatine bone

b　Bones of the cranium
   23　Frontal bone
   　23'　Its zygomatic process
   24　Frontal sinus
   25　Parietal bone
   26　Bregma
   27　Presphenoid bone
   28　Interparietal bone
   29　Sagittal crest
   30　Occipital bone
   31　External occipital protuberance
   32　Nuchal crest
   33　Occipital condyle
   34　Paracondylar process
   35　Internal occipital protuberance
   36　Foramen magnum
   37　Temporal bone, squamous part
   　37'　Its zygomatic process
   38　Retroarticular process
   39　Mandibular fossa
   40　Temporal bone, tympanic part

41　Tympanic bulla
42　External acoustic meatus
43　Temporal bone, petrosal part (petrous temporal bone)
44　Mastoid process
45　Jugular foramen
46　Tympanooccipital fissure
47　Basisphenoid bone
48　Hypophyseal fossa
49　Dorsum sellae
50　Oval foramen
51　Round foramen
52　Orbital fissure
53　Sphenoid sinus
54　Optic canal
55　Pterygoid bone
56　Hamulus of the pterygoid bone
57　Rostral cranial fossa
58　Middle cranial fossa
59　Caudal cranial fossa
60　Zygomatic arch
61　Dens of axis
62　Body of axis

c　Mandible
   14　Body of mandible
   15　Ramus of mandible
   16　Masseteric fossa
   17　Mental foramina
   18　Angular process
   19　Condylar process
   20　Coronoid process
   21　Mandibular foramen
   22　Mandibular symphysis

   63　Mandible
   64　Tympanic bulla
   65　Septum bullae

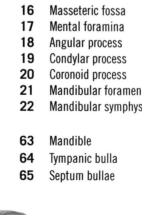

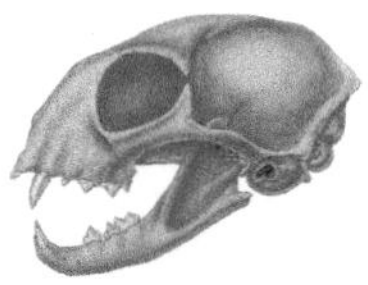

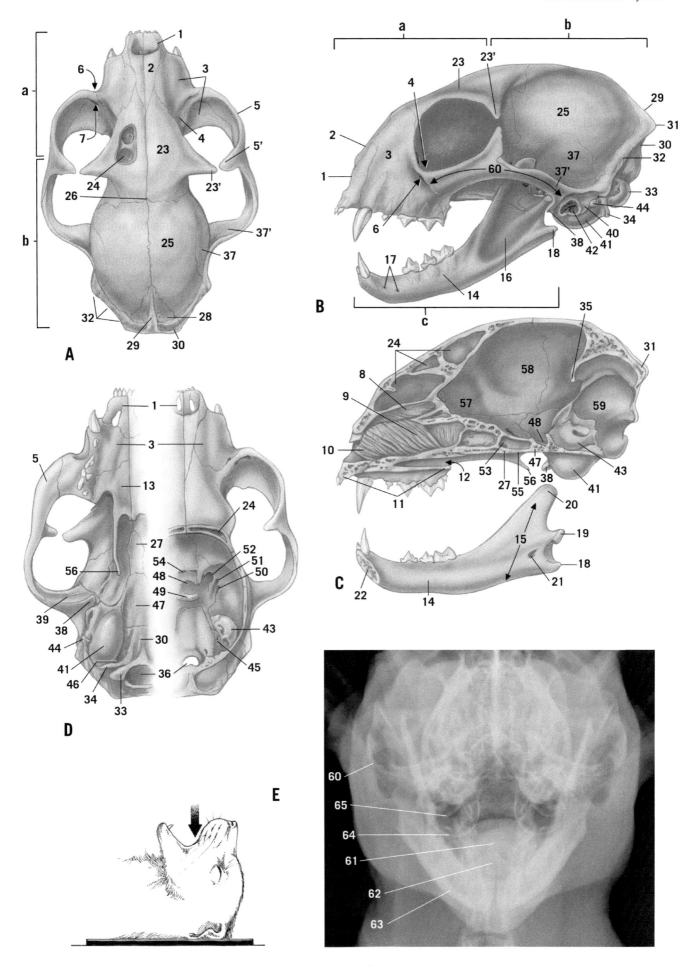

Vertebrae

The feline vertebral formula is $C_7 T_{13} L_7 S_3 Cd_{18-20}$[a]. A typical vertebra has a cylindrical body with various bony processes extending from it. The presence and prominence of the processes changes in the different body regions. The vertebrae of the different regions of the cat display the typical characteristics found in the same regions of other domestic mammals.

The atlas and axis show the most specialization and least resemble the other vertebrae. The first cervical vertebra (atlas or C_1) has large, palpable transverse processes commonly called wings. The second cervical vertebra (axis or C_2) has a long dorsal spinous process and a prominent dens on the cranial body. All the cervical vertebrae except C_7 have transverse foramina in the transverse processes. C_6 vertebra has larger, ventrally projecting transverse processes than is seen on adjacent vertebrae, a feature that can distinguish the C_6 vertebrae on lateral radiographs. In the cervical region, the articulations between caudal and cranial articular processes of adjacent vertebrae are close to the dorsal plane.

The cat lacks the nuchal ligament extending between the cranial thoracic vertebrae and the atlas or skull seen in some other mammals.

The cranial thoracic vertebrae have tall dorsal spinous processes as their most distinguishing feature. The height of these dorsal processes gradually decreases caudally through this region of the spine. The direction of the thoracic dorsal spines changes from caudal to cranial at T_{11} - the anticlinal vertebra. The thoracic vertebrae also have distinguishable mamillary processes.

The lumbar vertebrae are relatively long in the craniocaudal axis and have long, cranially-directed transverse processes. Mamillary processes and accessory processes are readily seen in vertebrae of this region. In the lumbar region, the articulations between caudal and cranial articular processes of adjacent vertebrae are in a more sagittal plane, almost a 90° shift from the articulations of these same processes in the cervical region.

The three sacral vertebrae are fused postnatally into the sacrum. The original sacral dorsal spinous processes remain individually distinct even after fusion of the bodies and transverse processes.

The caudal vertebrae vary in number, generally 18 to 20, and gradually lose all processes until elongate bodies are all that remain. Manx cats may fail to develop a large portion or all of their caudal vertebrae (agenesis), as well as some of the sacral vertebrae due to a genetic mutation. (Significant neurological dysfunctions may also occur in such "tailless" animals.)

[a] Frequently, a shorthand method for designating vertebrae, spinal cord segments, and spinal nerves is used. It consists of a capital letter followed by a single Arabic number or a range of Arabic numbers. The letters indicate the region - C for cervical, T for thoracic, L for lumbar, S for sacral, and Cd (or Ca) for caudal. The single number can represent an individual structure or, in this case, the maximum number of structure in that region. The range of numbers indicates more than one specific structure or, in this case, a variable maximum number of structures.

At the borders between regions, vertebrae with characteristics of both regions may be seen (transitional vertebrae). For example, the T_{13} (L_1?) vertebrae may have an associated rib on one side and a transverse process on the opposite side. It is also possible for the number of vertebrae in a given region to vary such as eight lumbar vertebrae instead of the usual seven.

Intervertebral discs consisting of a gelatinous center and the surrounding connective tissue anulus fibrosus are found between the bodies of adjacent vertebrae except at C_{1-2}. The articulations between caudal and cranial articular processes of adjacent vertebrae, between the skull and C_1, and between the ventral arch of C_1 and cranial articular surface of C_2 are synovial joints.

Ribs

There are normally 13 pairs of ribs in the cat. They tend to be short but rather broad at the cranial thorax becoming longer and less broad in the midthorax and finally shorter but still not broad at the caudal thorax. The shape of the enclosed thorax is roughly a cone.

The head and tubercles of the ribs articulate with thoracic vertebrae. The head and tubercle of the first rib articulates only with T_1. The head of the second rib articulates with the caudal body of T_1 and the cranial body of T_2 while its tubercle articulates with the transverse process of T_2. Successive ribs 3-10 articulate similarly on successive vertebrae. Ribs 11-13 articulate only with the body and transverse process of T_{11-13}, respectively.

Left and right rib pairs are connected by intercapital ligaments found dorsal to the intervertebral discs.

The costal cartilages of ribs 1-9 (sternal ribs) articulate directly with the sternum. The cartilages of ribs 10-12 (asternal ribs) unite to form the costal arch of the caudal thorax. The cartilage of the last rib (floating rib) remains separate from the others.

Sternum

The sternum has 8 bony elements (sternebrae); the first is the manubrium sterni (readily palpable), and the last is the xiphoid process that is continued caudally by the xiphoid cartilage.

With the exception of the first costal cartilage that articulates directly with the manubrium sterni, the costal cartilages of sternal ribs articulate with cartilage located between sternebrae.

Plate 3-3

Figure A   Dorsal (top) and ventral (bottom) view of atlas
Figure B   Left lateral view of axis
Figure C   Caudal view of C_5
Figure D   Craniolateral view of T_4 and left lateral view of T_1
Figure E   Right lateral view of L_6
Figure F   Ventral, dorsal, and left lateral views of sacrum
Figure G   Dorsal view of Cd_6
Figure H   Cranial view of left 13th, 8th, and 1st ribs
Figure I   Ventral view of sternum

1	Dorsal arch	19	Wing of sacrum
2	Ventral arch	20	Ventral sacral foramen
3	Ventral tubercle	21	Median sacral crest
4	Transverse process	22	Intermediate sacral crest
5	Transverse foramen	23	Dorsal sacral foramen
6	Alar notch	24	Promontory
7	Lateral vertebral foramen	25	Lateral sacral crest
8	Vertebral canal	26	Auricular face
9	Cranial articular fovea	27	Head
10	Caudal articular fovea	28	Tubercle
11	Dens	29	Body of rib
12	Cranial articular surface	30	Costochondral junction
13	Spinous process	31	Costal cartilage
14	Body	32	Manubrium sterni
15	Cranial articular process	33	3rd Sternebra
16	Caudal articular process	34	Intersternal cartilage
17	Costal fovea	35	Xiphoid process
18	Accessory process	36	Xiphoid cartilage

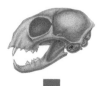

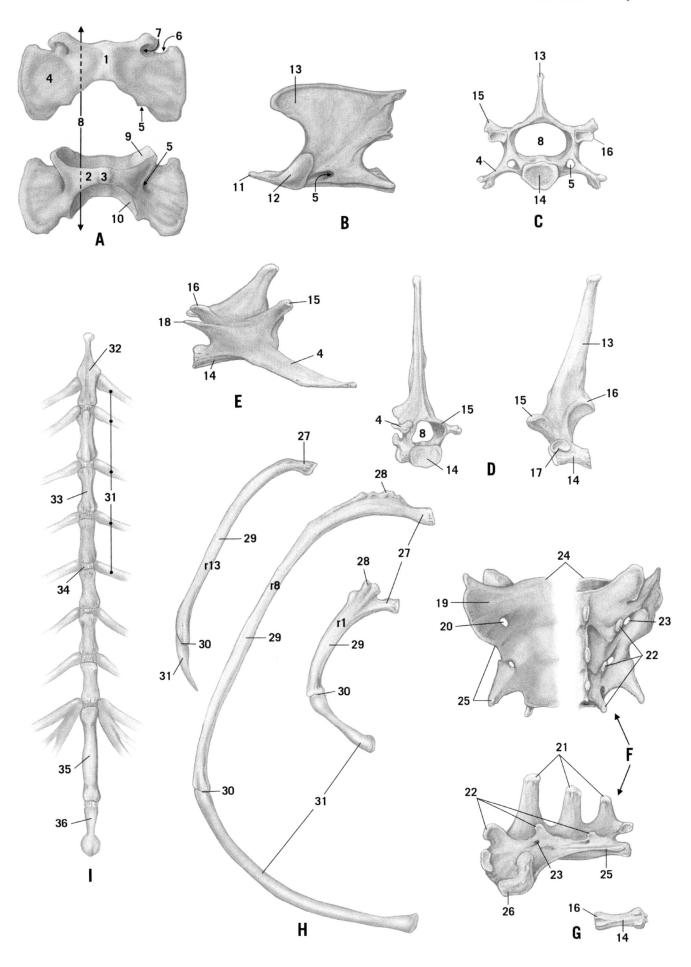

Appendicular Skeleton

The appendicular skeleton is composed of those bones located in the limbs. In general, the long bones of the cat limbs are straighter than the same bone in the dog. Also, many of the processes and bony ridges of the appendicular bones may not be very obvious due to the small size of the domestic cat.

Thoracic Limb

The clavicle (collarbone) is found in cats and can be appreciated radiographically. However, it does not articulate with the sternum or shoulder region as it does in human beings. Instead, the clavicle is located at the intersection of the m. cleidocephalicus, pars cervicalis and pars mastoideus, and the m. cleidobrachialis in the shoulder region.

The skeleton of the thoracic limb has no bony articulation with the axial skeleton. Musculature and connective tissue hold this limb in proper alignment with the vertebrae and ribs.

The dorsal border of the scapula is positioned dorsal to the thoracic spinous processes in the cat. This can be especially appreciated when watching a stalking cat - as the animal moves its forelimb, a ridge of bone is seen moving at the top line. This feature may not be appreciated in a non-weight-bearing cat as is encountered in positioning a cat for lateral radiographs. The acromion of the distal scapula is more complex than in other domestic mammals and has a hamate and suprahamate process. A rather pointed coracoid process is visible on the supraglenoid tubercle of the scapula.

The glenohumeral joint has rather weak ligaments, so the supraspinatus, infraspinatus, and subscapularis mm. act as collateral ligaments for this joint as they do in other domestic species.

The humerus is a rather long and robust bone. In the cat, it possesses a supracondylar foramen on the distomedial aspect.

The median n. and brachial a. (but not vein!) pass through this foramen. (Rarely, this foramen may be absent.) On the craniodistal aspect, a coronoid fossa, medial to the radial fossa, is present and receives the medial coronoid process of the ulna during flexion of the elbow. The supratrochlear foramen is not present.

The radius and ulna of the antebrachium remain as separate bones in their entirety. Proximally, the radius is positioned cranial and slightly lateral to the ulna. Distally, the radius is positioned medially to the ulna. The presence of 2 complete bones and their orientation in the antebrachium are responsible for the cat's ability to supinate and pronate the forelimb. When the distal antebrachium is viewed directly cranially, a relatively wide, but normal, space between the adjacent surfaces of the radius and ulna can be appreciated. The most common congenital limb deformity is radial agenesis.

The carpus consists of seven bones: intermedioradial, ulnar, and accessory carpal bones in the proximal row as well as carpal bones 1-4 in the distal row. An inconstant sesamoid bone in the tendon of the m. abductor pollicis longus may be seen on the medial aspect of the carpus.

The forelimb typically has five metacarpal bones and five digits numbered from medial to lateral. The first digit (pollex) has two phalanges and the remaining digits have three phalanges each. Digits II-V have a pair of small proximal sesamoid bones located on the palmar surface of the metacarpophalangeal joint. In the cat, the distal ends of the middle phalanges are oblique and beveled. The distal phalanges of digits II-V have become slightly modified so that a cat at rest places this bone into a position just lateral to the middle phalanx. Therefore, the resting position of the distal interphalangeal joint is greatly hyperextended. This orientation of middle and distal phalanges is passively maintained by a pair of dorsal elastic ligaments and allows the animal to sheath the claw during movement or rest if so desired. Unsheathing the claw requires sufficient contraction of the deep digital flexor m. to overcome the power of the dorsal elastic ligaments.

The distal phalanx of all digits has an unguicular crest and an unguicular process on its distal end. The claw arises from this area. The claw is shaped to the surfaces of the unguicular process, laterally compressed and drawn to a sharp point.

Some owners may elect to have their cat declawed to protect themselves or their furnishings from damage inflicted by the territorial marking proclivities of their pets (commonly referred to as "sharpening the claws"). Correct declawing (onychectomy) requires removal of the entire unguicular crest where the germinal cells of the claw are located. The more common error is to leave a part of the dorsal unguicular crest with subsequent regrowth of a malformed claw. (A proper incision line of one method is illustrated.) Declawing does not necessarily require removal of the entire distal phalanx, although this is one surgical method. If the entire phalanx is removed, it will require transecting the common digital extensor m. on the dorsal surface and the deep digital flexor m. on the palmar surface. Cutting the digital pad during surgery will extend the recovery time.

Extra digits (polydactyly) can be seen occasionally on both forepaw and hindpaw.

Pelvic Limb

Unlike the forelimb, the hind limb does have a bony articulation with the axial skeleton between the sacrum and the pelvis (sacro-iliac joint).

The pelvis is formed by the left and right ossae coxarum (joined at the pelvic symphysis), which, in turn, are formed by the fusion of the ilium, ischium, pubis, and acetabular bones postnatally. The lateral parts of the os coxae are essentially parallel to the longitudinal axis of the cat and ventrodorsal radiographs of this region show a pelvis outlined in a rectangle (box pelvis). The bony floor of the pelvis is V-shaped when viewed in a craniocaudal direction.

The femur is not markedly different from that of other carnivores. There is a ligament of the head of the femur present as an intracapsular ligament at the hip joint.

The patella should have the more pointed portion at the distal end- a mistake often present on commercially prepared skeletons available on the market. There is only one patellar ligament. The stifle joint has collateral ligaments, cranial and caudal cruciate ligaments, medial and lateral menisci, transverse ligaments, and meniscofemoral ligament present. Ruptures of the cranial cruciate ligament are known to occur in cats but repair of this is not generally attempted. Occasionally, the menisci may ossify. Each head of the m. gastrocnemius has a sesamoid bone (formerly called fabellae) that is located at the caudodistal femur. A sesamoid bone in the tendon of origin of the popliteus m. may also be seen in the caudolateral area of the stifle.

In the crus, the tibia and fibula remain separate throughout life. As with the femur, they are not markedly different from the same bones of other carnivores. The distal ends of these bones articulate at the tarsocrural joint, which is the major site of movement of the tarsal region.

The pes or foot consists of the tarsus, metatarsal bones, and digits. The tarsus is formed by seven bones: the talus, calcaneus, central tarsal bone, and tarsal bones 1-4. There are four complete metatarsal bones that are approximately twice as long as the corresponding metacarpal bones and a rudimentary first metatarsal bone. Digits II-V are present on the hindlimb and have the same arrangement of phalanges and proximal sesamoid bones as the digits of the forepaw.

Plate 3-4

Figure A   Bones of the thoracic limb, cranial view
Figure B   Distal humerus, craniolateral view
Figure C   Bones of the thoracic limb, lateral view
Figure D   Bones of the distal antebrachium and manus, dorsal view

a   Clavicle

b   Scapula
   1   Scapular spine
   2-3 Acromion
     2 Hamate process
     3 Suprahamate process
   4   Supraspinous fossa
   5   Infraspinous fossa
   6   Supraglenoid tubercle
   7   Coracoid process
   8   Infraglenoid tubercle
   9   Glenoid cavity

c   Humerus
   10 Head
   11 Lesser tubercle
   12 Greater tubercle
   13 Crest of greater tubercle
   14 Teres minor tuberosity
   15 Tricipital line
   16 Deltoid tuberosity
   17 Brachial groove
   18 Shaft
   19 Supracondylar foramen
   20 Medial epicondyle
   21 Lateral epicondyle
   22 Lateral supracondylar crest
   23 Coronoid fossa
   24 Radial fossa
   25 Trochlea
   26 Capitulum

d   Radius
   27 Head
   28 Radial tuberosity
   29 Shaft
   30 (Medial) styloid process

e   Ulna
   31 Tuber olecranon
   32 Anconeal process
   33 Trochlear notch
   34 Medial coronoid process
   35 Lateral coronoid process
   36 Body of ulna
   37 Articular circumference
   38 (Lateral) styloid process

f   Manus

g   Carpal bones
   39 Sesamoid bone for m. Abductor
      pollicis longus (inconstant)
   40 Intermedioradial carpal bone
   41 Ulnar carpal bone
   42 Accessory carpal bone
   43 Carpal bone I
   44 Carpal bone II
   45 Carpal bone III
   46 Carpal bone IV

h   Metacarpal bones
   47 Metacarpal bones I to V
   48 Base of metacarpal bone III
   49 Head of metacarpal bone III
   50 Proximal sesamoid bones of digit II
   51 Proximal phalanges of digits I to V
   52 Middle phalanges of digits II to V
   53 Distal phalanges of digits I to V
   54 Unguicular process

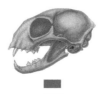

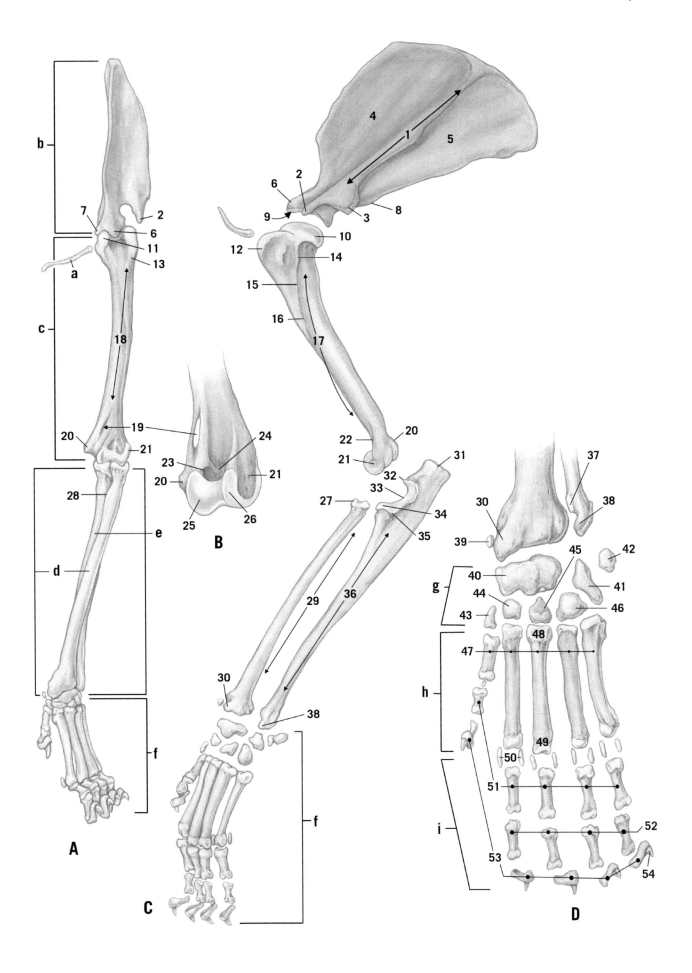

Plate 3-5

Figure A   Bones of the pelvic limb, lateral view
Figure B   Pelvis, dorsal view
Figure C   Bones of the tarsus, medial, plantar, and dorsal views

a   Os coxae (1/2 pelvis)
   1-2   Acetabulum
      1   Acetabular fossa
      2   Acetabular notch
   3   Obturator foramen

b   Ilium
   4   Iliac crest
   5   Gluteal surface
      6-7   Tuber sacrale
   6   Cranial dorsal iliac spine
   7   Caudal dorsal iliac spine
      8-9   Tuber coxae
   8   Cranial ventral iliac spine
   9   Alar spine
  10   Greater ischiatic notch
  11   Tuberosity for psoas minor

c   Ischium
  12   Ischiatic spine
  13   Lesser ischiatic notch
  14   Ischiatic tuberosity
  15   Ischiatic arch
     16-17 Pelvic symphysis
  16   Symphysis ischii

d   Pubis
  17   Symphysis pubis
  18   Body of pubis
  19   Caudal ramus of pubis
  20   Pecten

e   Femur
  21   Head
  22   Neck
  23   Greater trochanter
  24   Lesser trochanter
  25   Trochanteric fossa
  26   Intertrochanteric crest
  27   Third trochanter
  28   Shaft
     29-31 Trochlea
  29   Medial trochlear ridge
  30   Trochlear groove
  31   Lateral trochlear ridge

32   Extensor fossa
33   Lateral condyle
34   Lateral epicondyle
35   Patella
36   Sesamoid bones of medial and lateral heads of m. Gastrocnemius
37   Sesamoid bone of m. Popliteus

f   Tibia
  38   Medial condyle
  39   Lateral condyle
  40   Extensor sulcus
  41   Tibial tuberosity
  42   Shaft
  43   Medial malleolus

g   Fibula
  44   Head
  45   Shaft
  46   Lateral malleolus

h   Pes

i   Tarsal bones
  47   Talus
  48   Trochlea
  49   Calcaneus
  50   Tuber calcanei
  51   Sustentaculum tali
  52   Tarsal canal
  53   Central tarsal bone
  54   Tarsal bone I
  55   Tarsal bone II
  56   Tarsal bone III
  57   Tarsal bone IV

j   Metatarsal bones
  58   Metatarsal bones I to V

k   Digital bones
  59   Proximal sesamoid bones of digit V
  60   Proximal phalanx of digit V
  61   Middle phalanx of digit V
  62   Distal phalanx of digit

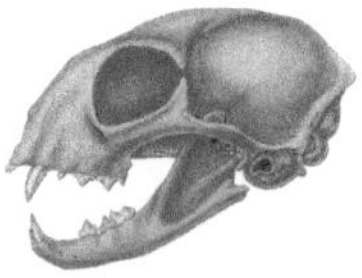

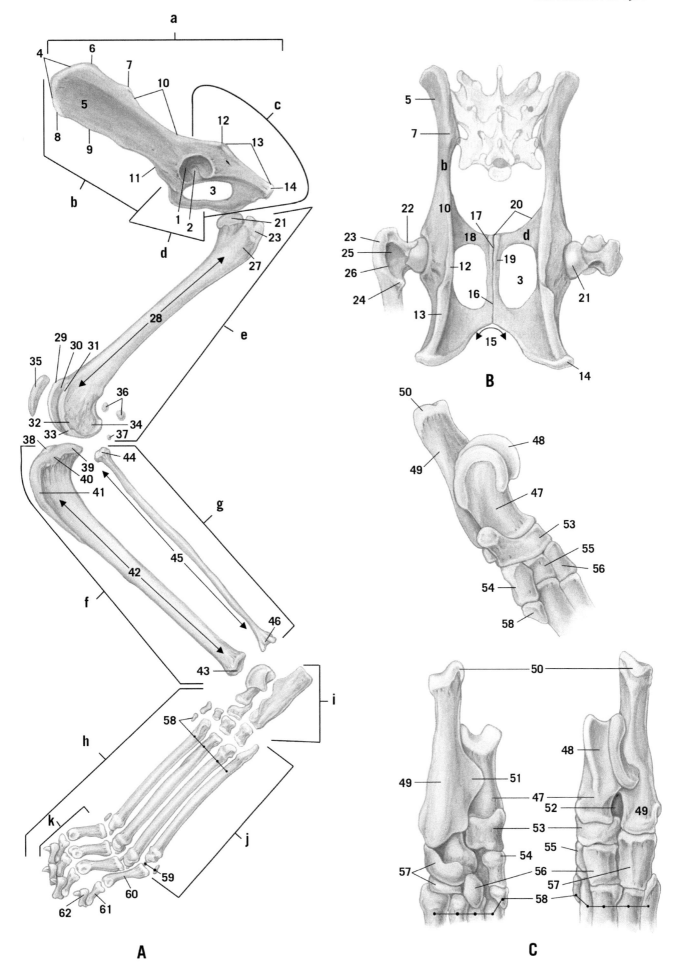

A

B

C

Articulations

The cat exhibits the 3 basic types of articulations or joints. The fibrous joint is seen with sutures of the skull and implantation of the teeth in the alveoli of the skull and mandible. These joints are immobile in the adult. The cartilaginous joint shows very limited movement. Some are temporary such as the physes of growing long bones; others persist such as the costochondral junction, pelvic symphysis, and intervertebral disc. These articulations utilize either hyaline cartilage or fibrocartilage.

The synovial articulation is what is most commonly thought of as a "joint." It is very mobile and is characterized by the presence of a joint cavity, joint capsule, synovial fluid, and articular cartilage on the contact surfaces. Such joints may involve only 2 bones (simple joint) or multiple bones (complex joint). The joints of the limbs, with the exception of the pelvic symphysis, are the synovial type. As some of these articulations lack stability, many also have extra-capsular ligaments such as the collateral ligaments. A few have intracapsular ligaments or menisci to further increase stability.

Skeletal Muscles

The majority of muscles of the head, trunk, and limbs are similar in position and action to muscles of the dog. Skeletal muscles are all bilaterally symmetrical, striated, under control of the "voluntary" nervous system, and have attachments (origin and insertion) on bone or cartilage (with a few exceptions). Their function is locomotion of the body. Any given muscle must have its attachments on either side (*i.e.,* proximal and distal, cranial and caudal, etc.) of a joint in order to act on that joint. (Note, muscles do NOT act on bones- the cat should not be able to flex its humerus.) Some limb muscles can act on 2 or more joints. In these, the major action is generally the more distal joint(s) that are involved. It should also be kept in mind that muscles can only contract; they cannot "actively" relax. Therefore, muscles are generally arranged in opposing groups, agonists and antagonists, with opposite actions, *e.g.,* flexors and extensors of the elbow joint.

Skeletal muscles are invested in a layer of connective tissue called the epimysium that is the actual anchor for suture material in surgery involving any of these muscles. However, most surgeries are designed to approach structures between muscles, or to transect relatively avascular tendons, rather than incise the fleshy portions of muscles.

The names of muscles often reflect some characteristic of them such as the attachments (m. sternocephalicus - from sternum to head), action (m. extensor carpi radialis - to extend the carpus), number of bellies (m. quadriceps femoris - 4 headed muscle of the thigh), shape (m. deltoideus - outline of a triangle), or location (m. interspinalis - located between dorsal spines of vertebrae). Muscles can be appropriately named in English or Latin/Greek. There is no particular reason why some muscles traditionally use their English form (common digital extensor m.) while the muscle immediately adjacent is referred to in Latin (m. extensor carpi radialis). Although directional terms in veterinary nomenclature differ from those of human medical nomenclature, many muscles have the same name in both areas even when not technically correct (e.g., m. triceps brachii - 3 headed muscle of the arm - of humans has 3 heads, m. triceps brachii of carnivores has 4

heads). This is to avoid confusion over identification when working across species lines.

The muscles of embalmed feline cadavers are often thin and small and, therefore, tend to shred easily with much manipulation.

Cutaneous Muscles

The mm. platysma, sphincter colli, and cutaneous trunci are closely attached to the skin of the head, cranial neck, and thorax/abdomen, respectively, in the cat and are usually reflected with the skin in dissection or surgery.

Plate 3-6

Figure A   Kitten (growing) elbow, medial and lateral view
Figure B   Kitten (growing) lumbar vertebra, lateral view
Figure C   Pelvis of few-days-old kitten, craniolateral view

1   Humerus
2   Epiphysis of different bones
3   Physis (epiphyseal plate) of different bones
4   Apophysis of different bones
5   Radius
6   Ulna
7   Ilium
8   Pubis
9   Ischium
10   Acetabular bone

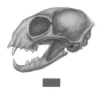

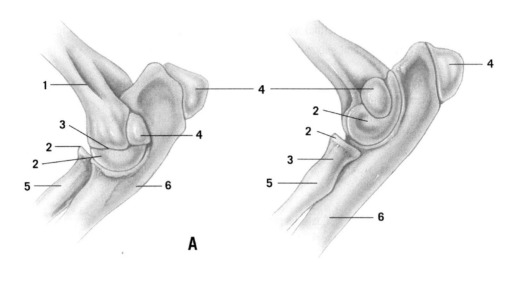

A

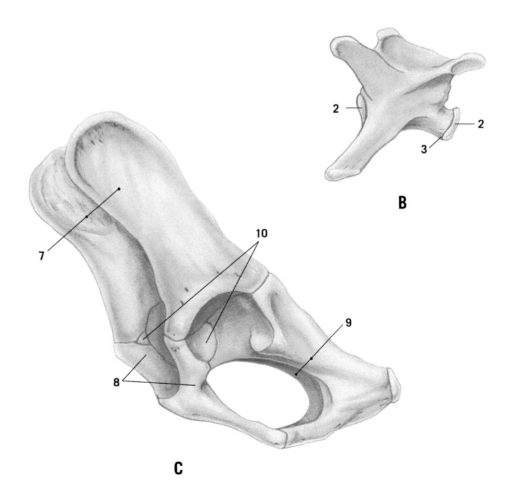

B

C

Plate 3-7

Figure A   Cartilaginous joint (intervertebral disc), cranial view
Figure B   Cartilaginous joint (intervertebral disc), ventral view
Figure C   Fibrous joint (skull suture), caudal view
Figure D   Synovial joint (stifle) with capsule removed, cranial left and caudal right views
Figure E   Synovial joint (elbow) with capsule removed, medial view

1	Anulus fibrosus	13	Caudal cruciate lig
2	Nucleus pulposus	14	Medial meniscus
3	Ventral longitudinal ligament	15	Lateral meniscus
4	Sagittal suture	16	Transverse lig
5	Parietal bone	17	Meniscofemoral lig
6	Medial and lateral femoral condyles	18	Medial collateral lig
7	Tibial tuberosity	19	Lateral collateral lig
8	Fibula	20	Humerus
9	Sesamoid bones of m. Gastrocnemius	21	Tuber olecranon
10	Sesamoid bone with cut and retracted tendon of m. Popliteus	22	Radius
		23	Cut tendon of m. Biceps brachii
11	Cut tendon of m. Extensor digitorum longus	24	Cut tendon of m. Brachialis
		25	Olecranon lig
12	Cranial cruciate lig	26	Medial collateral lig

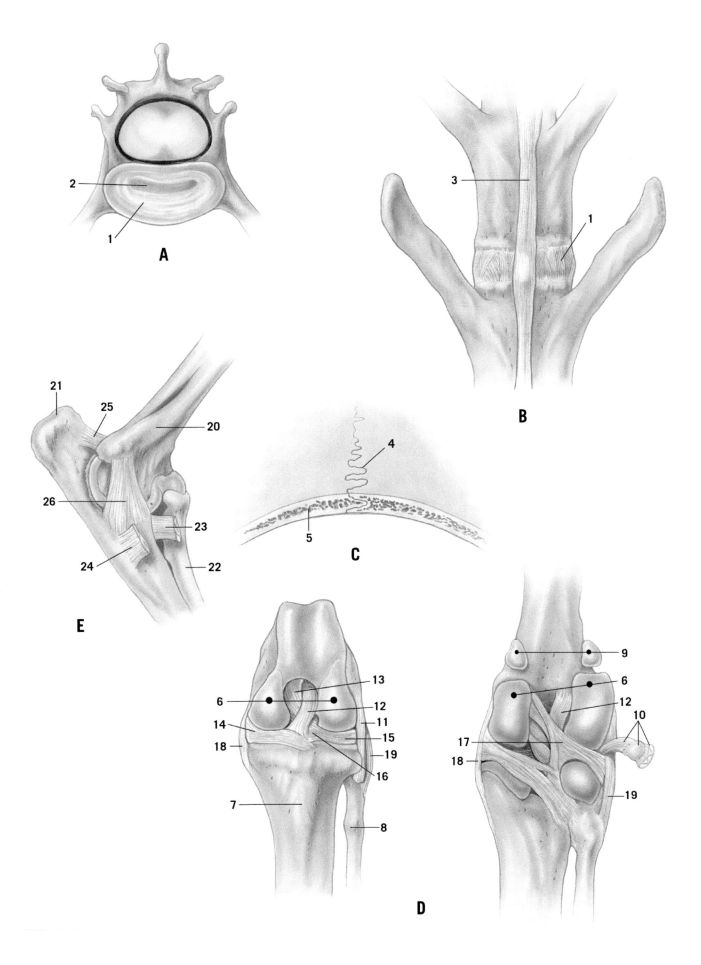

Plate 3-8

Superficial musculature with cutaneous muscle removed, lateral view

1   M. orbicularis oculi
2   M. frontalis
3   M. temporalis
4   M. digastricus
5   M. masseter
6   M. sternohyoideus
7   M. sternocephalicus, pars occipitalis
    (M. sternocephalicus, pars mastoidea not shown)
8-9   M. brachiocephalicus
8   M. cleidocephalicus, pars cervicalis
    (M. cleidocephalicus, pars mastoidea not shown)
9   M. cleidobrachialis
10   Clavicle
11   M. omotransversarius
12   M. trapezius, cervical and thoracic parts
13   M. latissimus dorsi
14   M. pectoralis profundus
15   M. obliquus externus abdominis
16   M. sacrocaudalis dorsalis lateralis
17   M. sacrocaudalis ventralis lateralis
18   M. deltoideus
19   M. triceps brachii, lateral head

20   M. triceps brachii, long head
21   M. brachioradialis
22   M. extensor carpi radialis
23   M. extensor digitorum communis
24   M. abductor pollicis longus
25   M. extensor digitorum lateralis
26   M. extensor carpi ulnaris (M. ulnaris lateralis)
27   M. flexor carpi ulnaris
28   M. satorius
29   M. tensor fasciae latae
30   M. gluteus medius
31   M. gluteus superficialis
32   M. gluteofemoralis (m. caudofemoralis)
33   M. coccygeus
34   M. semitendinosus
35   M. biceps femoris
36   M. cranialis tibialis
37   M. extensor digitorum longus
38   M. peroneus longus
39   M. extensor digitorum lateralis
40   M. flexor digitorum profundus, lateral head
41   M. peroneus brevis
42   M. gastrocnemius, lateral head
43   M. soleus

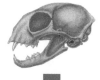

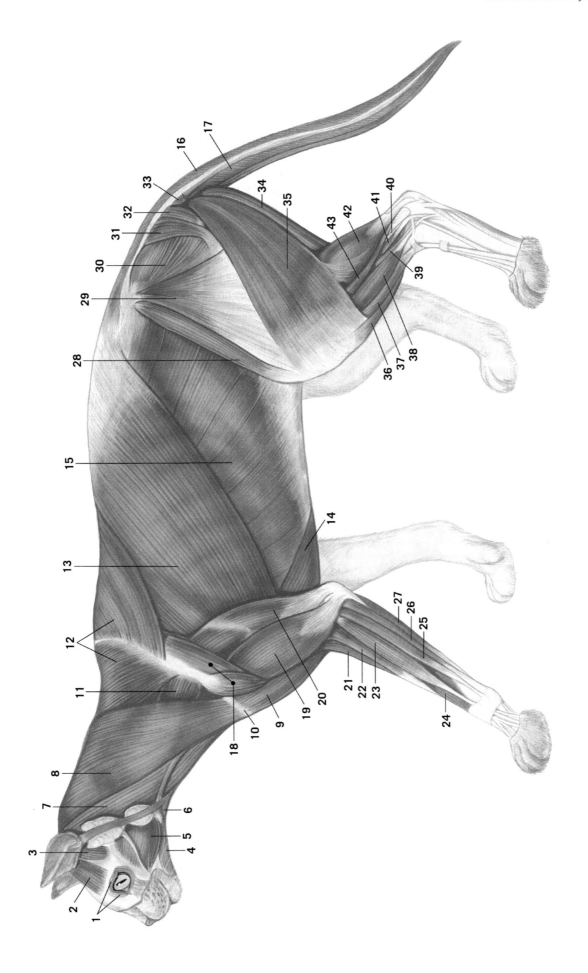

Axial Muscles

These muscles are responsible for locomotion of the axial skeleton. Their attachments are located on some part of the skull, hyoid apparatus, larynx, vertebrae, ribs, or sternum.

Head Muscles

The muscles of facial expression (innervated by the facial n.) are thin and often difficult to separate from one another particularly on the muzzle where the tactile hairs (whiskers) pass through them. This group includes the auricular (ear) muscles, eyelid muscles, and muscles surrounding the lips and nose.

The muscles of mastication (innervated by the mandibular branch of the trigeminal n.) are well developed. The m. temporalis and m. masseter are associated with the lateral temporal region of the skull and the caudolateral surface of the mandible respectively. The medial and (smaller) lateral pterygoid mm. extend from the medial side of the mandible to the pterygopalatine fossa of the lateral skull. The temporalis, masseter, and pterygoid mm. are relatively large and powerful. They act to close the jaw and can produce an astounding amount of pressure on the sharp borders of the teeth. The m. digastricus, attaching to the angular process of the mandible and the paracondylar process of the skull is the only muscle acting to open the jaw (the caudal part of the digastricus m. receives additional innervation from the facial n.). The mylohyoid mm. are innervated by the same cranial nerve as other muscles of mastication but are frequently included in the hyoid muscle group. The mylohyoid mm. form a sling for the tongue in the intermandibular space.

Extraocular muscles (innervated by oculomotor, trochlear, and abducens nn.) include the dorsal, medial, ventral, and lateral rectus mm., the dorsal and ventral oblique mm., 4 bellies of a m. retractor bulbi, and a m. levator palpebrae superioris (see Chapter 11 also).

The muscles of the tongue (innervated by the hypoglossal n.) include the mm. genioglossus, hyoglossus, styloglossus, and lingualis proprius.

The major pharyngeal muscles (innervated by glossopharyngeal and vagus nn.) include the m. cricopharyngeus, m. thyropharyngeus, and m. hyopharyngeus. These muscles are named for their respective origins and can be difficult to separate from each other. The mm. pterygopharyngeus and stylopharyngeus are included in this group but are difficult to dissect and visualize.

The major intrinsic laryngeal muscles (innervated by cranial laryngeal and caudal laryngeal nn.) include the m. cricoarytenoideus dorsalis, which is the only muscle to abduct the glottis, the m. cricoarytenoideus lateralis, m. thyroarytenoideus, and m. cricothyroideus. A major extrinsic laryngeal muscle is the m. sternothyroideus.

There are also several muscles that are associated with the tongue, pharynx, or larynx and have one attachment on some part of the hyoid apparatus. These include the m. geniohyoideus, m. thyrohyoideus, and other small weak muscles. The m. sternohyoideus extends between the sternum and basihyoid bone.

Epaxial Muscles

The epaxial muscles are associated with the dorsal and dorsolateral surfaces of the vertebrae. Superficially, the epaxial musculature of the neck and trunk is covered by extrinsic muscles of the forelimb and hindlimb as well as the thoracolumbar fascia. Once these are reflected, however, portions of the 3 epaxial systems- iliocostalis, longissimus, and transversospinalis - can be seen. These muscle groups, when contracting bilaterally, will extend the vertebral column. When acting unilaterally, they cause a lateral flexion. They are segmentally innervated by the dorsal branches of cervical, thoracic, and lumbar nerves.

The most lateral system is the mm. iliocostalis with its lumbar and thoracic parts. The lumbar portion arises in part from the neighboring m. longissimus lumborum and may be difficult to separate from it.

Medial to the mm. iliocostalis is the longissimus system extending from the sacrum and ilium to the skull making it literally the longest muscle in the body. The muscle is divided into lumbar, thoracic, cervical, and capital parts according to the major insertions of various muscle slips.

Medial to the longissimus system is the transversospinalis system. This includes mm. spinalis, mm. semispinalis, mm. multifidi, mm. interspinalis, and long and short rotator mm. Parts of this system are best seen in the deep areas of the dorsal neck where the m. spinalis et semispinalis and m. semispinalis capitis (poorly divided into mm. biventer cervicis and complexus) are located. The mm. intertransversalis are considered part of this system and are best seen in the cervical region. But even here they can be confused with the mm. scalenus and longus capitis.

Muscles seen in close approximation to the 3 epaxial systems but not strictly part of them are the muscles moving the specialized atlantooccipital and atlantoaxial joints. The m. rectus capitis, and mm. obliquus capitis, are deeply located on the dorsal and lateral surfaces of C_1 and C_2 vertebrae.

The m. splenius is located superficially to the m. semispinalis capitis and deep to the more cranial portions of the m. rhomboideus.

Plate 3-9

Figure A   Superficial musculature of the head, neck, and thoracic girdle, left lateral view
Figure B   Deep musculature of the head-neck junction, left lateral view
Figure C   Superficial and deep musculature of the head and neck, ventral view

1	M. orbicularis oculi		24-25	M. triceps brachii
2	M. frontalis		24	Lateral head
3	M. temporalis		24'	Its tendon
4	M. masseter		25	Long head
5	Parotid salivary gland		25'	Its tendon
5'	Its duct		26	M. pectoralis profundus
6	M. digastricus		27	M. obliquus externus abdominis
7	Sublingual salivary gland		28	M. hyopharyngeus
8	Mandibular salivary gland		29	Lateral retropharyngeal ln
9	M. sternohyoideus		30	M. thyropharyngeus
10	External jugular v.		31	Medial retropharyngeal ln
11	M. parotidoauricularis		32	M. cricopharyngeus
12	M. sternocephalicus, pars occipitalis		33	Esophagus
13	M. cleidocephalicus, pars cervicalis		34	Trachea
14	M. omotransversarius		35	M. styloglossus
15-16	M. trapezius		36	M. geniohyoideus
15	Pars cervicalis		37	M. hyoglossus
16	Pars thoracica		38	M. thyrohyoideus
17	Spine of scapula		39	M. sternothyroideus
18	M. infraspinatus		40	Mandible
19	M. latissimus dorsi		41	M. mylohyoideus
20	Clavicle		42	Linguofacial v
21	M. cleidobrachialis		43	Mandibular lln
22-23	M. deltoideus		44	Maxillary v
22	Pars acromialis		45	M. sternocephalicus, pars mastoidea
23	Pars scapularis		46	M. pectoralis transversus
			47	Venous hyoid arch
			48	Basihyoid bone
			49	Carotid sheath

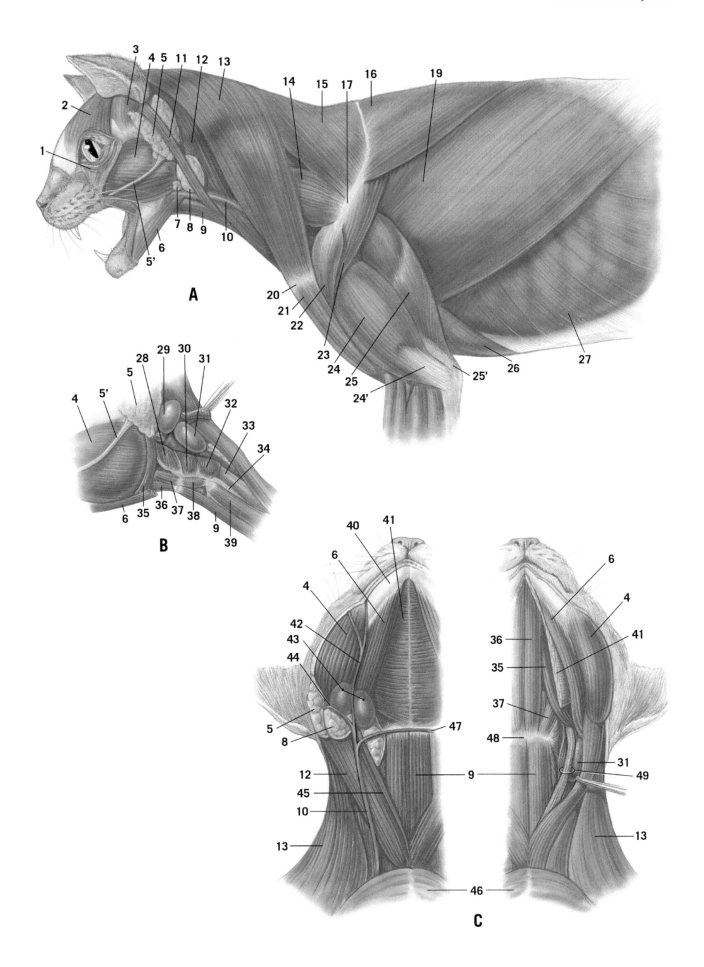

A

B

C

Plate 3-10

Figure A   Superficial musculature of the dorsum, dorsal view
Figure B   Deep musculature of the dorsum, dorsal view

1	M. brachiocephalicus	13	Spines of thoracic vertebrae
2	M. trapezius	14	M. serratus ventralis
3	M. latissimus dorsi	15	M. longissimus thoracis
4	M. obliquus externus abdominis	16	M. iliocostalis thoracis
5	M. gluteus medius	17	M. spinalis et semispinalis
6	M. gluteus superficialis	18	M. iliocostalis lumborum
7	M. gluteofemoralis (m. caudofemoralis)	19	M. longissimus lumborum
8	M. biceps femoris	20	Mm. transversospinalis
9	M. semitendinosus	21	M. sacrocaudalis dorsalis medialis
10-12	M. rhomboideus	22	M. sacrocaudalis dorsalis lateralis
10	M. rhomboideus capitis	23	Mm. intercostales externi
11	M. rhomboideus cervicis	24	M. intercostalis internus
12	M. rhomboideus thoracis	25	Ribs

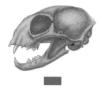

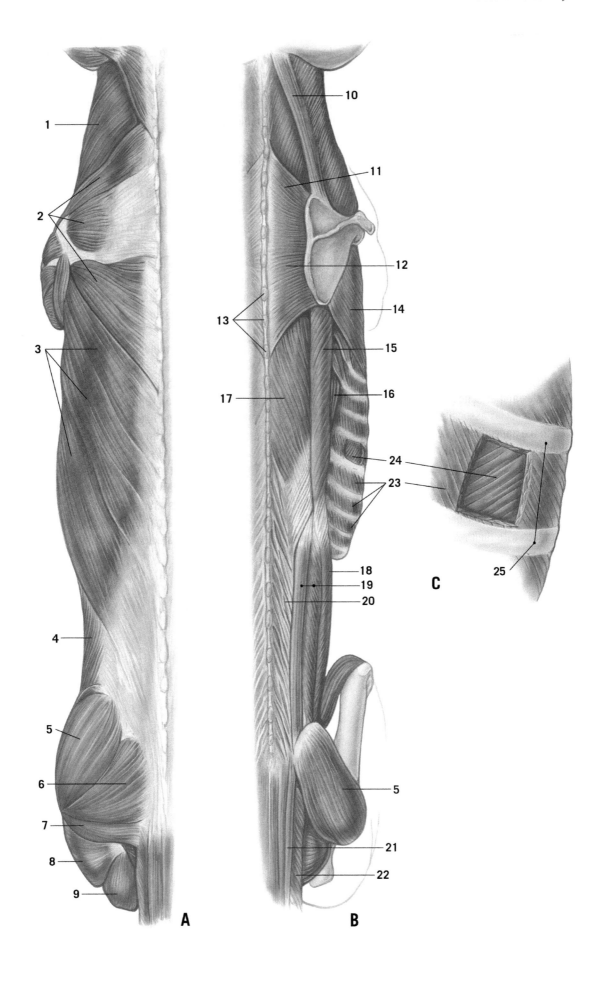

Hypaxial Muscles

Hypaxial musculature is associated with the ventral and ventrolateral surfaces of the vertebrae and tends to run in a craniocaudal direction. They are ventral to the vertebral body and transverse processes and act to flex the spinal column when acting bilaterally. Unilateral action will flex the appropriate vertebrae laterally. They are segmentally innervated by the ventral branches of cervical, thoracic, and lumbar nerves.

In the cervical region, the left and right mm. longus colli are found immediately adjacent to each other in an inverted "V" pattern directly ventral to the cervical and cranial thoracic vertebral bodies. Just lateral to the longus colli is the m. longus capitis that inserts on the basal portion of the skull. In the caudal thoracic and lumbar areas are the mm. psoas major, psoas minor, and quadratus lumborum. Each has one attachment to the ventral surfaces of thoracic and lumbar vertebrae. The m. psoas minor is the most ventral of these muscles and has a long slender tendon attaching to the ventrolateral pelvis. The m. psoas major joins with the m. iliacus caudally to form the m. iliopsoas that inserts on the lesser trochanter of the femur, acting as a major flexor of the hip. The m. quadratus lumborum is the deepest (most dorsal) of these sublumbar muscles and attaches to the medial ilium.

There are other muscles associated with the axial skeleton that do not attach to the appendicular skeleton. These include some ventral neck muscles, thoracic wall muscles, and abdominal wall muscles. These are technically hypaxial muscles.

In the ventral neck, with one attachment to the sternum are the mm. sternocephalicus, sternohyoideus, and sternothyroideus. The m. sternocephalicus can be divided into mastoid and occipital parts in accordance with their respective insertions. The m.

sternohyoideus is directly on the midline ventral to the trachea and inserts on the basihyoid bone. The m. sternothyroideus inserts on the lateral thyroid cartilage of the larynx. The mm. sternothyroideus and sternohyoideus cannot usually be separated at the sternal attachment and may be referred to as the m. sternothyrohyoideus, unofficially.

Thoracic Wall (Respiratory) Muscles

The m. scalenus medius of cats is mostly covered by the m. scalenus dorsalis and so may not be appreciated. The m. scalenus dorsalis attaches to the 3rd or 4th rib. Note that the brachial plexus passes just ventral to this muscle.

The mm. serratus dorsalis cranialis and serratus dorsalis caudalis are located on the dorsal parts of the ribs and cover portions of the mm. iliocostalis thoracis and iliocostalis lumborum. The fiber direction of these 2 muscles is divergent; the cranial muscle fibers run craniodorsal and caudal muscle fibers run caudodorsal.

The intercostal mm. lie in the intercostal spaces extending between the caudal edge of a more cranial rib and the cranial edge of the next, more caudal rib. The external intercostal m. fibers are oriented caudoventrally and cover the internal intercostal m. The internal intercostal m. fibers run caudodorsally. Along the more ventral parts of the intercostals spaces, only the internal intercostal muscles may be seen.

The m. rectus thoracis is located ventral to the mm. scalenus, superficial to external intercostal mm. on the cranioventral area of the thorax. The transversus thoracis mm. (not illustrated), which is located on the internal surface of the ventral thorax, covers the sternum and associated costal cartilages.

The diaphragm separates the thoracic and abdominal cavities. It is often described as a domed muscle (the tip of the dome pushing into the thorax). The center is tendinous, and the more peripheral fleshy parts attach to the caudal sternum (sternal part), along the 8th costal cartilage and near costochondral junctions of ribs 9-13 (costal part). Dorsally, the left and right crura (lumbar part) of the diaphragm attach to the 3rd lumbar vertebra (right) and the 4th lumbar vertebra (left). The crura and tendinous center have passageways located in them to allow structures to pass between the thorax and abdomen (see Chapter 7 also).

Abdominal Muscles

The abdominal muscles, external abdominal oblique m., internal abdominal oblique m., m. transversus abdominis, and m. rectus abdominis - form the soft tissue wall of the abdominal cavity and support much of the weight of abdominal viscera, including fetuses during pregnancy. The muscles fibers run in 4 directions, caudoventral (external abdominal oblique m.), cranioventral (internal abdominal oblique m.), dorsoventral (m. transversus abdominis), and craniocaudal (m. rectus abdominis). This evidently reduces strain and inherent weakness in any one direction. The external abdominal oblique m. also covers a large portion of the caudal ribs and costal arch. The m. rectus abdominis covers the caudal sternum and associated costal cartilages.

In both female and male cats, the caudoventral abdominal wall includes natural "defects," the superficial and deep inguinal rings, which allows passage of the vaginal tunic and associated structures such as the testes. The deep inguinal ring is formed by the lateral edge of the m. rectus abdominis, the caudal edge of the internal abdominal oblique m., and the inguinal ligament. The inguinal ligament is itself the caudal edge of the aponeurosis of the external abdominal oblique m. extending from the tuber coxae to the pubis, *i.e.,* connective tissue from bone to bone, a ligament. The superficial inguinal ring is a slit in the caudal aponeurosis of the external abdominal oblique m. Despite their names, "rings," neither inguinal ring is round or even oval in shape. The deep inguinal ring is triangular, and the superficial ring is ellipsoid.

The junction of the aponeuroses of these left and right abdominal muscles on the ventral midline results in a relatively wide, relatively avascular linea alba extending from the xiphoid to the pubis. The linea alba is the most frequent location for incisions in surgeries of any abdominal organ. The linea alba is also associated with the umbilicus, which can be hard to appreciate in the cat.

Tail Muscles

The dorsal muscles of the tail, the mm. sacrocaudalis dorsalis lateralis and medialis, are caudal continuations of the longissimus system and transversospinalis system, respectively, upon the sacral and caudal vertebrae. These act to extend or lift the tail.

The ventral tail muscles, which act to depress or tuck the tail, are similar to the elongate muscles found on the ventral surfaces of the cervical and lumbar vertebrae. The mm. sacrocaudalis ventralis lateralis and medialis do not appear to be direct continuations of the sublumbar muscles, however.

The mm. intertransversarius are located on the lateral surfaces of the sacral and some caudal vertebrae.

The m. coccygeus and m. caudofemoralis are included in the pelvic limb muscles.

Plate 3-11

Figure A   Superficial musculature of the neck and thorax with thoracic limb removed, lateral view

Figure B   Musculature of the abdominal wall, ventral view

1	M. trapezius, cut
2	M. rhomboideus, cut
3	M. latissimus dorsi, cut in Fig. A
4	M. pectoralis superficiales, cut in Fig A
5	M. pectoralis profundus, cut in Fig A
6	M. splenius
7-8	M. semispinalis capitis
7	M. biventer cervicis
8	M. complexus
9	M. longissimus capitis
10	M. longissimus cervicis
11	M. longissimus thoracis
12	M. spinalis et semispinalis thoracis
13	M. serratus dorsalis cranialis
14	M. serratus dorsalis caudalis

15	M. obliquus externus abdominis
15'	Its aponeurosis
16	M. serratus ventralis thoracis
17	M. serratus ventralis cervicis, cut
18	M. scalenus medius
19	M. scalenus dorsalis
20	M. rectus thoracis
21	Mm. intertransversarii
22	M. longus capitis
23	M. sternothyroideus
24	M. transversus abdominis
25	M. rectus abdominis
26	M. obliquus internus abdominis
26'	Its aponeurosis
27	Linea alba
28	M. sartorius
29	M. gracilis

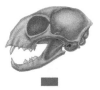

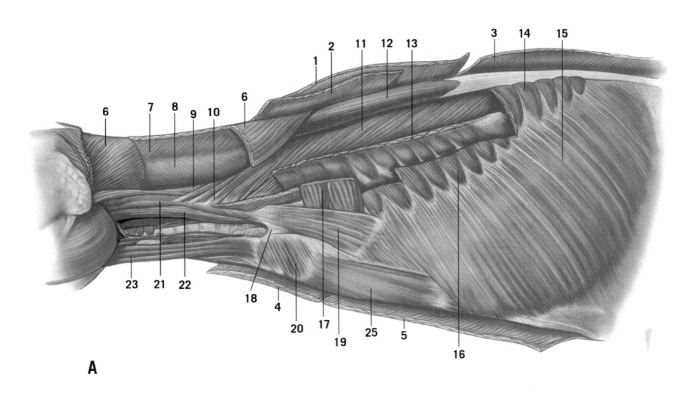

A

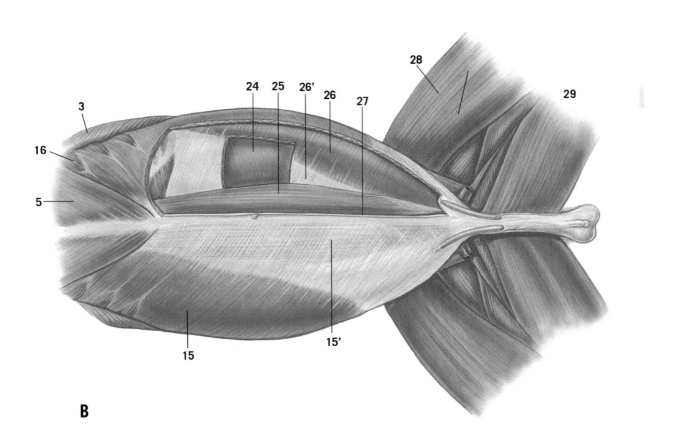

B

Plate 3-12

Figure A   Deep musculature of the vertebral column (sublumbar), ventral view
Figure B   Superficial and deep musculature of the inguinal region, ventral view

1	Central tendon of the diaphragm	16	M. sacrocaudalis ventralis medialis
2	Costal part, diaphragm	17	M. sacrocaudalis ventralis lateralis
3	Lumbar part, diaphragm	18	M. externus abdominis obliquus
4	Left crus, diaphragm	**18'**	its aponeurosis
5	Right crus, diaphragm	19	M. rectus abdominis
6	Esophageal hiatus	20	M. internus abdominis obliquus
7	Aortic hiatus	21	Superficial inguinal ring
8	M. retractor costae	22	Deep inguinal ring
9	M. transversus abdominis	23	External pudendal a, v, genitofemoral n
10	M. psoas minor	24	Spermatic cord (males only)
11	M. psoas major	25	Inguinal ligament (caudal edge of aponeurosis of m. externus abdominis obliquus)
11'	Its tendon		
12	M. quadratus lumborum	26	Scrotal branches
13	M. levator ani	27	Caudal superficial epigastric a, v
14	M. gracilis	28	M. sartorius
15	M. rectococcygeus (cut)		

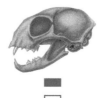

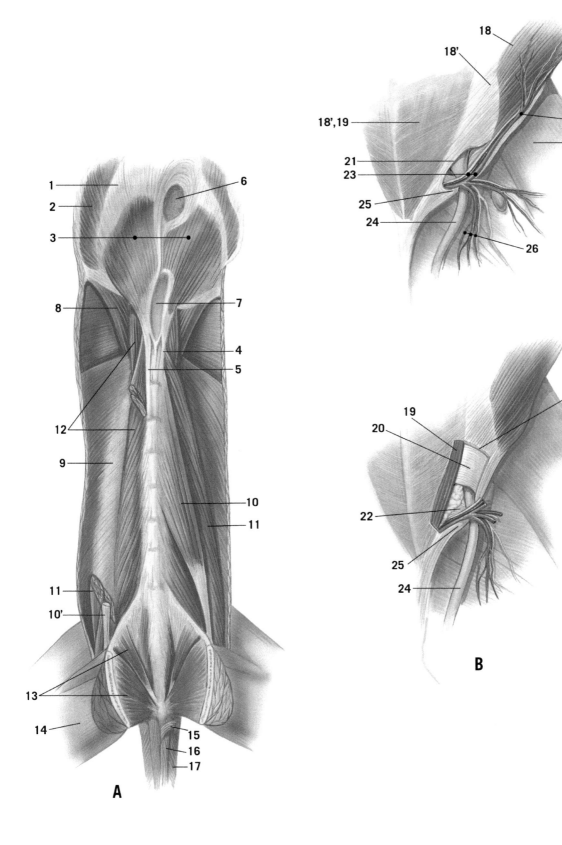

A

B

Appendicular Muscles

The musculature of the limbs of cats does not vary greatly from that of other carnivores except for a few specific points. Therefore, detailed descriptions will not be provided in the interest of space. Particular muscles may have several actions, some of which are opposite to each other. This seeming contradiction is usually explained by whether the limb is weight-bearing or non-weight-bearing.

Thoracic Limb Muscles

Extrinsic Muscles

Because the thoracic limb does not have a bony connection to the axial skeleton, the muscles that hold the limb apposed to the trunk have relatively large importance. Amputations of the entire forelimb will include transection of all these extrinsic muscles. These are the superficial pectoral m., deep pectoral m., m. brachiocephalicus, m. omotransversarius, m. trapezius, m. rhomboideus, m. latissimus dorsi, and m. serratus ventralis.

The superficial pectoral m. cannot always be readily separated into descending and transverse parts. Additionally, the superficial pectoral m. extends to an insertion on the ulna. The deep pectoral m. consists of several different slips of muscle but all pass deep to the superficial pectoral m. near their insertion on the humerus. The m. brachiocephalicus can be divided into m. cleidobrachialis, and m. cleidocephalicus, pars mastoideus and pars cervicalis. In the cat, a constant bony clavicle is located at the junction of these three muscles and serves as the origin. The m. cleidobrachialis, despite the indications of its name, inserts on the ulna in the cat.

Intrinsic Muscles

The intrinsic muscles of the forelimbs (all attachments on the appendicular skeleton) can be arranged into functional groups based on similar location, action, and innervation.

• Extensors of the shoulder (glenohumeral) joint (suprascapular and subscapular nn.): m. supraspinatus, m. infraspinatus, and m. subscapularis. These muscles also serve to stabilize the shoulder joint, supplementing the weak glenohumeral ligaments.

• Flexors of the shoulder joint (axillary n.): m. deltoideus, m. teres major, m. teres minor,

• Extensors of elbow (cubital) joints (radial n.): m. triceps brachii, m. anconeus, m. tensor fasciae antebrachii. The m. triceps brachii of the cat actually has 4 heads. There is also an additional short part of the medial head on the distal medial brachium.

• Flexors of the elbow joint (musculocutaneous n): m. coraco-brachialis, m. biceps brachii, and m. brachialis. The mm. biceps brachii and brachialis each have their insertion only on one bone; the radius and ulna, respectively. The m. coracobrachialis is included in this group because of its location and innervation even though it does not actually act on the elbow.

• Extensors of the carpal and digital joints (radial n.): m. brachio-radialis, m. extensor carpi radialis, common digital extensor m., lateral digital extensor m., m. abductor pollicis longus, m. extensor digit I et digiti II (not illustrated), and m. supinator. On the cranial antebrachium, the superficially located m. brachioradialis is well developed and contributes to the supination ability of the cat. The m. extensor carpi radialis has a long and short part present. The common and lateral digital extensor mm. insert on digits II-V. These antebrachial muscles are bound down as they cross the carpus by extensor retinaculum, which is a visible thickening of the fascia in this area. The tendon of the common digital extensor m., which is joined by other tendons, will insert on the extensor process of the distal phalanges. The m. supinator is included in the group because of its location and innervation even though it does not act on the carpus or digits.

• Flexors of the carpal and digital joints (median and ulnar nn.): m. flexor carpi radialis, superficial digital flexor m., m. flexor carpi ulnaris, m. extensor carpi ulnaris (m. ulnaris lateralis), deep digital flexor m., m. pronator teres, and m. pronator quadratus. On the caudal antebrachium, the deep digital flexor m. has the 3 heads seen in other carnivores, but the relative size of these heads is roughly equal in the cat. The m. m. extensor carpi ulnaris (ulnaris lateralis), acts as a carpal flexor despite its name, but retains its phylogenetic innervation by the radial n. The deep digital flexor m. inserts on the palmar surface of the distal phalanges and will also act to unsheath the claw in cats. The mm. pronator teres and pronator quadratus are included in this group because of their location and innervation even though they do not act on the carpus or digits.

The small muscles with origin and insertion on the palmar surface of the manus are not individually listed although some are illustrated.

The tendons of flexors of the carpal and digital joints are bound down by thickening of fascia called flexor retinaculum (carpus), palmar annular ligament (metacarpophalangeal joint), proximal digital annular ligament (proximal phalanx) and distal digital annular ligament (middle phalanx).

Plate 3-13

Deep (viewer's left) and superficial (viewer's right) musculature of the neck and thorax, ventral view

1	Mandibular lln	8	M. pectoralis transversus
2	External jugular v	9	M. pectoralis descendens
3	M. sternohyoideus	10	Trachea
4	M. sternocephalicus	11	Esophagus
5-7	M. brachiocephalicus	12	M. longus capitis
5	M. cleidocephalicus, pars cervicalis	13	M. longus colli
6	M. cleidocephalicus, pars mastoidea	14	M. latissimus dorsi
		15	M. pectoralis profundus
7	M. cleidobrachialis	16	M. serratus ventralis
		17	M. obliquus externus abdominis

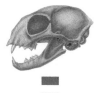

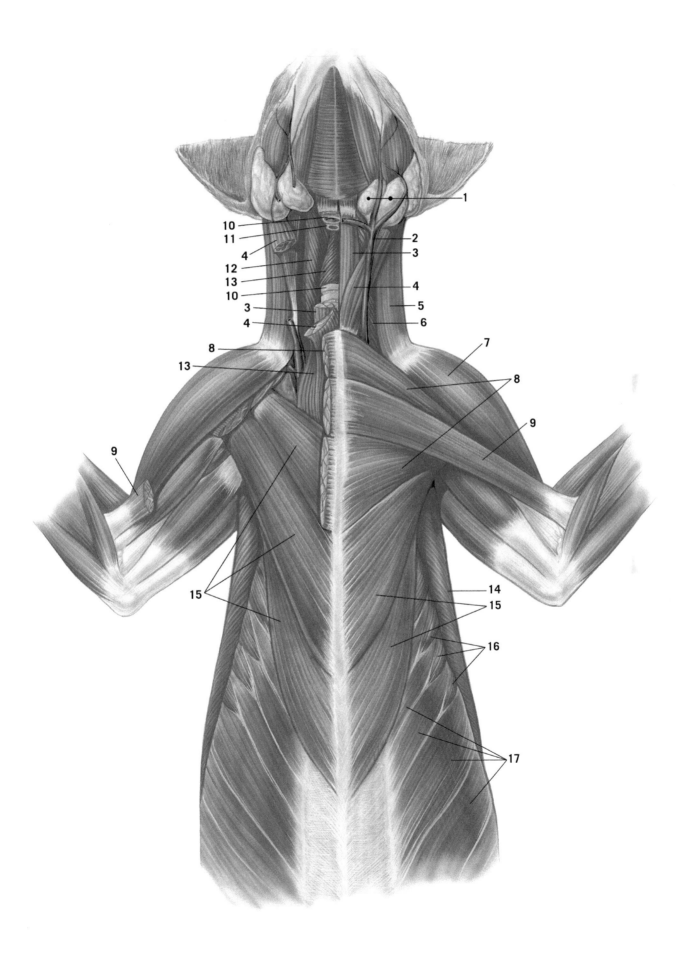

Plate 3-14

Figure A   Intrinsic musculature of thoracic limb with deep musculature of antebrachium, lateral view

Figure B   Intrinsic musculature of thoracic limb with deep musculature of antebrachium, medial view

Figure C   Superficial and deeper musculature of the manus, palmar view

Figure D   Deep musculature of the manus, palmar view

1 M. trapezius, cut	21 M. extensor carpi ulnaris (m. ulnaris lateralis)
2 M. omotransversarius, cut	**21'** Its tendon
3 M. supraspinatus	22 M. supinator
4 M. infraspinatus	23 M. abductor pollicis longus
5 M. teres major	**23'** Its tendon
6-7 M. deltoideus	24 M. extensor pollicis et digiti II
6 Pars scapularis	25 M. flexor carpi ulnaris
7 Pars acromialis	26 M. pronator teres
8 M. subscapularis	27 M. flexor carpi radialis
9 M. coracobrachialis	28 M. flexor digitorum superficialis
10-13 M. triceps brachii	**28'** Its tendon
10 Long head	29 M. flexor digitorum profundus
11 Lateral head	**29'** Its tendon
11' Its tendon	30-32 Heads of m. flexor digitorum profundus
12 Accessory head	**30** Radial head
13 Medial head	**31** Humeral head
13' Its short part	**32** Ulnar head
14 M. tensor fasciae antebrachii, cut	33 M. interflexorius
15 M. biceps brachii	34 Extensor retinaculum
16 M. brachialis	35 M. abductor pollicis brevis
17 M. brachioradialis	36 M. flexor pollicis brevis
18 M. extensor carpi radialis	37 M. adductor pollicis
18' Its tendon	38 M. adductor digiti II
19 M. extensor digitorum communis	39 M. abductor digiti II
19' Its tendon	40 M. adductor digiti V
20 M. extensor digitorum lateralis	41 M. abductor digiti V
20' Its tendon	42 Mm. interossei
	43 Proximal digital annular ligament
	44 Distal digital annular ligament

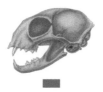

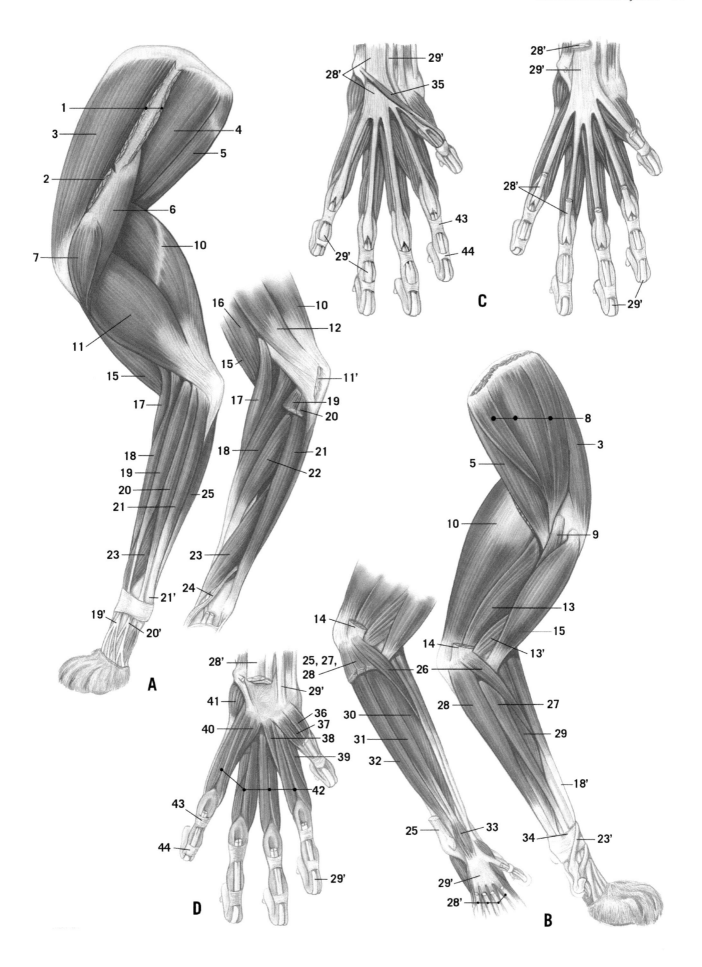

Pelvic Limb Muscles

Extrinsic Muscles

The pelvic limb, unlike the thoracic limb, has an articulation between appendicular skeleton and axial skeleton at the sacroiliac joint. There are relatively few true extrinsic muscles. The mm. psoas major, psoas minor, and. quadratus lumborum, with attach- ments on the femur or pelvis, have been previously mentioned under hypaxial muscles. More laterally on the pelvis are the m. piriformis, which some authorities consider a part of the middle gluteal m., and the m. gluteofemoralis (m. caudofemoralis or cranial crural abductor m.), m. coccygeus, and m. levator ani which can be considered as lateral tail muscles. The m. gluteofemoralis is located between the superficial gluteal and biceps femoris mm. The m. gluteofemoralis originates on Ca_{2-4} vertebrae and inserts via an aponeurosis into the fascia lata. Its action is abduction of the hip joint or lateral movement of the tail. Innervation is via the caudal gluteal n. The mm. coccygeus and levator ani extend from the lateral and ventral surfaces of specific caudal vertebrae to the medial surface of the ilium and pelvic symphysis. These muscles are part of the pelvic diaphragm. Although perineal hernias are fairly rare in the cat, surgical protocols utilizing the sacrotuberous ligament as described in some small animal surgery texts cannot be performed in this way because there is no sacrotuberous ligament in the cat.

Plate 3-15

Figure A Superficial musculature and tendons of the distal antebrachium and manus, dorsal view

Figure B Superficial musculature of the distal antebrachium and manus, lateral view

Figure C Single digit with associated tendons and ligaments, medial view

Figure D Retracted and extended claw, medial view

Figure E Schematic illustration of incision for one method of onchyectomy (declaw).

1	M. extensor carpi radialis	13	Tendon of deep digital flexor m.
2	M. abductor pollicis lingus	14	Tendon of superficial digital flexor m.
3	M. extensor carpi ulnaris (m. ulnaris lateralis)	15	Metacarpal bone
4	Lateral digital extensor m.	16	Proximal phalanx
4'	Its tendon	17	Middle phalanx
5	Common digital extensor m.	18	Distal phalanx
5'	Its tendon	19	Plantar annular lig
6	Tendon of m. extensor digiti I and II	20	Proximal digital annular lig
7	Extensor bands of mm. interossei	21	Distal digital annular lig
8	Combined extensor tendons	22	Dorsal elastic lig
9	Claw covering unguicular process	23	Extensor process
10	Extensor retinaculum	24	Flexor tubercle
11	M. flexor carpi ulnaris	25	Unguicular crest
12	M. interossei	26	Unguicular process
		27	Skin of claw sheath
		28	Digital pad

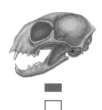

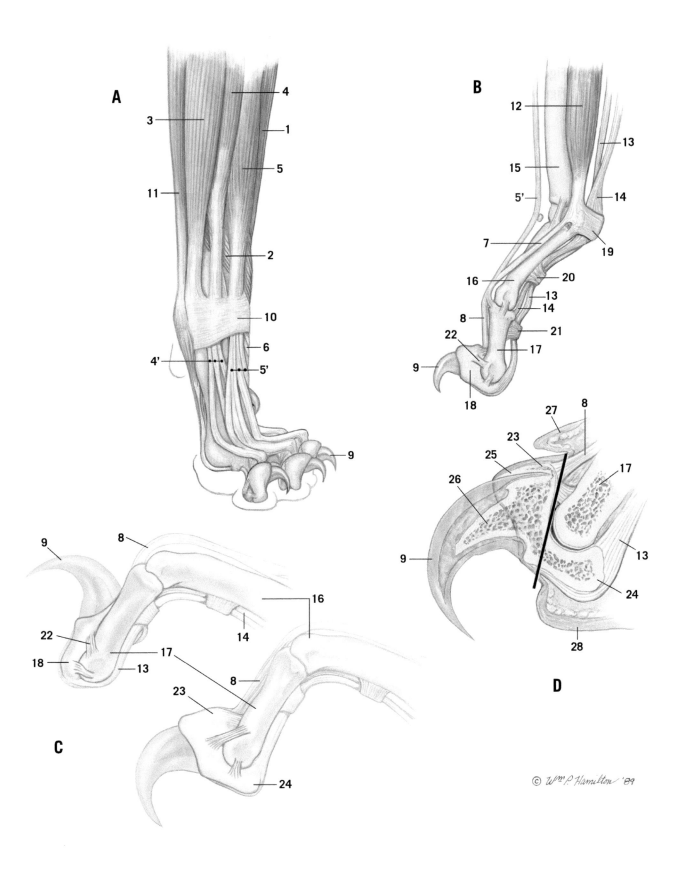

© Wm. P. Hamilton '89

Plate 3-16

Figure A   Superficial musculature of the pelvic limb, lateral view
Figure B   Deep musculature of the pelvic limb, lateral view
Figure C   Deep musculature of the pelvis, dorsocaudolateral view
Figure D   Superficial and deep musculature of the pes, plantar view

1	M. gluteus medius	**23**	M. levator ani
2	M. gluteus superficialis	**24**	M. tibialis cranialis
3	M. gluteofemoralis (m. caudofemoralis)	**25**	M. extensor digitorum longus
4	M. coccygeus	**25'**	Its tendon
5	M. sacrocaudalis dorsalis lateralis	**26**	M. peroneus (fibularis) longus
6	M. sacrocaudalis ventralis lateralis	**26'**	Its tendon
7	M. sartorius	**27**	M. extensor digitorum lateralis
8	M. tensor fasciae latae, cut in Fig B and C	**27'**	Its tendon
9	Fascia lata, cut in Fig B and C	**28**	M. peroneus (fibularis) brevis
10	M. biceps femoris	**28'**	Its tendon
11	M. semitendinosus	**29**	M. gastrocnemius, lateral head
12-14	M. quadriceps femoris	**29'**	Its tendon
12	M. vastus medialis	**30**	M. soleus
13	M. rectus femoris	**31**	M. flexor digitorum profundus, lateral head
14	M. vastus lateralis	**31'**	Its tendon
15	M. adductor	**32'**	Tendon of m. flexor digitorum superficialis
16	M. semimembranosus	**29'+32'**	Common calcanean tendon
17	M. abductor cruris caudalis	**33**	M. flexor digitorum brevis
18	M. gluteus profundus	**34**	M. abductor digiti V
19	M. piriformis	**35**	M. adductor digiti V
20	M. quadratus femoris	**36**	M. adductor digiti II
21	Mm. gemelli	**37**	M. abductor digiti II
22	M. obturatorius internus	**38**	Mm. interossei

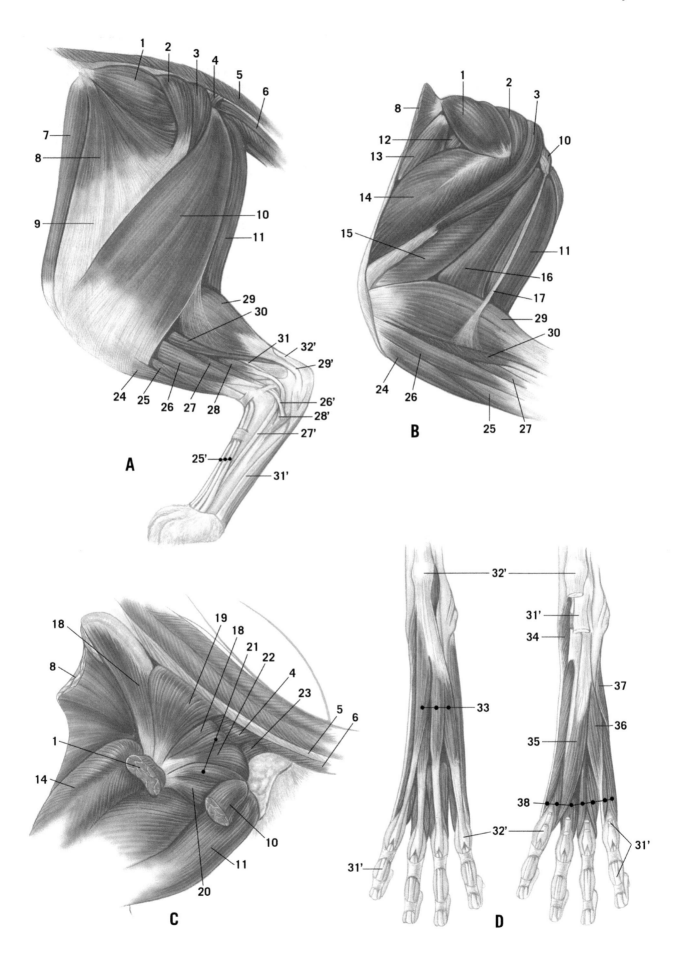

Intrinsic Muscles

Separation of intrinsic pelvic limb muscles into functional groups is a more difficult task than on the thoracic limb due to the multiple actions of some proximal muscles such as the m. biceps femoris.

• Flexors of the hip (coxal) joint (femoral n. and cranial gluteal n.) (The iliopsoas m., an extrinsic muscle, is the most important flexor of the hip): m. rectus femoris and m. tensor fasciae latae.

• Extensors and abductors of the hip joint (cranial and caudal gluteal nn): superficial gluteal m., middle gluteal m., deep gluteal m.

• Adductors of the hip joint (obturator n.): m. gracilis, m. pectineus, m. adductor, and external obturator m. On the medial aspect of the thigh, the m. pectineus is quite small and may be difficult to separate from the mass of the adductor m.

• Outward rotators of the hip joint (sciatic n.): Internal obturator m., mm. gemelli, m. quadratus femoris. These muscles are included in a group known as pelvic association muscles. The tendon of the internal obturator m. may be completely enveloped by the mass of the mm gemelli in the cat. Some authorities consider the external obturator m. as part of the pelvic association group.

• Extensors of the stifle (genual) joint (femoral n.): m. quadriceps femoris - rectus femoris, vastus lateralis, vastus medialis, vastus intermedius-, and m. satorius. The m. satorius is not divided into cranial and caudal parts in the cat.

• Flexors of the stifle joint (sciatic n.): m. biceps femoris, m. semitendinosus, and m. semimembranosus. This group of muscles also acts to extend the stifle when the limb is weight-bearing. A small tendon of the mm. biceps femoris and semitendinosus joins the common calcanean tendon; these parts act to extend the tarsal joints.

• Flexors of the tarsal joints and extensors of the digital joints (superficial and deep peroneal nn.): m. cranialis tibialis, long digital extensor m., m. peroneus longus, lateral digital extensor m., m. peroneus brevis, m. extensor digiti I longus (not illustrated). The long digital extensor m. inserts on the extensor process of the distal phalanges.

• Extensors of the tarsal joints and flexors of the digital joints (tibial n.): m. gastrocnemius: medial and lateral heads, superficial digital flexor m., m. soleus, deep digital flexor m., m. tibialis caudalis, m. popliteus. The m. soleus is well developed in the cat and is found on the lateral surface of the crus. It originates on the head of the fibula and its tendon joins with the tendon of the lateral head of the gastrocnemius to insert on the tuber calcaneus. The medial and lateral heads of the m. gastrocnemius plus the m. soleus may be termed m. triceps surae. The m. triceps surae and the superficial digital flexor m. are the major contributors to the common calcanean tendon. The lateral part of the deep digital flexor m. is relatively large and its tendon remains separate from that of the medial part until about halfway through the length of the metatarsal region. The deep digital flexor m. inserts on the plantar surface of the distal phalanges. The caudal tibial m. has a relatively robust tendon that joins with the tendon of the lateral head of the deep digital flexor m. The m. popliteus does not act on either the tarsal joint or digital joints but is included here due to its innervation. The m. popliteus acts to rotate the limb medially.

• The small muscles with origin and insertion on the pes are not listed although some have been illustrated.

• Similar to the carpal region, tendons crossing the tarsus are bound down by retinacula. Dorsally, the extensor retinaculum is divided into more proximal and distal parts. The single flexor retinaculum at the level of the tarsus is located plantarly and primarily binds the tendon of the lateral head of the deep digital flexor m. There are ligaments binding tendons over the metatarsal bones and phalanges analogous to the forepaw.

Plate 3-17

Figure A   Superficial musculature of the pelvic limb, medial view
Figure B   Deep musculature of the pelvic limb, medial view
Figure C   Deep musculature of the pelvis, ventral view

1   M. iliopsoas
2   M. rectus femoris
3   M. pectineus
4   M. vastus medialis
5   M. adductor
6   M. gracilis
7   M. semitendinosus
   7'   Tendinous contribution to common calcanean tendon
8   M. sartorius
9   M. semimembranosus
10   M. obturatorius externus
11   M. quadratus femoris

12   M. gastrocnemius, medial head
   12' Its tendon
13   Tendon of m. flexor digitorum superficialis
14   M. flexor digitorum profundi, medial digital flexor
   14' Its tendon
15   M. flexor digitorum profundi, lateral digital flexor
   15' Its tendon
16   M. cranialis tibialis
   16' Its tendon
17   M. extensor digitorum brevis
18   Tendon of m. extensor digitorum longus
19   Extensor retinaculum
20   Flexor retinaculum

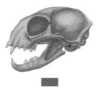

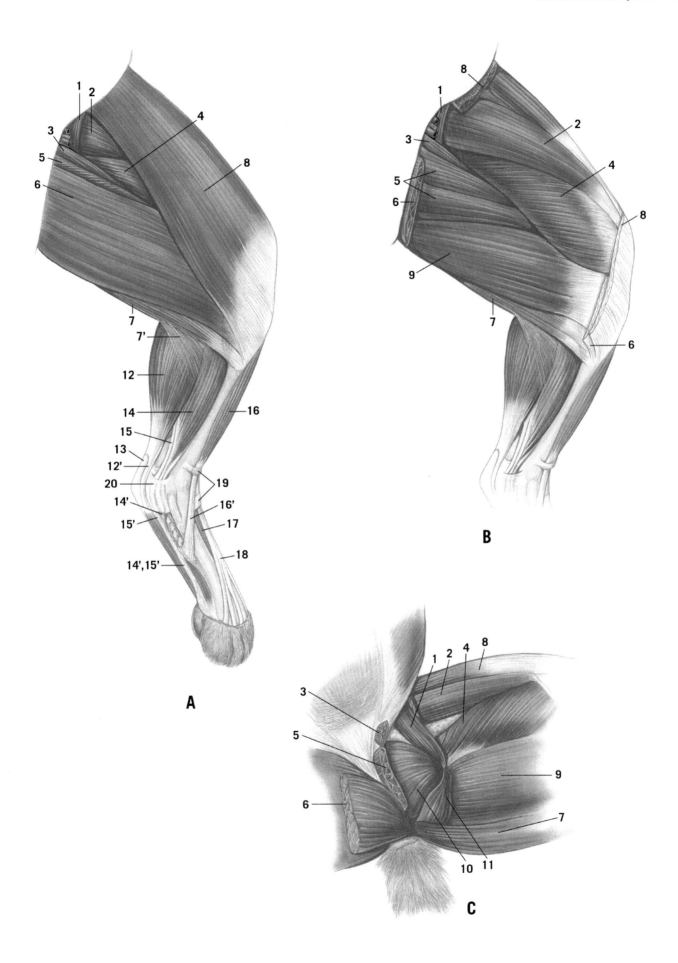

A

B

C

Plate 3-18

Figure A Muscle attachment sites on the left lateral and right medial thoracic limbs. Attachments distal the radius and ulnar are not shown due to size constraints. Red numbers indicate attachment of extrinsic muscles. Prime symbol indicates the distal (typically insertion) site of intrinsic muscles.

Figure B Muscle attachment sites on the left lateral and right medial pelvic limbs. Attachments distal the radius and ulnar are not shown due to size constraints. Red numbers indicate attachment of extrinsic muscles. Prime symbol indicates the distal (typically insertion) site of intrinsic muscles.

1   M. rhomboideus
2   M. trapezius
3   M. omotransversarius
4   M. serratus ventralis
5,5'   M. supraspinatus
6,6'   M. deltoideus
       a   Pars scapularis
       b   Pars acromialis
7,7'   M. infraspinatus
8,8'   M. subscapularis
9,9'   M. teres major
10,10' M. teres minor
11,11' M. triceps brachii
       a   Long head
       b   Intermediate head
       c   Lateral head
       d   Medial head
12,12' M. biceps brachii
13,13' M.coracobrachialis
14,14' M.brachialis
15   M. pectoralis superficialis
16   M. pectoralis profundus, m. latis-
       simus dorsi
17,17' M. aconeus
18   M. brachioradialis
19   M. extensor carpi radialis
20   Common digital extensor m.
21   Lateral digital extensor m.

22   M. extensor carpi ulnaris
       (m. ulnaris lateralis)
23,23' M. supinator
24   M. flexor digitorum produndus
       a   Humeral head
       b   Radial head
       c   Ulnar head
25   M. flexor digitorum superficialis
26   M. flexor carpi ulnaris
       a   Humeral head
       b   Ulnar head
27   M. flexor carpi ulnaris
28,28' M. pronator teres
29   M.extensor digiti II
30   M. abductor pollicis longus
31   M. m. pronator quadratus
32,32' M. sartorius
33   M. tensor fasciae latae
34,34' Deep gluteal m.
35,35' Middle gluteal m.
36   Mm. gemelli
37   M. quadratus femoris
38,38' M. biceps femoris
39,39' M semitendinosus
40   External obturator m.
41,41' M. adductor
42,42' M. gracilis

43,43' M. pectineus
44   Internal obturator m.
45,45' M. iliacus
46   M. psoas major
47,47' M. semimembranosus
48'   Superficial gluteal m.
49,49' M. quadriceps femoris
       a   Rectus femoris
       b   Vastus lateralis
       c   Vastus medialis
       d   Vastus intermedius
50   M. gluteofemoralis
       (m. caudofemoralis)
51,51' Superficial digital flexor m.
52,52' M. m gastrocnemius
       a   Lateral head
       b   Medial head
53   Long digital extensor m.
54,54' M popliteus
55   Cranial tibial m.
56   M. peroneus (fibularis) longus
57   Lateral digital extensor m.
58   M. peroneus (fibularis) brevis
59,59' M. soleus
60   Caudal tibial m.
61   Deep digital flexor m.
       a   Lateral digital flexor
       b   Medial digital flexor

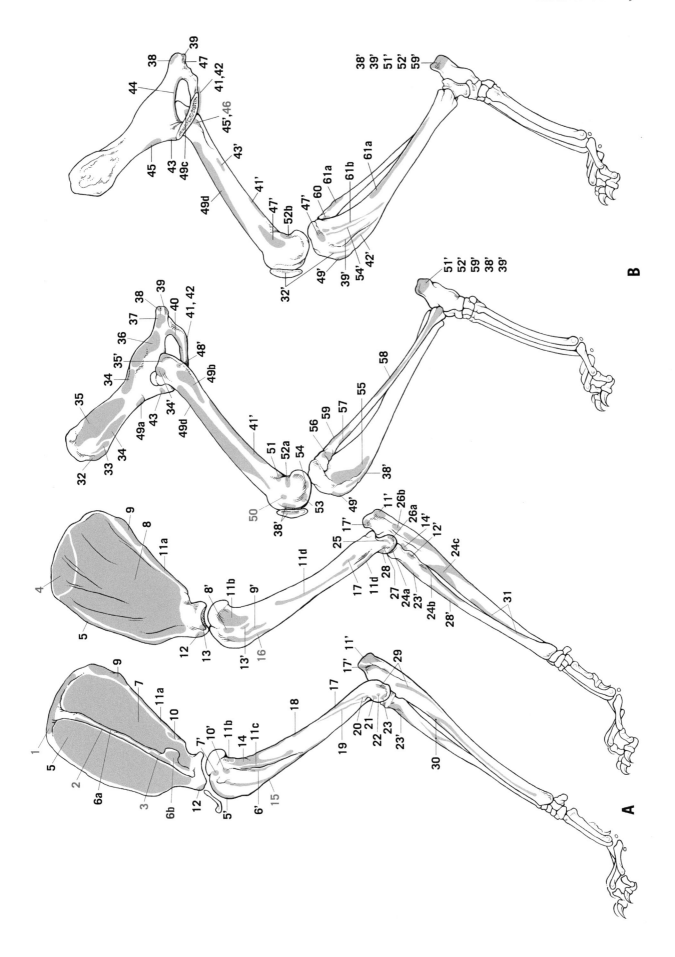

Selected References

1. Crouch JA. *Text-Atlas of Cat Anatomy.* Philadelphia, WB Saunders, 1969; 10, 80.

2. Evans HE. *Miller's Anatomy of the Dog.* 3rd Ed. Philadelphia, WB Saunders, 1993: 122, 219.

3. Gilbert SG. *Pictorial Anatomy of the Cat.* Seattle, University of Washington Press, 1968; 3, 16.

4. Hermanson JW, Evans HE. In: Evans HE (Ed). *Miller's Anatomy of the Dog.* 3rd Ed. Philadelphia, WB Saunders, 1993: 258.

5. Nickel R, et al. *The Anatomy of Domestic Animals,* Vol. 1. The locomotor system of the domestic mammals. New York, Verlag Paul Parey/Springer Verlag, 1986; 52, 75, 100, 267, 270, 278, 304.

6. Nickel R, et al. *The Viscera of the Domestic Mammals,* 2nd Ed. New York, Verlag Paul Parey/Springer Verlag, 1979; 248.

7. Shummer A, et al. *The Anatomy of Domestic Animals,* Vol. 3. The circulatory system, the skin, and the cutaneous organs of the domestic mammals. New York, Verlag Paul Parey/Springer Verlag, 1981; 493.

8. *Nomina Anatomica Veterinaria,* 5th edition. Hannover, Germany, published on line <http://www.wava-amav.org/nav_nev.htm> by the International Committee on Veterinary Gross Anatomical Nomenclature, 2005;32, 52, 62.

9. Richardson D. Radial agensis. *J Vet Orthopedics* 1(1979): 39.

10. Schaller O. Illustrated Veterinary Nomina Anatomica. Stuttgart, Enke Verlag, 1992: 10, 76, 98.

11. Schebitz H and Wilkens H. *Atlas of Radiographic Anatomy of the Cat,.* Stuttgart, Parey Verlag; 2004.

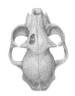

Chapter 4

Cardiovascular System

■ Jill A. Barnes

Modified from the original chapter by Martha Moon and Theresa Rowles

The cardiovascular system serves to supply and drain blood to all tissues of the body, thereby, supplying oxygen and nutrients and removing carbon dioxide and certain metabolites. The heart serves as the pump and all sizes of vessels serve as conduits. Arteries are basically open pipe, and blood can be pushed in either direction through an artery. Which direction is dependent upon the pressure produced by the heart's contraction. Arteries contain smooth muscle and elastic tissue in their walls that allow them to expand with the pulse and then return to their regular diameter and maintain the blood pressure. Veins, in contrast, contain much less smooth muscle in the wall (as pressures are much lower), but do contain valves resulting in unidirectional flow of blood. Arteries and veins that are consistently present are named but the branching patterns frequently vary.

Heart

The heart is the central organ of the cardiovascular system, serving as a pump for both the systemic and pulmonic circulatory systems. Reports vary somewhat as to the average weight of the heart in cats, with 9-12 grams in the adult female and 11-18 grams reported in the adult male.

Pericardium

The heart is encased within the pericardium, a fibroserous sac that also encloses the origin of the great vessels leaving the base of the heart. The fibrous pericardium is a tough connective tissue layer that forms the more superficial aspect of the pericardium and is, in turn, covered by the pericardial mediastinal pleura (see Chapter 7 also). The apex of the fibrous pericardium extends to the ventral portion of the muscular diaphragm, forming a short wide band called the sternopericardial ligament. The serous layer is actually a sac into which the heart is invaginated. The serous membrane is divided into a visceral pericardium (epicardium), which is in intimate contact with the heart muscle, and the parietal pericardium, which lies against the deep surface of the fibrous pericardium. The pericardium is not essential for life, as it can be surgically removed when diseased, but does protect the heart against external friction and inflammation from surrounding structures, stabilizes the heart position, and helps maintain cardiac shape.

A pericardial cavity is located between the visceral and parietal pericardium and normally contains a very small amount of fluid secreted by the serous surfaces. Pericardial effusion, an increase in the volume of this fluid, is uncommon in the cat but can be caused by pericarditis (as a result of bacterial infection, feline infectious peritonitis, cardiomyopathy, and cardiac neoplasia). Pericardiocentesis is indicated to remove excess fluid and/ or obtain samples for laboratory diagnosis. This procedure will reduce pericardial pressure around the heart and improve cardiac filling, relieving clinical signs. To perform this procedure, the cat is generally placed in left lateral recumbency, the site is aseptically prepared and a small gauge needle is used to penetrate the ventral portion of the 6th or 7th right intercostal space.

Persistent communication between the peritoneal and pericardial cavities is a congenital defect. These peritoneal-pericardial diaphragmatic hernias result in varying amounts of abdominal viscera (omentum, liver, spleen, stomach, large and small bowel) displaced into the pericardial sac. While clinical signs of respiratory distress or gastrointestinal upset may result, the cat can be asymptomatic for years, with the defect picked up as an incidental finding.

External Anatomy

The feline heart within its pericardial sac is surrounded laterally by the lungs except at the cardiac notch. This is a large V-shaped fissure between the right middle and right caudal lung lobes that leaves the right lateral surface of the heart in contact with the lateral surface of the thoracic wall. A smaller notch is located between the left cranial and caudal lung lobes.

The feline heart is somewhat pear-shaped, with a dorsocranially directed base and a caudoventrally directed apex. The apex deviates slightly to the left in the thoracic cavity. The external surface of the heart is marked by three grooves that indicate the division of the heart into four chambers (right and left atria and ventricles). A part of each chamber can be seen from the left or right lateral surface. At the base of the heart the coronary groove separates the atria from the ventricles. The paraconal interventricular groove marks the internal separation of the left and right ventricles (junction of interventricular septum with external wall) on the left craniolateral surface of the heart. It is named for its position adjacent to the conus arteriosus, or right ventricular outflow track. The paraconal interventricular groove originates at the coronary groove, just caudal to the origin of the pulmonary trunk, and then extends ventrally to the apex. The subsinuosal interventricular groove marks the junction of the interventricular septum with the external wall on the right caudolateral surface of the heart, originating at the coronary groove immediately ventral to the coronary sinus (located ventral to the entrance of the caudal vena cava into the right atrium). The subsinuosal interventricular groove extends to the apex, where it joins with the paraconal interventricular groove. These three grooves persist, even with heart enlargement.

Originating from the base of the heart are the pulmonary trunk and aorta. The pulmonary trunk originates from the conus arteriosus, the outflow tract of the right ventricle, on the left side of the heart base. It curves dorsally, then caudally, dividing into right and left pulmonary aa. The aorta originates from the left ventricle, at the center of the base of the heart. It extends cranially and dorsally (ascending aorta), then curves caudally and slightly to the left, forming the aortic arch. The descending aorta continues caudally from the aortic arch. The dorsomedial surface of the pulmonary trunk is in contact with the ventrolateral surface of the ascending aorta. At this close approximation of large vessels, the ductus arteriosus originates from the pulmonary trunk just proximal to the bifurcation of the pulmonary trunk, and joins the aorta. In the fetus, it serves as a conduit for blood from the pulmonary trunk to the aorta, bypassing the lungs.

After birth the duct closes, eventually completely obliterating the lumen, forming the remnant called the ligamentum arteriosum. The ductus arteriosus may remain open in some cats (patent ductus arteriosus) resulting in a left to right (high pressure to low pressure) shunting of blood. This causes a volume overload on the left heart and may eventually lead to left-sided congestive heart failure. A continuous, left basilar murmur is typically auscultated with patent ductus arteriosus. Although uncommon in cats, it is an important congenital defect, as it can be surgically corrected.

Entering the base of the heart are the cranial and caudal vena cava and the pulmonary vv. The cranial and caudal venae cavae terminate in the right atrium, which forms the right cranial portion of the base of the heart. A variable number of pulmonary vv. (5-7) bringing oxygenated blood from the lungs terminate in the left atrium, at the more caudal and left base of the heart.

Coronary Circulation

Blood circulating through the heart chambers does not completely supply the heart muscle, so a separate coronary circulation is necessary. Coronary aa. and vv. supply and drain the heart. The left and right coronary aa. originate from the ascending aorta, just distal to the aortic valve. The left coronary a., which is the larger, travels toward the left lateral surface and immediately divides into septal, paraconal interventricular, and circumflex branches. In some cats, a fourth branch, the angular a. supplying a portion of the left ventricle, is present. The septal branch supplies the interventricular septum. The paraconal interventricular branch extends ventrally from its origin down the paraconal interventricular groove, to the apex of the heart, where it joins the subsinuosal interventricular branch. The paraconal inter-ventricular branch supplies arterial branches to portions of the left ventricle and wall of the conus arteriosus of the right ventricle. The circumflex branch proceeds caudally and then turns to the right within the coronary groove. It gives off branches to portions of the left ventricle and left atrium. When the circumflex branch reaches the right lateral surface of the heart, it turns ventrally into the subsinuosal interventricular groove as the subsinuosal inter-tricular branch, supplying the left and right ventricles. The right coronary a. is smaller, and initially reaches the cranial surface of the heart. It then courses to the right and caudally within the coronary groove. It supplies branches to the right ventricle and right atrium. Occasionally the artery in the subsinuosal groove may originate from the right coronary a. rather than the circumflex branch (from left coronary a.).

Most of the blood to the heart itself is returned to the right atrium via the coronary sinus. The sinus lies in the coronary groove ventral to the caudal vena cava, where it opens into the right atrium. The coronary sinus receives blood from the great cardiac v. that courses from the left side in the coronary groove. The great cardiac v. (v. cordis magna) originates in the paraconal inter-tricular groove and then proceeds caudally in the coronary groove. The coronary sinus also receives blood from the v. cordis media, which extends dorsally in the subsinuosal groove. Due to the heavier musculature of the left side of the heart, arteries and veins

supplying and draining the left side are larger than those on the right side.

Internal Anatomy

The right atrium lays dorsocranial to the right ventricle and receives all venous blood from the body except from the lungs. The right auricle, which extends cranially and ventrally, is a small ear-shaped, blind-ended projection off the right atrium.

The coronary sinus opens into the right atrium just ventral to the entrance of the caudal vena cava. The cranial vena cava enters the right atrium from its dorsocranial aspect. The right azygous v., returning blood from portions of the dorsal thoracic wall and lumbar region, usually empties into the cranial vena cava, but may enter the right atrium directly. Internally, a muscular ridge of tissue, the intervenous tubercle, projects from the dorsomedial wall between the cranial and caudal vena caval openings, directing the incoming blood towards the right ventricle. The right and left atria are separated by the interatrial septum. The fossa ovalis, a small depression, is present in the interatrial septal wall caudal to the intervenous tubercle. This is a remnant of the embryonic foramen ovale, which allowed blood to pass directly from the right to left atrium. The foramen functionally closes shortly after birth, and should fibrose within one week. The wall of the main portion of the right atrium is smooth; the wall of the right auricle is lined by branching muscular bands called pectinate muscles.

Blood from the right atrium empties into the right ventricle via the right atrioventricular (tricuspid) valve. This valve consists of a parietal cusp adjacent to the parietal (outer) wall, a septal cusp adjacent to the septum, and an angular cusp located between the other two. This valve is closed during ventricular systole (contraction), preventing regurgitation of ventricular blood into the right atrium. The valve cusps are stabilized by chordae tendineae, connective tissue strands that attach to the free border of the cusps. The chordae tendineae extend from the apices of papillary muscles, conical muscular projections that line the walls of the right ventricle.

The right ventricle is U-shaped, with a distinct inflow tract, extending from the right atrioventricular valve toward the apex, and an outflow tract, from the apex to the conus arteriosus. The conus arteriosus is the funnel shaped portion of the right ventricle that extends dorsally towards the pulmonic valve. It is located adjacent to the paraconal interventricular groove. The interventricular septum separates the right and left ventricles. Congenital lesions of the interatrial and interventricular septa can occur as small, insignificant defects, or result in more marked anomalies such as a common atrioventricular canal. The interventricular septum and the parietal wall of the right ventricular are lined with protruding muscular ridges called trabeculae carneae. The trabecula septomarginalis is a muscular strand that extends across the lumen of the ventricle, from septum to free wall, near the apex. It carries Purkinje fibers across the lumen of the right ventricle aiding in the conduction system of the heart. More than one trabecula septomarginalis may be present.

During right ventricular contraction blood is pumped from the

Plate 4-1

Figure A   Heart and great vessels, right lateral view
Figure B   Heart and great vessels, left lateral view
Figure C   Heart and great vessels, dorsal view
Figure D   Internal structures of heart and great vessels, sagittal section (pulmonic valve not seen)
Figure E   Schematic illustration of blood flow through heart chambers

l	Left surface	**15**	Auricle of left atrium
		16	Paraconal a. and great cardiac v. in paraconal interventricular groove
r	Right surface	**17**	Angular a. (inconstant)
1	Cranial vena cava	**18**	Left and right pulmonary aa.
2	Caudal vena cava	**19**	Ligamentum arteriosum
3	Azygous v.	**20**	Brachiocephalic trunk
4	Right atrium (covered by fat in fig A)	**21**	Left subclavian a.
5	Auricle of right atrium	**22**	Intercostal aa.
6	Right ventricle	**23**	Left atrium (covered by fat in fig C)
7	Left ventricle	**24**	Interventricular septum
8	Apex of heart	**25**	Right atrioventricular valve
9	Subsinuosal a., v. in subsinuosal interventricular groove	**26**	Left atrioventricular valve
		27	Chordae tendineae
10	Coronary sinus in coronary groove	**28**	Papillary muscle
11	Right coronary a.	**29**	Trabecula septomarginalis (may also be present in left ventricle, not shown)
12	Pulmonary vv.		
13	Pulmonary trunk	**30**	Trabeculae carneae
14	Aorta	**31**	Aortic valve

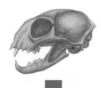

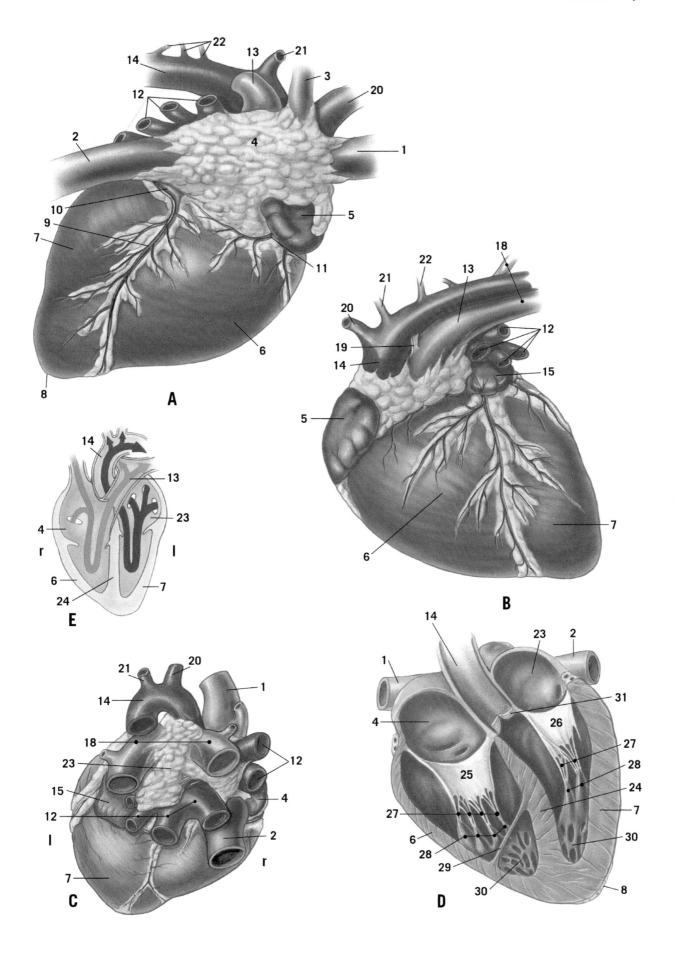

right ventricle to the pulmonic trunk, across the pulmonic valve. The pulmonic valve is located at the junction of the pulmonic trunk and conus arteriosus, and consists of three semilunar-shaped valvulae (right, left, and intermediate). Behind each valvula, on the pulmonary trunk, small pouches are formed called the pulmonary sinuses. During ventricular systole, blood forces the valvulae open, and against the pulmonary trunk wall. During ventricular diastole (relaxation) backflow from the pulmonary trunk fills the pulmonary sinuses, closing the pulmonic valve.

The left atrium lies dorsal and caudal to the left ventricle, forming the left dorsocaudal base of the heart. Multiple pulmonary vv. enter the left atrium bringing oxygenated blood from the lungs. The left auricle is similar in shape to the right auricle, and pectinate muscles are present in both. The auricles lie near each other on the left lateral surface of the heart separated by the pulmonary trunk.

Blood from the left atrium passes through the left atrioventricular (mitral, bicuspid) valve into the left ventricle. This valve consists of two cusps, septal and parietal. The valve cusps are stabilized by chordae tendineae attached to papillary muscles as in the right ventricle. Congenital dysplasia of the left and right atrioventricular valves in cats causing regurgitation into the respective atria is among the most common cardiac malformations in the cat. Left AV valve dysplasia appears to be more prevalent in males and commonly seen in the Siamese breed.

The left ventricle wall is approximately three times as thick as that of the right ventricle, and is conical in shape. Trabeculae carneae and trabecula septomarginalis may be present. The left ventricle pumps blood through the aortic valve and into the systemic circulation via the aorta. The aortic valve, like the pulmonic valve, has three valvulae, but due to greater pressures present in systemic circulation, the aortic valvulae are better developed. Aortic sinuses are formed behind each aortic valvula, with the left and right coronary aa. originating from the left and right sinuses. Congenital stenosis of both the pulmonic and aortic valves has been reported in cats.

While numerous congenital heart defects can occur in the cat, acquired heart disease is a more common clinical problem. Cardiomyopathy (disease of the myocardium) occurs in several forms in the cat; dilated cardiomyopathy (DCM) and hypertrophic cardiomyopathy (HCM) are the best defined. DCM is characterized by dilation of the left ventricle and left atrium and reduced left ventricular function. The right atrium and ventricle may also be dilated, resulting in generalized cardiomegaly. The diagnosis of DCM is best made by echocardiography where left ventricular dilation and reduced function can be directly visualized. It has been shown that many cases of DCM were associated with low plasma taurine levels and were improved with taurine supplementation, which led to increased taurine in modern commercial cat foods. HCM in cats is characterized by marked hypertrophy of the left ventricular free wall, interventricular septum, and papillary muscles, along with left atrial dilation. The left ventricle is increased in weight based on heart weight to body weight ratios. Unlike DCM, left ventricular function is normal. Aortic thrombosis can occur with both DCM and HCM. The thrombus can lodge anywhere, but commonly lodges at the aortic bifurcation into iliac arteries, causing acute pelvic limb paresis/paralysis (ischemic neuronomyopathy).

Cardiac auscultation is used to detect abnormal heart sounds and murmurs caused by either congenital or acquired heart disease. The point of maximal intensity of the apex beat (apical impulse) in the cat is low in the left fifth intercostal space. Each valve also has a punctum maximum but auscultation of individual valves is difficult because the standard stethoscope bell covers several feline intercostal spaces at once.

Radiographic Anatomy

Thoracic radiographs are invaluable in the assessment of heart size as well as other intrathoracic pathology. The cardiac silhouette visualized radiographically also includes the pericardium and the origin of the aorta and pulmonary trunk. Details such as the coronary groove are smoothed out by the pericardium and its contents. On the lateral view the heart extends for about two and one half intercostal spaces, between the 4th and 6th ribs. Radiographically, feline cardiac silhouette has a more horizontal position, with more sternal contact, when compared to the canine cardiac silhouette. The convex cranial border is formed by the right ventricular outflow tract, the right auricle, and the ascending aorta. The right ventricle lies in the cranial and ventral portions of the cardiac silhouette. The caudodorsal border of the heart is formed by the left atrium, while the left ventricle forms the caudal border, ending in the cardiac apex. On the ventrodorsal (VD) or dorsoventral (DV) radiographic view, the right side of the heart silhouette is formed by the right atrium cranially, and right ventricle caudally. The left auricle forms the left cranial and lateral border of the heart, with the left ventricle forming the remainder of the left border, down to the apex (usually located just to the left of midline). The left atrium is superimposed over the caudal border of the heart, on the midline, between the left and right main stem bronchi. The right auricle does not form a border on the VD/DV view. The pulmonary trunk lies at about the 1:00 position (using a clock-face analogy) on the left cranial border. The aortic arch lies between 11:00-1:00, and the descending aorta can be followed as it extends past the heart to the left of midline. Peripheral pulmonary arteries are seen dorsal to pulmonary veins as they extend into cranial lung lobes on the lateral view. Pulmonary vessels are best visualized in the caudal lung lobes on VD/DV views, where the arteries lie lateral to the veins (see Chapter 7 also). The arteries can be traced to their origin on the more cranial aspect of the heart, while the veins terminate more caudally in the left atrium.

Plate 4-2

Figure A   Radiograph of thorax, left lateral view

Figure B   Radiograph of thorax, ventrodorsal view

Radiographs provided courtesy of Diagnostic Imaging (Radiology) Service, Veterinary Teaching Hospital, North Carolina State University College of Veterinary Medicine

1	11th Thoracic vertebra	**9**	Pulmonary vessels (associated with caudal lung lobe)
2	Sternum	**10**	Thoracic aorta
3	Ribs 13	**11**	Pulmonary trunk
4	Spine of scapula	**12**	Right atrium
5	Diaphragm		**12'** Right auricle
	5' Crura of diaphragm	**13**	Left atrium
6	Liver		**13'** Left auricle
7	Trachea	**14**	Right ventricle
8	Caudal vena cava	**15**	Left ventricle
		16	Apex of heart

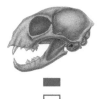

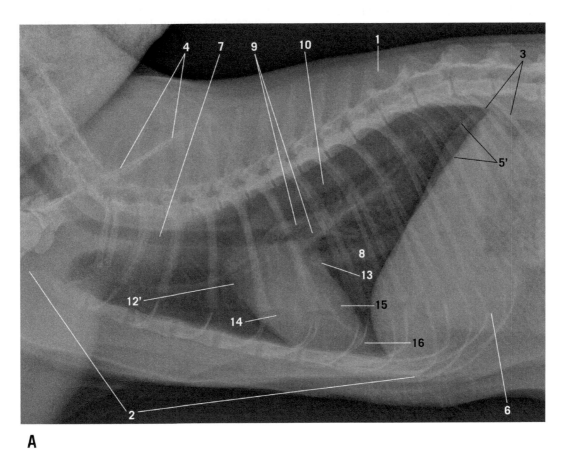

A

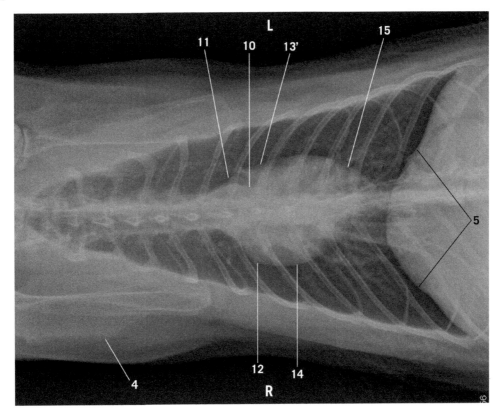

B

Vessels of the Thorax

The brachycephalic trunk is the first large artery to arise from the aortic arch, and it extends cranially, just ventral to the trachea. This trunk immediately divides into a bicarotid trunk and a right subclavian a. From the bicarotid trunk, the right and left common carotid aa. proceed cranially on the ventrolateral aspect of the trachea. The right subclavian a. has four major branches, and then continues as the axillary a. supplying the right thoracic limb.

The vertebral a. is usually the first to arise from the subclavian a., on its dorsal surface. It proceeds cranially and dorsally, eventually entering the transverse foramina of the cervical vertebrae. The costocervical trunk branches next from the subclavian a., and courses dorsally, sending smaller branches to cervical and thoracic musculature. In the cat, a supreme inter-costal artery often arises from the costocervical trunk and gives rise to the dorsal intercostal arteries II and III. The third main branch of the subclavian a. is the superficial cervical a., which arises from the cranial surface, and proceeds cranially supplying musculature of the neck and scapula. The fourth main branch is the internal thoracic a., which arises ventrally from the subclavian

a. very close to the origin of the superficial cervical a. The internal thoracic a. proceeds caudally and ventrally, lying along the internal surface of the sternum. This artery gives off numerous branches that extend dorsally along both sides of the thoracic wall (ventral intercostal aa.). It then terminates as the musculophrenic a. that supplies the diaphragm, and the cranial epigastric a., that supplies the middle portion of the m. rectus abdominis and the cranial abdominal mamma.

The left subclavian a. is the second branch off the aortic arch, and branches in a similar fashion to the right subclavian a., termi-nating in the left axillary a.

Arising from the dorsal surface of the thoracic aorta are numerous paired dorsal intercostal aa. These arteries pass down the thoracic wall on each side, close to the caudal border of each rib, eventually joining the ventral intercostal branches of the internal thoracic a. The location of these arteries should be kept in mind and avoided when performing procedures which penetrate the intercostal space, such as pericardiocentesis, thoracocentesis, etc. The bronchoesophageal a. usually arises from right fifth dorsal intercostal a. The bronchoesophageal a. in turn, branches into bronchial aa. that supply the bronchial structures, and esophageal branches which supply the thoracic esophagus. It should be noted that the origin of the broncoesophageal, bronchial and esophageal aa. is quite variable.

Persistent right aortic arch (PRAA) is a congenital vascular ring anomaly in which the aorta arises from the right fourth embryonic aortic arch rather than the left fourth aortic arch. The ligamentum arteriosum continues to develop from the left side, forming a band that crosses over the esophagus to connect the pulmonary trunk and the aorta. This results in partial esophageal obstruction and regurgitation, typically noted following weaning and ingestion of solid food.

Venous blood is returned to the heart via the cranial vena cava, caudal vena cava, and the azygous v. The cranial vena cava receives blood from the head, neck, thoracic limbs, and ventral thorax. It is formed by the convergence of the right and left brachiocephalic vv. at the thoracic inlet, and then enters into the cranial part of the right atrium. The azygous v. lies adjacent to the descending aorta (on the right), ventral to the thoracic vertebrae, and returns venous blood from the vertebral venous plexus and the dorsal intercostal veins. The azygous v. terminates in the cranial vena cava just before the latter vessel enters the right atrium. The caudal vena cava returns venous blood from the abdomen, pelvis, and pelvic limbs, entering the more caudal portion of the right atrium.

The pulmonary trunk (from the right ventricle) divides into right and left pulmonary aa. The right pulmonary a. leaves the trunk at a right angle, coursing to the right side, and then branches into smaller arteries that carry relatively unoxygenated blood to the right lung lobes. The left pulmonary a. divides into two or more branches carrying blood to the left lung lobes. Heartworm disease, Dirofilaria immitis infection, can affect the pulmonary arteries, especially those going to the caudal lung lobes. Adult heartworms residing in the right ventricle and pulmonary arteries cause endothelial damage and intimal proliferation, eventually resulting in enlarged and tortuous pulmonary arteries. Right heart enlargement also occurs. The incidence of heartworm disease in cats is lower than in dogs, and is also harder to detect due to increased resistance to infection and lower numbers of adult heartworms during infection.

Plate 4-3

Figure A   Vessels of the thorax, left lung removed, left lateral view
Figure B   Vessels of the thorax, right lung removed, right lateral view
Figure C   Vessels of the thorax and axilla; sternum, thymus, and ventral lung removed, ventral view

1	Heart in pericardium	23	Caudal vena cava
2	Thymus	24	External jugular v.
3	Sternum	25	Internal jugular v.
4	First rib	26	Axillary v.
5	Trachea	27	Axillary a.
6	Esophagus	28	External thoracic a.
7	Thoracic aorta	29	Lateral thoracic a.
8	Brachiocephalic trunk	30	Subscapular a.
9	Bicarotid trunk	31	Cranial circumflex humeral a.
10	Right subclavian a.	32	Brachial a.
11	Left subclavian a.	33	Ramus communicans
12	Vertebral a.	34	Sympathetic trunk ganglion
13	Costocervical trunk	35	Sympathetic trunk (not shown in b but also present in the right thorax)
14	Internal thoracic a.	36	Cervicothoracic ganglion
15	Superficial cervical a	37	Vertebral n.
16	Dorsal intercostal aa.	38	Ansa subclavia
17	Pulmonary trunk	39	Vagosympathetic trunk
18	Brachiocephalic vv.	40	Left (a) and right (b) vagus n.
19	Internal thoracic v.	41	Left recurrent laryngeal n.
20	Cranial vena cava	42	Dorsal vagal trunk
21	Azygous v.	43	Ventral vagal trunk
22	Dorsal intercostal vv.	44	Left (a) and right (b) phrenic n.

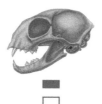

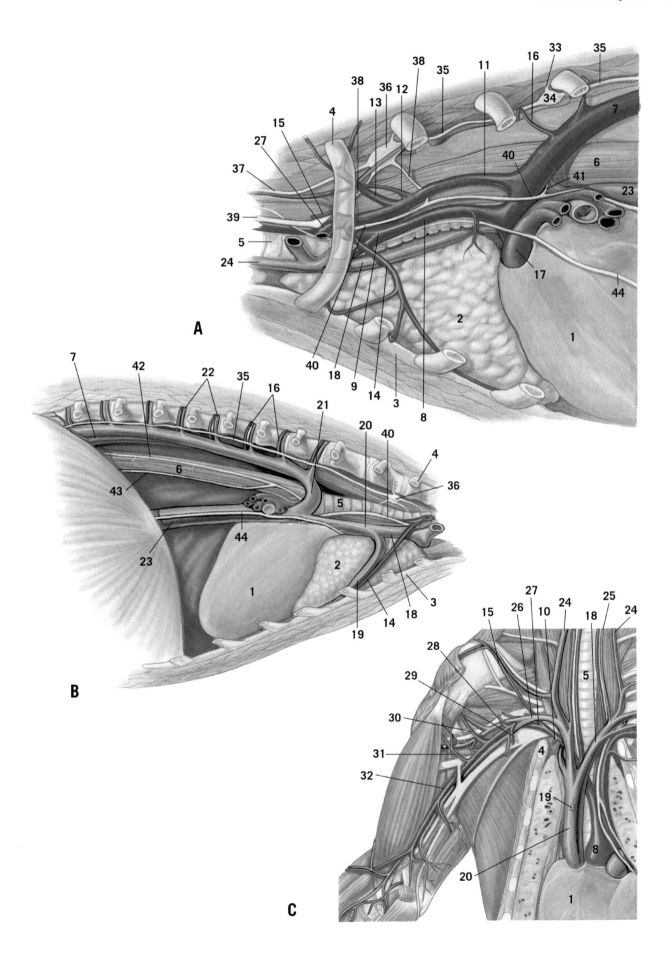

Vessels of the Head and Neck

The principal arterial supply to the head is via the right and left common carotid aa., although the vertebral a. contributes blood to the occipital and cerebral circulation. Each common carotid a. courses in the ventrolateral neck adjacent to the vagosympathetic trunk within the carotid sheath. Along this course the common carotid a. supplies the thyroid gland and larynx and then terminate at the angle of jaw by dividing into internal carotid and external carotid aa. At the bifurcation lies the carotid body, and the carotid sinus is in a bulge at the origin of internal carotid a. The extracranial internal carotid a. becomes reduced in size or ligamentous past the level of the carotid sinus. Extracranial head structures receive blood via the external carotid a. through the following branches. The occipital a. supplies the occipital region and anastomoses with the vertebral a. The ascending pharyngeal a. supplies the pharynx. The lingual, facial, and caudal auricular aa. arise next from the external carotid a. and supply the tongue and palate, superficial face, and caudal ear, respectively. The final two branches of the external carotid a. are the superficial temporal a., which supplies the rostral ear, m. masseter, lateral face, and temporal region, and the maxillary a., which supplies the deep structures of the face and nasal cavity and the rete mirabile maxillaris. From the rete, branches enter the orbital fissure and provide blood to the cerebral circulation.

Venous drainage of the head is by satellite veins which drain into the linguofacial v. (from tongue and superficial face) and maxillary v. (from deep face and venous sinuses of the brain). These merge at the caudal angle of the mandible to form the external jugular v. The external jugular v. is a main venipuncture site in the cat. These right and left veins run parallel, but not satellite, to the common carotid aa. The external jugular vv. unite with the subclavian vv. to form the right and left brachiocephalic vv. which then join to form the unpaired cranial vena cava.

Vessels of the Central Nervous System

On the base of the feline brain is an arterial circle. The rostral cerebral aa., rami retis, caudal communicating aa. and basilar a. interconnect to form the circle. The distal portions of the rostral cerebral aa., the middle cerebral aa., the caudal cerebral aa., and the rostral cerebellar aa. leave the circle to supply large areas of brain parenchyma. The feline internal carotid a., which degenerates in the perinatal period, does not enter the arterial circle as it does in some other species. Instead, multiple branches of the maxillary a. form a rete mirabile maxillaris; in turn, rami retis leave the rete and enter the arterial circle at the base of the brain. The rami retis join the feline arterial circle at a position analogous to where the canine internal carotid a. enters the canine arterial circle. The caudal cerebellar aa. and pontine aa. are usually branches of the basilar a. caudal to the arterial circle.

The basilar a. is continuous with the ventral spinal a. that runs near the ventral fissure on the longitudinal axis of the spinal cord. There are also a pair of longitudinally oriented dorsal spinal arteries on the spinal cord. At each intervertebral foramen, radicular branches of spinal arteries enter the vertebral canal, following the spinal nerve roots and anastomosing with the dorsal spinal and ventral spinal arteries. They form a collateral circulation through an arterial plexus on the surface of the spinal cord. Series of branches from the arterial plexus, and from the dorsal and ventral spinal arteries penetrate and supply the spinal cord parenchyma. The central branches of the ventral spinal artery are especially important in nourishing the gray matter of the spinal cord.

The veins of the brain are rather complex and the larger vessels do not usually travel as satellites of the supplying arteries. The dorsal sagittal sinus on the midline drains the dorsal aspect of the cerebral hemispheres. It is joined by the straight sinus, also on the midline but at a deeper level, which drains the area of the corpus callosum and the dorsal part of the rostral brain stem. The dorsal sagittal sinus enters a foramen in the caudal cranial vault and divides into left and right transverse sinuses within the occipital bone. The transverse sinuses travel laterally in the transverse canals and grooves. They will each branch off a sigmoid sinus and then continue to travel ventrolaterally until they leave the skull

through the retroarticular foramina as the retroarticular veins. Each sigmoid sinus travels along a sinuous route in the caudolateroventral skull and further divides into a condyloid sinus and ventral petrosal sinus. The condyloid sinus exits via the condyloid canal. The ventral petrosal sinus travels rostrally to enter the large cavernous sinus in the base of the cranial vault. The left and right cavernous sinuses have interconnections with each other across the midline. These sinuses also have multiple connections with veins draining ophthalmic region, olfactory region, and structures of the pterygopalatine fossa. These connections could allow hematogenous spread of infections from head structures (eye, nose, etc.) to the brain resulting in a meningitis and/or encephalitis.

The condyloid sinuses continue caudally as the basilar sinuses which, in turn, are connected with the ventral vertebral venous plexi associated with the spinal cord. The vertebral plexi are located in the epidural space of the ventrolateral vertebral canal. They are longitudinally oriented, but have a scalloped appearance. When viewed together, the plexi approach each other at midbody of the vertebra and are furthermost apart at intervertebral spaces. There are inconstant interconnections across the midline between the plexi and there are also connections with intervertebral veins at each intervertebral space.

Plate 4-4

Figure A   Superficial vasculature of the head, lateral view

Figure B   Deep vasculature of the head with zygomatic arch removed, lateral view.
Inset: detail of area of rete mirabile maxillaris

Figure C   Schematic illustration of head vasculature, lateral view

Figure D   Arterial circle of brain and major branches, ventral view

Figure E   Major venous sinuses of brain, caudolateral view

1	Facial a., v.	30	Inferior alveolar n.
2	Linguofacial v.	31	Lingual n.
3	Transverse facial a. v.	32	Buccal n.
4	Rostral auricular v.	33	Auriculotemporal n.
5	Maxillary v.	34	Maxillary n.
6	External jugular v.	35	Zygomatic n.
7	M. masseter	36	Lacrimal n.
8-10	Facial n. (cranial nerve VII)	37	Occipital a.
8	Ventral buccal branch	38	Cranial laryngeal a.
9	Dorsal buccal branch	39	Lingual a.
10	Auriculopalpebral n.	40	Rostral and caudal auricular aa.
11	Transverse facial branch (cranial nerve V)	41	Palpebral a.
12	Parotid salivary gland	42	Mental a.
12'	Its duct	43	Malar a.
13	Mandibular salivary gland	44	Infraorbital a.
14	Great auricular n.	45	Tympanic bulla
15	Ramus of mandible, cut	46	Rami retis
16	Zygomatic arch, cut and removed	47	Rostral cerebral a.
17	Temporal fossa (m. Temporalis cut and removed)	48	Middle cerebral a.
18	Common carotid a.	49	Caudal cerebral a.
19	Caudal auricular v.	50	Caudal communicating branch
20	External carotid a.	51	Rostral cerebellar a.
21	Superficial temporal a.	52	Caudal cerebellar a.
22	Maxillary a.	53	Basilar a.
23	Caudal deep temporal a.	54	Dorsal sagittal sinus
24	Inferior alveolar a.	55	Straight sinus
25	Rete mirabile maxillaris	56	Transverse sinus
26	Rostral deep temporal a.	57	Temporal sinus
27	External ophthalmic a., V.	58	Retroarticular v.
28	Buccal a.	59	Condyloid v.
29-33	Branches of mandibular n. (Cranial nerve v)	60	Basilar sinus
29	Mylohyoid n.	61	Internal jugular v.
		62	Ventral petrosal sinus
		63	Cavernous sinus
		64	Intercavernous sinus

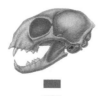

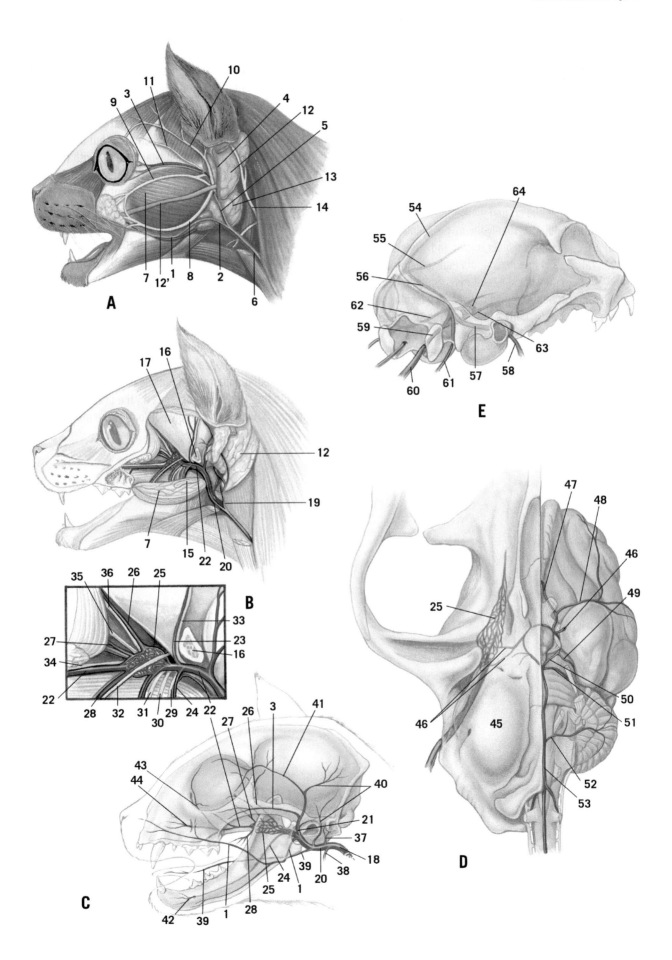

Vessels of the Thoracic Limb

The thoracic limb is mainly supplied by branches of the axillary a. which is the continuation of the subclavian a. The axillary a. begins at the cranial border of the first rib and becomes the brachial a. at the caudal border of m. latissimus dorsi. It typically gives rise to four major branches: external thoracic a., which supplies the superficial and deep pectoral mm.; lateral thoracic a., which travels caudally and supplies the latissimus dorsi, cutaneous trunci, and deep pectoral mm.; subscapular a., which supplies the scapulohumeral region; and cranial circumflex humeral a. which supplies the cranial glenohumeral joint. Specific branches of the subscapular a. supply the m. latissimus dorsi (thoracodorsal a.), caudal glenohumeral joint and humerus (caudal circumflex humeral a.), and caudal scapula (subscapular a.). Surgical approaches to the shoulder joint must contend with these branches. The cranial scapular region derives its vascular supply from the suprascapular a. (usually a branch of the superficial cervical a.).

The axillary a. is continued as the brachial a. that supplies the brachium, the elbow region and proximal antebrachium. The brachial a. is continued by the median a. in the proximal antebrachium at the point where the caudal interosseous a. is released. The brachial a. usually gives rise to several arteries.

The deep brachial a. courses caudally with the radial n. to the m. triceps brachii. The superficial brachial a. supplies the mm. biceps brachii and brachialis, then gives rise to the collateral ulnar a., which courses caudally across the caudal surface of the medial epicondyle The superficial brachial a. continues onto the cranial antebrachium as the cranial superficial antebrachial a. At this point on the distal humerus the brachial a. (but not the brachial v.) passes through the supracondylar foramen with the median n. This artery may be damaged in distal humeral fractures or surgical approaches to this area. Distal to this point the transverse cubital a. arises and courses laterally across the cranial antebrachium to supply the craniolateral antebrachial muscles. Two or more deep antebrachial aa. next arise and supply the caudomedial antebrachial muscles. The final two branches are the cranial and caudal interosseous aa. These usually arise separately in the cat. The cranial interosseous a. passes laterally through the interosseous space to supply the craniolateral antebrachial muscles. The caudal interosseous a. gives rise to the ulnar a. and then continues deep distally to supply the caudomedial antebrachial muscles. The larger ulnar a. travels deep to the m. flexor carpi ulnaris to supply the caudomedial antebrachial muscles and portions of the manus.

Distal to the caudal interosseous a., the brachial a. continues as the median a. which will supply portions of the manus. The median

a. continues distally on the medial side of the radius giving rise to the radial a. in the distal 1/3 of the antebrachium. The radial a. is larger than the continuation of the median a. and will be a main channel of blood to the manus.

The arterial supply to the manus involves anastomosing arches fed by several branches. The cranial superficial antebrachial a. unites with the dorsal carpal branch of the ulnar a. to form the dorsal superficial carpal arch that gives rise to the dorsal common digital and dorsal proper digital aa. The radial a. and cranial interosseous a. anastomose to form the dorsal carpal rete from which the dorsal metacarpal aa. arise. The largest of these, dorsal metacarpal a. II, has a large branch (proximal perforating branch) that penetrates between metacarpal bones II and III to emerge on the palmar side. A palmar branch of the ulnar a. gives rise to the abaxial palmar digital a. V and also anastomoses with the proximal perforating branch to form the deep palmar arch from which the palmar metacarpal aa. arise. The median a. supplies the palmar common digital aa. II, III, IV from the superficial palmar arch.

The anastomotic blood supply of the manus is important in such an accident-prone area allowing multiple alternate routes for blood flow. Onychectomies (declaw) involve the palmar and dorsal proper digital aa. on axial and abaxial surfaces of each digit.

The main channel of blood to the paw is via axillary a., brachial a., median a., radial a., perforating brachial arches, deep palmar, palmar metacarpal and palmar proper digital aa.

Most of the arterial pathways described above have satellite veins bearing the same name as the accompanying artery, i.e., brachial a., brachial v. The superficially located, non-satellite venous return is the cephalic system. The cephalic v. begins with subcutaneous drainage of the medial palmar manus as a continuation of the superficial palmar venous arch. It courses proximally and moves dorsally to join, at the distal radius, with the accessory cephalic v., which drains the dorsum of the manus. The cephalic v. then continues to the elbow subcutaneously on the cranial border of the antebrachium adjacent to and parallel with the superficial branch of the radial n., superficial antebrachial a., and the m. brachioradialis. At this level the cephalic v. is a site for venipuncture. The cephalic v. has a branch at the elbow, the median cubital v., which communicates with the brachial v. on the medial side. The cephalic v. then courses laterally to the brachium from which an axillobrachial v. goes deep to the m. deltoideus and caudal to the shoulder joint to communicate with the subscapular v. The cephalic v. continues its path deep to the m. brachiocephalicus and terminates by joining with the superficial cervical v. or, more commonly, by joining the external jugular v.

Plate 4-5

Figure A   Schematic illustration of the vasculature of the forelimb, medial view with satellite veins (not labeled) and cephalic system (labeled)

Figure B   Superficial and deep vasculature of the forepaw, dorsal view, (all veins not shown)

Figure C   Superficial (top) and deep vasculature of the forepaw, palmar view (veins not shown)

m	Medial	**14**	Collateral radial a.
		15	Thoracodorsal a.
l	Lateral	**16**	Cranial circumflex humeral a.
		17	Deep brachial a.
1-8	Main channel arteries	**18**	Superficial brachial a.
1	Axillary a.	**19**	Collateral ulnar a.
2	Brachial a.	**20**	Cranial superficial antebrachial a.
3	Median a.	**21**	Transverse cubital a.
3'	Median a., Not main channel	**22**	Deep antebrachial a.
4	Radial a.	**23**	Cranial interosseous a.
5	Proximal perforating branch II	**24**	Ulnar a.
6	Deep palmar arch	**25**	Caudal interosseous a.
7	Palmar metacarpal aa. II-IV	**26**	Cephalic v.
8	Axial/abaxial palmar proper digital aa. I-V	**27**	Accessory cephalic v.
9	Suprascapular a.	**28**	Median cubital v.
10	External thoracic a.	**29**	Axillobrachial v.
11	Lateral thoracic a.	**30**	Dorsal carpal rete
12	Subscapular a.	**31**	Dorsal common digital aa. I-IV
13	Caudal circumflex humeral a.	**32**	Axial/abaxial dorsal proper digital aa. I-V
		33	Palmar common digital aa. I-IV

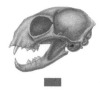

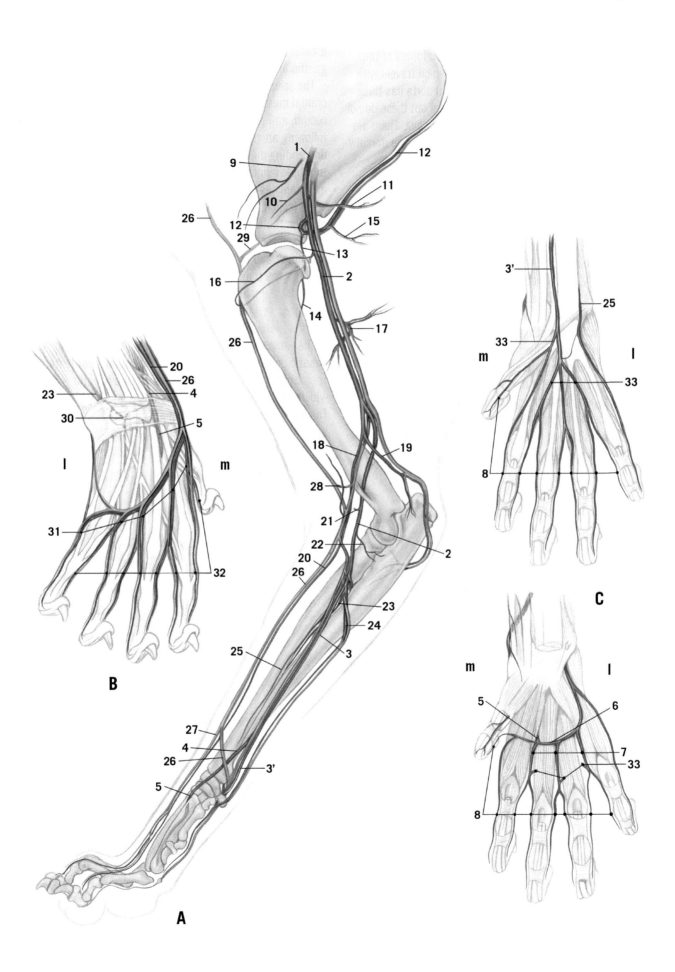

Vessels of the Abdomen

The descending aorta passes through the aortic hiatus of the diaphragm and becomes the abdominal aorta which travels with the abdominal caudal vena cava. The abdominal aorta has three unpaired vessels that supply the digestive system but these do not have satellite veins draining into the caudal vena cava. There are seven pairs of lumbar aa. (with satellite veins) that travel dorsally toward the lumbar intervertebral spaces and epaxial muscles. The aorta also has four paired arterial branches (with satellite veins) which supply the abdominal wall or paired viscera, paired external iliac aa. (with satellite veins) which supply the pelvic limbs, paired internal iliac aa. (with satellite veins) which supply the pelvic structures, and one median sacral a. (with satellite vein) which supplies the region of the sacral vertebrae. This last artery is continued caudally as the median caudal a. to supply the tail.

The first unpaired branch of the aorta is the celiac a. which supplies the cranial abdominal digestive tract. The celiac a. has three major branches: hepatic a., left gastric a. and splenic a. The hepatic a. supplies the liver (hepatic branches), gall bladder (cystic a.), right lesser curvature of the stomach (right gastric a.), right greater curvature of the stomach (right gastroepiploic a.), and cranial portions of the right lobe of the pancreas and descending duodenum (cranial pancreaticoduodenal a.). The left gastric a. supplies the left lesser curvature of the stomach and the esophagus (left gastric a.). The splenic a. supplies the spleen, left greater curvature of the stomach (left gastroepiploic a. and short gastric aa.), and left lobe of pancreas (pancreatic branches).

The second unpaired branch of the abdominal aorta is the cranial mesenteric a. supplying most of the small intestine, the cecum, and part of the colon. This artery generally supplies the following areas: caudal portion of right lobe of the pancreas and descending duodenum (caudal pancreaticoduodenal a.), jejunum (multiple jejunal aa.), ileum, cecum and ascending colon (ileocolic a.). Branches of the ileocolic a. supply the proximal ascending colon (colic br.), the cecum (cecal a.), antimesenteric portion of ileum (antimesenteric ileal a.) and mesenteric surface of ileum (mesenteric ileal a.). The right colic a. supplies the distal ascending and proximal transverse colon. The middle colic a. supplies the transverse and proximal descending colon.

The third unpaired branch of the abdominal aorta, the caudal mesenteric a., supplies the distal descending colon (left colic a.) and the proximal rectum (cranial rectal a.).

The venous drainage from the digestive viscera forms the hepatic portal system, a non-satellite system near its termination. The viscera drain via several veins into the hepatic portal v. which enters the liver at the hilus (adjacent to the gall bladder). The blood filters through the hepatic sinusoids and re-enters the systemic circulation (caudal vena cava) via the hepatic vv. Portosystemic shunts are a congenital or acquired anomaly in which venous blood from the gastrointestinal, splenic, or pancreatic vessels bypasses the liver, entering directly into the central venous system, usually the caudal vena cava. Central nervous system signs, such as blindness and stupor, and gastrointestinal signs, such as vomiting and excess salivation, may result due to toxins or metabolites that are not adequately filtered by the bypassed liver. Partial or complete ligation of the shunt vessel may increase hepatic circulation and allow remission of clinical signs.

The paired lateral branches of the abdominal aorta, which have satellite veins emptying into the caudal vena cava, are (in order, cranial to caudal) the phrenicoabdominal, renal, ovarian or testicular, and deep circumflex iliac aa. The phrenicoabdominal a. supplies the caudal diaphragm, craniolateral abdominal wall, and the adrenal gland. The right phrenicoabdominal a. may arise from the renal a. rather than as a separate branch. This vessel is closely associated with the adrenal gland and will be approached in adrenal surgeries. The renal aa. arise near the level of lumbar vertebrae 1 and 2, and the right renal a. usually arises cranial to the level of the left renal a. The right renal a. passes ventral to the caudal vena cava. The ovarian or testicular aa. usually arise caudal to the renal aa. and supply the ovary, uterine tube, and cranial uterine horn in the queen and the testis and epididymis in the tom. The deep circumflex iliac aa. arise near the level of the sixth lumbar vertebra to supply the caudolateral abdominal wall.

Paired lumbar aa. with satellites veins leave the aorta dorsally. They will supply the lumbar vertebrae and associated muscles and contribute to the circulation of the caudal spinal cord.

The descending aorta terminates by branching into paired external iliac aa., paired internal iliac aa., and unpaired median sacral a. The external iliac and internal iliac aa. will be described later. The median sacral a. travels caudally to supply the tail region.

The caudal vena cava originates as the right and left common iliac vv. come together (at the region of the lumbar vertebra 7-sacral vertebra 1). The common iliac v. is formed by the joining of the external and internal iliac vv. on one side. The caudal vena cava receives drainage from deep circumflex iliac, ovarian or testicular, renal, phrenicoabdominal, and lumbar vv. before passing dorsal to the liver to receive the hepatic vv. The kidneys have a capsular venous plexus that empties into the renal vv. (may be one or two per side) and then into the caudal vena cava. The left ovarian or testicular v. often enters the left renal v. The caudal vena cava then passes through the caval foramen of the diaphragm to enter the thoracic cavity and terminates in the right atrium.

Plate 4-6

Figure A   Branches of celiac artery to abdominal viscera, ventral view
Figure B   Branches of cranial mesenteric and caudal mesenteric arteries to abdominal
viscera, ventral view
Figure C   Schematic illustration of paired lateral and unpaired ventral branches of
abdominal aorta, ventral view

l	Left	20	Cecum
		21	Ascending colon
r	Right	22	Transverse colon
		23	Descending colon
1	Stomach	24	Cranial mesenteric a.
2	Spleen	25	Caudal pancreaticoduodenal a.
3	Pancreas	26	Jejunal aa.
4	Descending duodenum	27	Middle colic a.
5	Abdominal aorta	28	Ileocolic a.
6	Celiac a.	29	Right colic a.
7	Left gastric a.	30	Cecal a.
8	Splenic a.	31	Antimesenteric ileal a.
9	Left gastroepiploic a.	32	Mesenteric ileal a.
10	Pancreatic branch	33	Caudal mesenteric a.
11	Hepatic a.	34	Left colic a.
12	Hepatic branches	35	Cranial rectal a.
13	Right gastric a.	36	Phrenicoabdominal a.
14	Gastroduodenal a.	37	Renal a.
15	Cranial pancreaticoduodenal a.	38	Testicular/ovarian a.
16	Right gastroepiploic a.	39	Deep circumflex iliac a.
17	Ascending duodenum	40	External iliac a.
18	Jejunum	41	Internal iliac a.
19	Ileum	42	Median sacral a.

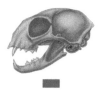

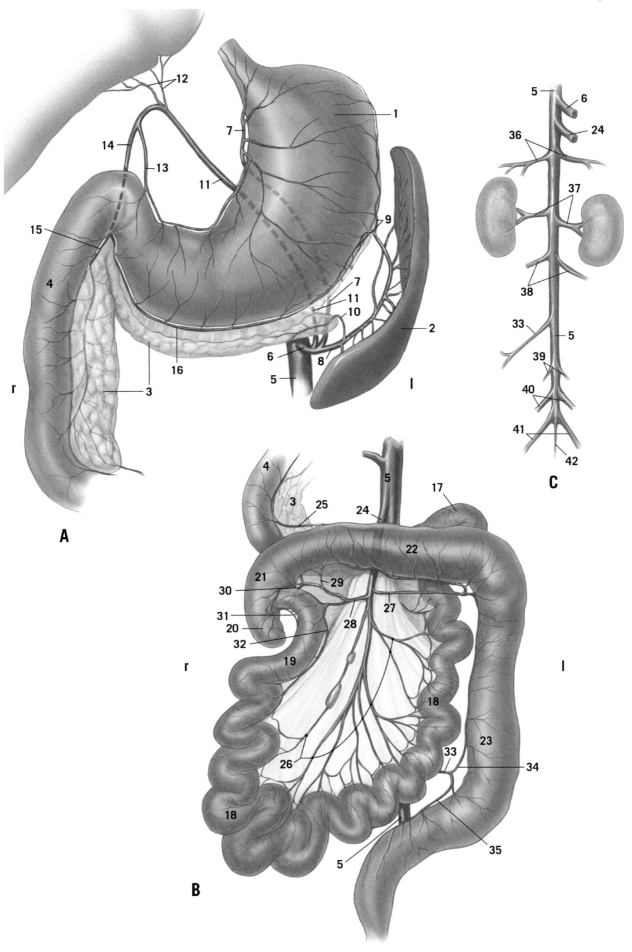

Plate 4-7

Figure A   Schematic illustration of the hepatic portal blood flow associated with the liver, lateral view

Figure B   Tributaries of the hepatic portal system, ventral view

1	Heart	13	Duodenum
2	Diaphragm	14	Jejunum
3	Liver	15	Ascending colon
4	Hepatic portal v.	16	Descending colon
5	Hepatic sinusoids	17	Jejunal vv.
6	Hepatic vv.	18	Caudal pancreaticoduodenal v.
7	Caudal vena cava	19	Cranial mesenteric v.
8	Cranial vena cava	20	Caudal mesenteric v.
9	Aorta	21	Splenic v.
10	Stomach	22	Gastroduodenal v.
11	Spleen	23	Cranial pancreaticoabdominal v.
12	Pancreas	24	Right gastric v.

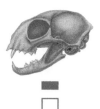

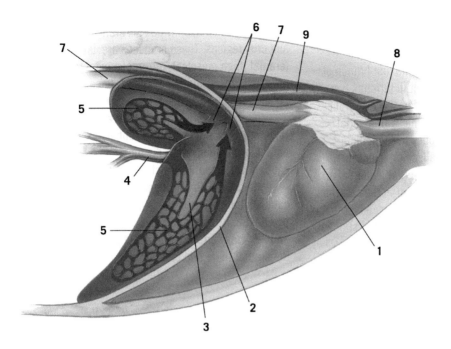

A

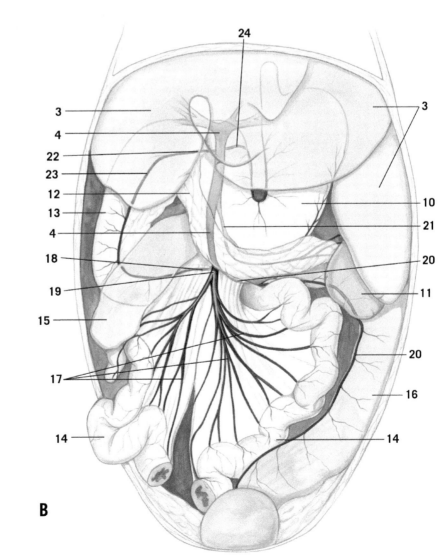

B

Vessels of the Pelvic Limb

The external iliac a. supplies the main distal portion of the pelvic limb. The extrinsic pelvic mm. are supplied in part by branches of the internal iliac a. (to be described later). The first branch of the external iliac a. is the deep femoral a. that in turn has two small branches. The first branch of the deep femoral a. supplies the deep surface of the caudoventral abdominal wall (caudal epigastric a.) and the second branch supplies the superficial surface of the caudoventral abdominal wall, scrotum or labia, caudal mammary glands or cremaster m. (external pudendal a.). A common pudendoepigastric trunk is inconstant in the cat, thus these branches usually come off separately. The deep femoral a. is then continued as the median circumflex femoral a. that supplies the proximal medial and caudal thigh muscles. After the deep femoral a. leaves, the external iliac a. continues distally as the femoral a. which usually has six branches supplying the thigh and crus regions. These branches are: lateral circumflex iliac a. (cranial thigh muscles), proximal caudal femoral a. (medial thigh muscles), descending genicular a. (medial thigh muscles and stifle), saphenous a. (medial crus and pes), middle caudal femoral a. (caudal thigh muscles), and distal caudal femoral a. (caudal thigh muscles and crus). The saphenous a. is the most and lengthy branch of the femoral a., dividing into two branches, cranial and caudal, which continue distally to supply the pes.

The femoral a. is continued as the popliteal a., which courses caudodistally between the two heads of the gastrocnemius m. The popliteal a. is short and gives off various small crural, muscular and genicular arteries. The popliteal a. terminates by dividing into the cranial tibial and caudal tibial arteries. The caudal tibial a.

is small and supplies the deep digital flexor m. The cranial tibial a. passes through the interosseous space between the tibia and fibula to the craniolateral surface of the tibia and supplies the craniolateral crural muscles. The cranial tibial a. continues on the dorsal tarsal joint as the dorsal pedal a.

Similar to the manus, the arterial supply to the pes involves anastomosing arches fed by several branches. The pes is supplied dorsally by the cranial branch of the saphenous a. and cranial branch of the cranial tibial a., which together form the superficial dorsal arch from which the dorsal common digital aa. are derived. The dorsal pedal a. gives rise to the arcuate a. from which the dorsal metatarsal aa. arise. A perforating branch of dorsal metatarsal a. II goes to the plantar surface to join the deep plantar arch from which the plantar metatarsal aa. arise. The

caudal branch of the saphenous a. supplies the medial and lateral plantar aa. that supply the superficial plantar surface of the digits (plantar common digital aa.). The plantar metatarsal aa. join with the plantar common digital aa. then redivide to supply the plantar proper digital aa. The main channel of blood supply to the paw is via: external iliac a., femoral a., popliteal a., cranial tibial a., dorsal pedal a., perforating branch, deep plantar arch, plantar metatarsal aa., and plantar proper digital aa.

Venous return of the pelvic limb is by way of satellite veins for deep drainage and by way of the medial and (non-satellite) lateral saphenous veins for superficial drainage. The medial saphenous v. is commonly used for venipuncture; and a lateral saphenous v. is present but small.

Plate 4-8

Figure A   Schematic illustration of vasculature of hindlimb, medial view with satellite veins (not labeled) and saphenous system (labeled).

Figure B   Superficial and deep vasculature of the hindpaw, dorsal view (veins not shown)

Figure C   Superficial (top) and deep vasculature of the hindpaw, plantar view (veins not shown)

m	Medial	**18**	Medial circumflex femoral a.
		19	Lateral circumflex femoral a.
l	Lateral	**20**	Superficial circumflex iliac a.
		21	Proximal caudal femoral a.
1-10	Arteries of main channel	**22**	Descending genicular a.
1	Abdominal aorta	**23**	Saphenous a.
2	External iliac a.	**24**	Cranial branch, saphenous a.
3	Femoral a.	**25**	Caudal branch, saphenous a.
4	Popliteal a.	**26**	Middle caudal femoral a.
5	Cranial tibial a.	**27**	Distal caudal femoral a.
6	Dorsal pedal a.	**28**	Caudal tibial a.
7	Proximal perforating branch II	**29**	Superficial branch, cranial tibial
8	Deep plantar arch	**30**	Cranial branch, medial saphenous v.
9	Plantar metatarsal aa. II-IV	**31**	Caudal branch, medial saphenous v.
10	Axial/abaxial plantar proper digital aa. II-V	**32**	Medial saphenous v.
		33	Lateral saphenous v.
11	Internal iliac a.	**34**	Dorsal common digital aa. II-IV
12	Cranial gluteal a.	**35**	Axial/abaxial dorsal proper digital aa. II-V
13	Caudal gluteal a.		
14	Internal pudendal a.	**36**	Plantar common digital aa. II-IV (cut in deep orientation of C)
15	Deep femoral a.		
16	Caudal epigastric a.	**37**	Medial plantar a.
17	External pudendal a.	**38**	Lateral plantar

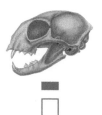

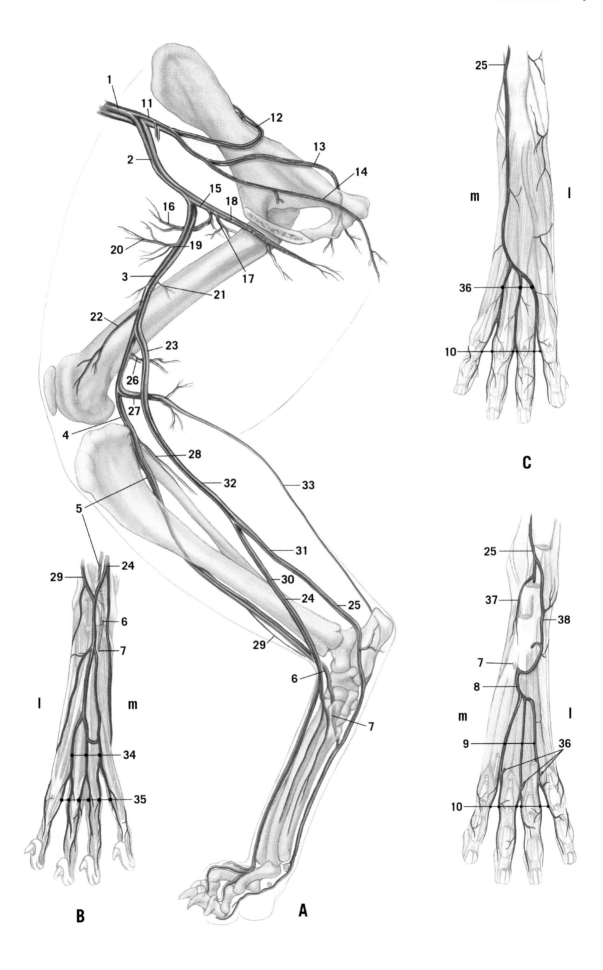

Vessels of the Pelvis

The pelvic viscera and pelvic muscles are supplied by branches of the bilateral internal iliac aa. The first branch of the internal iliac a. is the umbilical a. Although very prominent in the fetus, this artery decreases in size and remains patent in part as the cranial vesicular a. to supply the urinary bladder. Distal to the urinary bladder the fibrosed artery remains as a remnant called the round ligament of the bladder. The cranial gluteal a. is the next branch of the internal iliac a. This artery gives rise to the obturator and iliolumbar aa., which supply the cranial and medial thigh muscles, then passes through the greater ischiatic foramen, and terminates laterally in the middle gluteal and deep gluteal muscles. The internal iliac a. terminates (within the pelvic cavity) by dividing into the caudal gluteal and internal pudendal aa. The caudal gluteal a. travels through the lesser ischiatic foramen and supplies the gluteal and hamstring muscles, tail muscles and the dorsal perineum external to the pelvic cavity. The internal pudendal a. supplies most of the pelvic viscera as described in the following branches. The vaginal (or prostatic a.), through its branches, supplies the uterus (or ductus deferens), rectum, ureter, caudal bladder, vagina (or prostrate). This artery courses lateral to the rectum before branching. Venous drainage of this region is via satellite veins.

The continuation of the internal pudendal a. gives off middle rectal aa (rectum), and urethral a. (urethra), ventral perineal a. (caudal rectum, labia or scrotum, anal sphincters, skin of perineum). The termination of the internal pudendal a. is the artery of the clitoris (penis) supplying erectile tissue of the clitoris (penis) and associated muscles.

Plate 4-9

Figure A   Vasculature of the male (left) and female pelvic region, ventral view. The pelvic symphysis is split and retracted; pelvic viscera are retracted to the right.

Figure B   Vasculature of the gluteal region, dorsocaudolateral view

1	Rectum	19	Caudal vesicular a.
2	Bladder	20	Urethral branch
3	Urethra	21	Vaginal a.
4	Testis	22-24	Branches of vaginal a (female)
5	Penis	22	U terine branch
6	Ovary	23	Caudal vesicular a.
7	Uterine horn	24	Urethral branch
8	Vagina	25	Caudal rectal a.
9	Abdominal aorta, caudal vena cava	26	Artery of penis
10	Deep circumflex iliac a., v.	27	Artery of clitoris
11	External iliac a., v.	28	Iliolumbar a.
12	Femoral a., v.	29	Lateral caudal a.
13	Internal iliac a.	30	Sciatic n.
14	Umbilical a.	31	Crest of ilium
15	Cranial gluteal a.	32	M. tensor fasciae latae, cut and retracted
16	Caudal gluteal a.	33	Superficial and middle gluteal mm., cut and retracted
17	Internal pudendal a.	34	M. biceps femoris
18	Prostatic a.	35	Internal obturator m.
19-20	Branches of prostatic a (male)		

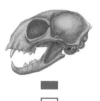

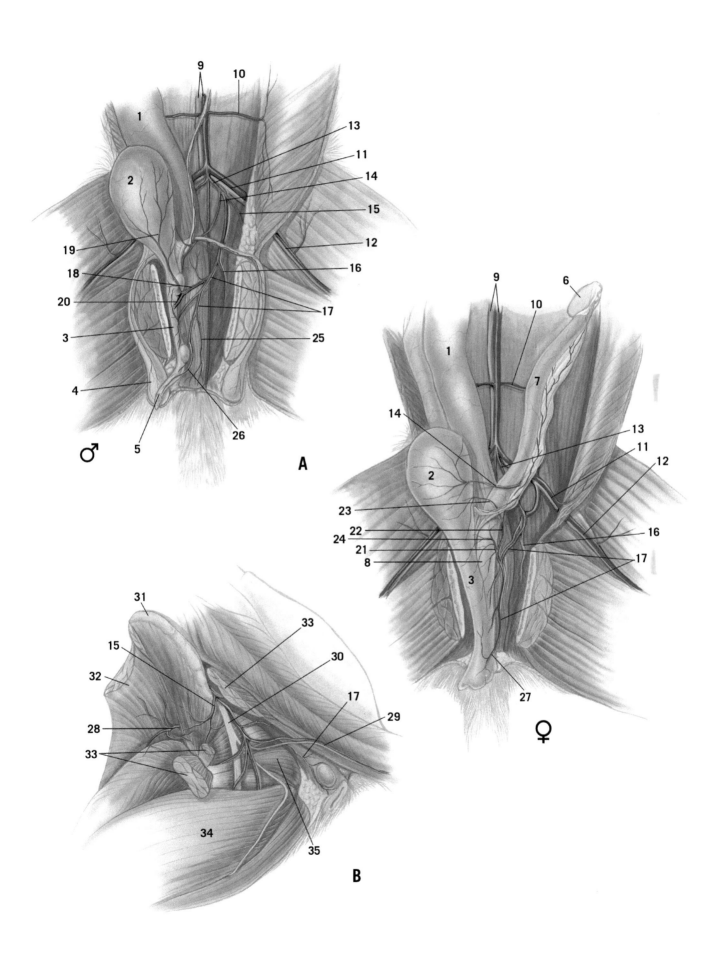

Selected References

1. Bonagura J. In: Sherding R (Ed): *The Cat: Diseases and Clinical Management.* New York, Churchill Livingstone, 1994:819.

2. Evans HE. Miller's Anatomy of the Dog. 3rd Ed. Philadelphia, WB Saunders, 1993; 586

3. Ghoshal NG. In: Getty R.(Ed) Sisson and Grossman's *The Anatomy of the Domestic Animals.* Philadelphia, WB Saunders, 1975: 1594

4. Kuman AJ, Hochwald GM, Kricheff I. An angiographic study of the carotid arterial and jugular venous systems in the cat. *Am J Anat* 145; 357-370.

5. McClure RC, Dallman MJ, Garrett PG. *Cat Anatomy.* Philadelphia, Lea and Febiger, 1973.

6. Rosenzeig LJ. *Anatomy of the Cat.* Iowa, Wm. C. Brown Publishers, 1990.

7. Rush JE, Keene BW, Fox PR. Pericardial disease in the cat: A retrospective evaluation of 66 cases. *J Am Anim Hosp Assoc* 1990;26:39.

8. Scavelli TD, Hornbuckle WE, Roth L, et al. Portosystemic shunts in cats: Seven cases (1976-1984). *J Am Vet Med Assoc* 189;1986:317.

9. Schummer A, Wilkens H, Vollmerhaus B, et al. The Anatomy of the Domestic Animals. Vol. 3. The Circulatory System, the skin, and the cutaneous organs of the domestic animals. Verlag Paul Parey - Springer Verlag 1981; 42, 71, 184.

10. Tillson DM, Winkler JT. Diagnosis and treatment of portosystemic shunts in the cat. *Vet Clinics North Am Small Anim Pract* 32, 2002: 881.

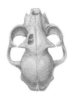

Chapter 5

Lymphoid System

Mary B. Tompkins and Kristina E. Howard

Modified from the original chapter by Mary Tompkins

The lymphoid system acts as a filtration system for blood and lymph to remove toxins and invading organisms thereby functioning as a host defense mechanism. Components of the lymphoid system are 1) primary lymphoid organs, consisting of the thymus and bone marrow, and 2) secondary lymphoid organs, consisting of spleen, lymph nodes, and aggregated lymphoid tissue such as tonsils. The secondary lymphoid organs are interconnected by a specialized vascular system called lymphatic vessels.

Primary Lymphoid Organs

The role of the primary lymphoid organs is to regulate the production and differentiation of lymphocytes. Lymphoid stem cells seed these organs during fetal development and become either T lymphocytes (in the thymus) or B lymphocytes (in the bone marrow).

Thymus

The thymus is a pale pink, lobulated organ located in the cranial mediastinum ventral to the trachea. It varies in size depending on the age of the cat, with it being largest on a relative basis in the neonate and largest in absolute size at puberty. In kittens, it extends cranial to the thoracic inlet and extends caudally between the brachiocephalic veins to the level of the fifth or sixth costal cartilage, where it lies against the ventral surface of the pericardium. At its caudal end, the right lobe is shorter than the left. The thymus begins to involute when the cat reaches sexual maturity and, in the adult cat, is a small remnant in the cranial mediastinum.

The function of the thymus is to "educate" and provide the circulation and secondary lymphoid organs with antigen responsive T lymphocytes. Lymphocytes populate the thymus by 40 days of gestation, where they develop the ability to distinguish self from nonself. The secondary lymphoid organs are then seeded with functional T cells, and in the cat this occurs prior to birth.

Recurrent infections in kittens can lead to premature thymic atrophy and an accompanying wasting syndrome. This occurs because T cells in the secondary lymphoid tissue as well as thymic lymphocytes are depleted. The most common cause of thymic atrophy is infection with feline leukemia virus (FeLV). On necropsy, little or no thymic tissue can be found in these kittens. FeLV also causes thymic lymphomas, which are typically seen in cats at 1-2-years old. In these cases the thymus enlarges, forming a mass that eventually compresses the lungs and heart against the dorsocaudal aspect of the thorax. The thymus is usually the only lymphoid organ involved in this type of tumor, so diagnosis can be difficult, with the first clinical signs being respiratory distress.

Bone Marrow

The bone marrow is the source of all lymphoid stem cells. While those that will mature into T cells migrate to the thymus, in mammals the bone marrow also serves as the site of development and maturation of B cells. Once they have matured into antigenic responsive cells, the B cells migrate from the marrow to the secondary lymphoid organs.

Secondary Lymphoid Organs

The secondary lymphoid organs are the location for trapping antigen and initiating an immune response.

The Lymphatic Vessels

The lymphatic vessels link the secondary lymphoid organs to one another and to the blood circulatory system. Lymphatic circulation is a one-way flow system in that lymph drains from the periphery toward the heart. Absorbed fat (from the small intestine lymphatic capillaries or lacteals) gives lymph a cloudy, milky appearance and is termed chyle. Lymph is driven through the vessels by a number of external forces such as contraction of neighboring muscles and limb movement. Larger lymphatic vessels contain muscle fibers. Retrograde flow is prevented by numerous valves.

The lymphatic vessels begin as extremely small capillaries that cannot be seen on gross dissection. These capillaries drain into larger vessels, several of which may enter a lymph node. These vessels are then referred to as vasa afferentia or afferent lymphatic vessels. The area through which these lymph capillaries and vessels have flowed, picking up fluid and cells, prior to entering the lymph node is the drainage area for that node. Although several afferent vessels will enter a single node, only one or two efferent vessels (vasa efferentia) will leave the node. Thus as the system flows toward the heart, the number of vessels is gradually reduced. The lymph vessels flow into larger lymphatic trunks or ducts. The trunks anastomose with the blood circulatory system at the point of confluence of the external jugular and subclavian veins (venous angle).

The lymphatic trunks are the only ones that can be seen on gross dissection. Unfortunately, other than the thoracic duct and cisterna chyli, there is very little description in the literature of the large lymphatic trunks in the cat. Therefore, the following descriptions, except for the thoracic duct and cisterna chyli, are drawn from other carnivores. It should be emphasized, however, that there is a great deal of individual variation in lymphatic vessel drainage patterns.

Tracheal Trunks

The lymphatic vessels of the head and neck flow into the left and right tracheal trunks, which arise from the efferent vessels of the medial retropharyngeal lln. The trunks lie along either side of the trachea as they enter the thorax. The left tracheal trunk usually enters the thoracic duct just prior to the left venous angle, or it may enter the venous angle on its own. The right tracheal trunk becomes the right lymphatic duct and terminates at the right venous angle.

Visceral and Lumbar Trunks

The visceral trunks arise from the efferent vessels of the mesenteric and celiac lymphocenters. They then enter the ventral aspect of the cisterna chyli. The lumbar trunks arise from the medial iliac lln. and run along the aorta into the caudal part of the cisterna chyli.

Cisterna Chyli

The cisterna chyli consists of two interconnected sac like structures: a large sac (dorsal cistern) on the dorsal aspect of the aorta that is connected to a smaller, ventral sac. The cistern is located between the crura of the diaphragm, ventral to the bodies of caudal thoracic and cranial lumbar vertebrae. The visceral trunks empty into the ventral cistern and the lumbar trunks usually empty into the most caudal part of the dorsal cistern. The thoracic duct arises from the cranial part of the dorsal cistern.

Thoracic Duct

The thoracic duct is the largest of the lymphatic trunks, receiving lymph from all the vessels caudal to the diaphragm. It contains many valves and may look beaded on dissection due to back flow of fluid against the valves. The duct arises cranially from the dorsal cistern and passes through the aortic hiatus of the diaphragm. In the caudal mediastinum, there is a single duct in most cats, which runs dorsal to the thoracic aorta and slightly left of midline. The duct then splits into several interconnecting ducts in the middle mediastinum. In about half these cases, the thoracic duct is again a single trunk in the cranial mediastinum. In 95% of cats examined, the duct lies on the left surface of the esophagus in the cranial mediastinum then terminates in the left venous angle.

Chylothorax is the clinical manifestation of effusion of chyle into the mediastinum or pleural cavity as a result of rupture, obstruction, or anomalous development of the thoracic duct. Chylothorax has developed in association with cardiomyopathy, tumors in the thorax, diaphragmatic hernias, and lung lobe torsion. In most cases, the chylothorax is not due to an actual rupture of the duct, but rather blockage of flow and subsequent lymphangiectasia. Although chylothorax is initially treated medically, if the effusion does not resolve, ligation of the duct should be undertaken.

Lymph Nodes

Lymph nodes are round or bean shaped structures scattered throughout the body. There are many nodes, most of which are small and embedded in fascia and fat. Lymph nodes are named primarily by location, and the numbers of nodes at a particular location varies from species to species. Nodes in a particular location across species lines are referred to as lymphocenters. There is a variation in number, size, and presence of some lymph nodes from cat to cat. Only lymph nodes in lymphocenters that have been identified in at least 50% of cats examined will be described here.

The role of the lymph node is to trap foreign material received from the lymphatic vessels and provide a site for the immune response to develop. Lymph nodes are surrounded by a connective tissue capsule and internally are divided into a peripheral cortex, a central medulla, and a paracortical zone between the two. Material "up stream" from the lymph node drains into the node via the afferent lymphatic vessels, which enter at various points around the node's periphery. The lymph then percolates through the node, where the antigen is trapped by dendritic cells in the cortex and macrophages in the medulla. Lymph leaves the node via efferent lymphatic vessels located in a depression or hilus, on one side of the node. Nodes draining a sight of infection will often enlarge as cells and fluid accumulate in response to antigenic stimulation. As the nodes enlarge, their capsules become stretched and the nodes become hot and painful.

Some peripheral nodes of the cat (parotid, retropharyngeal, axillary, caudal epigastric, superficial inguinal, and ischiatic) normally are difficult, if not impossible to palpate because they are small or in a deeper location. It is possible to palpate the popliteal and mandibular nodes and, with practice, the superficial cervical nodes, which will feel like small pebbles. It should be kept in mind that if a feline lymph node is easy to locate and palpate, it is probably abnormal, and reasons for its enlargement should be determined.

Focal sites of infection such as cat bite abscesses or upper respiratory infection will lead to enlargement of the local nodes draining those sites. Therefore, it is helpful from a clinical standpoint to have a general idea of lymph node locations and drainage sites. Tables 5-1 through 5-4 describe the location, afferent drainage sites, and efferent lymphatic routes of the lymph nodes identified in a majority of cats. In addition to focal enlargement, cats can be presented with generalized lymphadenopathy involving superficial and/or visceral nodes. A syndrome referred to as distinctive lymph node hyperplasia has been described in young cats infected with FeLV. The most commonly affected nodes are the mandibular and popliteal, but all the peripheral and visceral nodes can be involved. The lymphadenopathy may last only a few weeks then resolve. A marked and prolonged (5-9 months) generalized lymphadenopathy also occurs in the early stages of feline immunodeficiency virus (FIV) infection. Finally, lymphoma should be considered in any cat, especially an adult cat that has a generalized lymphadenopathy.

Plate 5-1

Figure A   Location of lymphoid structures of the thoracic cavity, left lateral view, lungs removed

Figure B   Location of abdominal lymph nodes associated with the abdominal aorta, ventral view

Figure C   Schematic illustration of a typical lymph node, external view and sagittal section

1	Body of thoracic vertebra	17	Kidney
2	Transected rib	18	Adrenal gland
3a	Thoracic aorta	19	Renal a,v,
3b	Abdominal aorta	20	Ovarian/testicular a,v
4	Esophagus	21	Deep circumflex a,v
5	Caudal vena cava	22	External iliac a
6	Diaphragm	23	Internal iliac a
7	Phrenic n.	24	Aortic lumbar lln
8	Heart within pericardium	25	Medial iliac ln
9	Transected bronchus and pulmonary vessels	26	Sacral lln
10	Sternum	27	Capsule of lymph node
11	Cranial mediastinal ln.	28	Hilus of lymph node
12	Thoracic (lymphatic) duct	29	Afferent lymphatic vessels
13	Aortic thoracic lln	30	Efferent lymphatic vessels
14	Cranial sternal ln.	31	Artery and vein to lymph node
15	Thymus (present in young cats, regressed in older cats)	32	Trabeculae
		33	Lymphatic sinus
16	Tracheobronchial lln	34	Lymphatic cortex
		35	Medulla

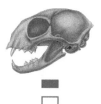

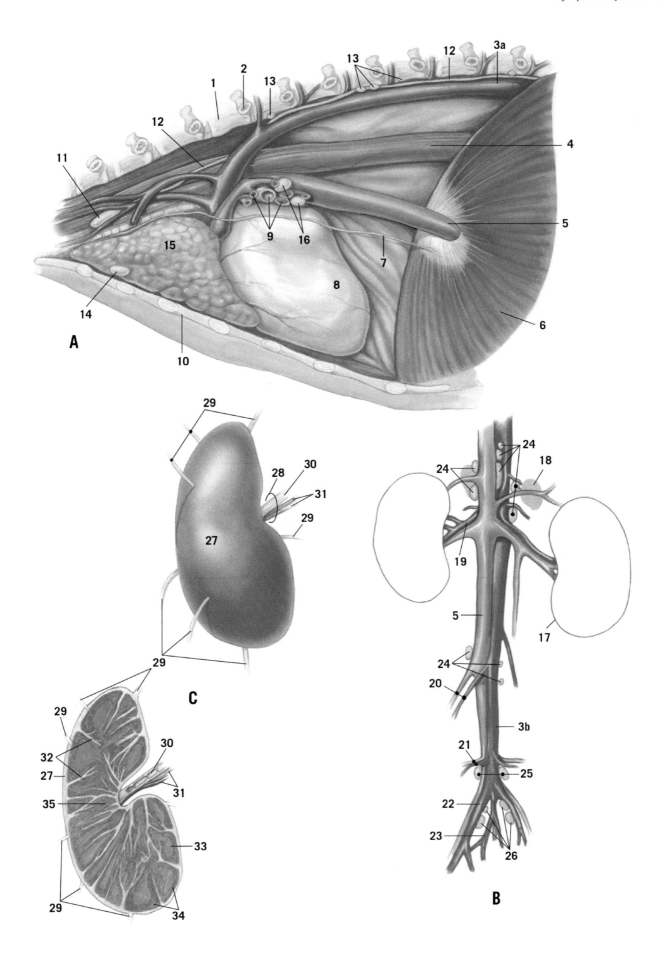

TABLE 5-1
Major Lymph Nodes of the Head and Neck

Lymph Nodes	No.	Location	Drainage
Parotid ln.	1-2	Cranial boarder of parotid salivary gland against the superficial temporal v.	**A:***Dorsal half of head, eyes, parotid salivary gland. **E:** Lateral retropharyngeal lln.
Mandibular lln.	2	Lying dorsal and ventral to facial v. at the angle of the mandible deep to the platysma muscle.	**A:** Lips, chin, lower jaw, eyelids. **E:** Medial retropharyngeal ln.
Retropharyngeal lateral lln.	1-7 (3-4)+	Caudal to parotid salivary gland along the caudal auricular v.	**A:** Ear and parotid salivary gland. **E:** Medial retropharyngeal ln.
medial ln.	1	Adjacent to carotid sheath at level of the atlas and bounded medially by pharyngeal musculature.	**A:** Tongue, oral and nasal passages, thyroid and mandibular salivary glands. **E:** Vessels form the tracheal trunk.
Superficial cervical dorsal lln.	1-3 (2)	Deep to the omotransversarius m. cranioventral to the trapezius m.	**A:** Dorsal part of the neck and forelimb. **E:** Tracheal trunk.
ventral ln.	1	On external jugular v. near the origin of the superficial cervical v.	**A:** Ventral part of neck, thoracic inlet. **E:** Tracheal trunk.
Caudal deep cervical lln.	1-6 (2-4)	Ventral surface of the trachea near the thoracic inlet.	**A:** Thyroid gland, trachea, esophagus. **E:** Venous angle.

***A** = afferent lymphatic drainage; **E** = efferent drainage routes.   +Numbers in parenthesis indicate the most common number of nodes.

TABLE 5-2
Major Superficial Lymph Nodes of the Limbs and Trunk

Lymph Node	No.	Location	Drainage
Axillary ln.	1	Medial surface of the forelimb between the axillary and lateral thoracic vv.	**A:** *Medial aspect of forelimb, lateral thoracic wall. **E:** Venous angle.
Accessory axillary lln.	1-7 (3-5)+	Medial to the latissimus dorsi m. between the 3rd and 6th intercostal space along the lateral thoracic v.	**A:** Medial and cranial aspect of forelimbs, skin of lumbar region, lateral chest wall, cranial half of mammary glands. **E:** Axillary ln.
Caudal epigastric lln.* *Name not recognized by NAV	1-5 (1-3)	On the ventral abdomen along the caudal epigastric a. and v.	**A:** Ventral, caudal aspect of abdominal wall, skin of thigh. **E:** Superficial inguinal ln. , thoracic lln.
Superficial inguinal ln.	1	In the femoral canal along the external pudendal a. and v.	**A:** Inguinal and gluteal regions, caudal half of mammary glands. **E:** Medial iliac lln.
Ischiatic ln.	1	Deep to the m. gluteofemoris along the caudal gluteal a. and v.	**A:** Hind limb, anal region, popliteal ln. **E:** Medial iliac lln.
Superficial popliteal ln.	1	Lies subcutaneously in the popliteal fossa.	**A:** Distal hindlimb. **E:** Ischiatic ln.

***A** = afferent lymphatic drainage; **E** = efferent drainage routes.   +Numbers in parenthesis indicate the most common number of nodes.

TABLE 5-3
Major Lymph Nodes of the Thoracic Cavity

Lymph Node	No.	Location	Drainage
Aortic thoracic lln.*	1-5	Ventral surface of the thoracic vertebrae.	A:+ Pleura. E: Thoracic duct.
Cranial sternal ln.	1	Along the internal thoracic a. and v. at the level of the 2nd costal cartilag e.	A: Diaphragm, pericardium, ventral thoracic and abdominal walls. E: Thoracic duct.
Cranial mediastinal lln.	2-8	Ventral and/or medial to the trachea in the cranial mediastinum at the level of the 1st and 2nd ribs.	A: Trachea, esophagus, heart, pericardium, pleura. E: Thoracic duct.
Tracheo-bronchial lln. (left, right, medial)	1-2 each	Lying left, right, and caudal, respectively, to the bifurcation of the trachea.	A: Lung. E: Cranial mediastinal lln.

*Inconsistently found but present in at least 50% of cats examined.   +A = afferent lymphatic drainage; E = efferent drainage routes.

TABLE 5-4
Major Lymph Nodes of the Abdominal Cavity

Lymph Node	No.	Location	Drainage
Aortic lumbar lln.	3-10	Cranial and caudal to the renal artery along the abdominal aorta.	A:* Dorsal wall of abdomen, diaphragm, kidneys, uterus or testes. E: Cisterna chyli.
Celiac splenic lln.+	1-3	Along the splenic v.	A: Spleen, stomach, pancreas. E: Visceral trunk, hepatic lln.
gastric lln.+	1-4	On the lesser curvature of the stomach.	A: Stomach, liver, esophagus. E: Visceral trunk, hepatic lln.
hepatic lln.	2-4	Around the junction of the portal, splenic, and gastroduodenal vv.	A: Liver, stomach, diaphragm, pancreas, cranial part of duodenum. E: Visceral trunk.
pancreatico-duodenal ln.	1	Along the cranial pancreaticoduodenal v.	A: Pylorus, duodenum, pancreas. E: Hepatic lln., cranial sternal ln.
Cranial Mesenteric jejunal lln.	2-20 (2-5)‡	From the root of the mesentery into the mesojejunum along either side of the jejunal aa. and vv.	A: All of the small intestine. E: Visceral trunk.
cecal lln.	1-3 (2)	Both sides of the cecum.	A: Cecum, ileum. E: Jejunal lln., lumbar trunks.
colic lln.	3-9	In the mesentery of the ascending and transverse colon.	A: Ileum, cecum, large colon. E: Lumbar trunks.
Caudal mesenteric lln.	1-5 (1-3)	In the mesentery of the descending colon near the bifurcation of the caudal mesenteric a.	A: Descending colon, rectum. E: Colic lln., lumbar trunks.
Iliosacral medial iliac lln.	2-4	Between the bifurcation of the aorta and the origin of the deep circumflex ileal aa. on both sides of the aorta.	A: Tail, pelvic wall and limbs, bladder, uterus. E: Form the lumbar trunks.
sacral lln.	1-6 (1-3)	Near the origin of the internal iliac aa. around the aorta.	A: Rectum, bladder, ureter, pelvic wall, tail, hind limbs. E: Medial iliac lln.

*A = afferent lymphatic drainage; E = efferent drainage routes.   †Inconsistently found but present in at least 50% of cats examined.   ‡Numbers in parenthesis indicate the most common number of nodes.

Plate 5-2

Figure A   Location and relative depth of peripheral lymph nodes. The darkest shade
denotes most superficially located nodes; the lightest shade is the most
deeply located nodes. Frequently, these nodes are not palpable in the normal
animal, but enlargement of any node may render it palpable at the indicated
site.

8   Accessory axillary ln. (medial to thoracic limb on thoracic wall)
9   Caudal epigastric ln. (on ventral abdomen)
10 Superficial inguinal ln. (on caudal ventral abdomen, medial to pelvic limb)
11 Ischiatic ln.
12 Popliteal ln.

1   Parotid ln.
2   Mandibular ln.
3   Lateral retropharyngeal ln.
4   Medial retropharyngeal ln.
5   Dorsal and ventral superficial cervical lln.
6   Caudal deep cervical lln.
7   Axillary ln. (medial to thoracic limb)

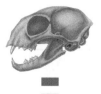

more superficial

middle depth

deep

Aggregated Lymphoid Tissue

In addition to well organized lymph nodes, throughout the body are discrete collections of lymphoid cells that vary in size and extent of organization. These collections of cells are not surrounded by a capsule as are lymph nodes, but rather by specialized epithelial cells that are capable of transporting antigen. Nor do these tissues filter lymph, although they are often surrounded by lymphatic capillaries. Their main role is host defense at mucosal surfaces. The most highly organized of these tissues are the tonsils, which are seen as a ring around the root of the tongue, palate, pharynx and entrance to the larynx. The most readily distinguished tonsil in the cat is the palatine tonsils located in small fossae in the lateral wall of the oropharynx. When inflamed and enlarged, they may protrude and be visible to an examiner. Located in (but much less obvious) the aryepiglottic folds of the larynx are the plate-like paraepiglottic tonsils, which are not present in other common domestic animals. The highest concentration of aggregated lymphoid tissue is in the ileum of the small intestine, also known commonly but unofficially as Peyer's patches. These white nodules can at times encompass the entire circumference of the ileum, and are seen along the mucosal surface. Isolated lymphoid follicles, which may be very small but measure as large as 1 cm x 1.5 cm, are found in the duodenum and jejunum of most cats. They typically appear as ovoid raised areas on the serosal surface, and also appear white on the mucosal surface. While Peyer's patches and isolated lymphoid follicles lack afferent lymphatics, efferent lymphatics drain these sites to various mesenteric lymph nodes (jejunal, cecal and colic lln). Intestinal leukocytes circulate via the thoracic duct to peripheral circulation and the spleen.

Spleen

The spleen is a dark, elongated organ located in the left cranial quadrant of the abdomen where it extends along the greater curvature of the stomach. The caudal half of the spleen is located caudal to the costal arch. The spleen is attached to the stomach by the greater omentum (gastrosplenic ligament). The spleen is designed to filter antigens and aged circulating cells from the bloodstream. In fact, in a 24 hour period, about 50% of circulating lymphocytes migrate through the spleen, in contrast to only about 10% reaching the blood via the thoracic duct. Thus, the spleen is the most important organ in lymphocyte migration. It also functions as a storage site for erythrocytes and platelets and can function as a site of extramedullary hematopoiesis. As a result, the splenic parenchyma is divided histologically into two parts; the red pulp, where erythrocyte storage and antigen trapping occur, and the white pulp, where the immune response occurs.

On a relative basis, the size of the spleen is smaller in the cat. It is possible to palpate the spleen in a relaxed adult cat. It is the last structure that can be "slipped" on abdominal palpation in the cranial quadrant and feels similar to an empty loop of small intestine. If, however, the spleen is easily palpated and identifiable as spleen, it is most likely enlarged. Splenomegaly in the cat is not nearly as common as in the dog. Neoplasia (myeloproliferative disease, lymphosarcoma, and mast cell tumor) is the most common cause of feline splenomegaly.

Plate 5-3

Figure A   Location of lymph nodes associated with the abdominal digestive system, ventral view. The stomach is retracted to the left, the liver is retracted to the right, and the jejunum is retracted caudally.

Figure B   Exposure of luminal surface of ileum

Figure C   Location of spleen and splenic lymph nodes. Spleen is retracted laterally and portions of the greater omentum are removed.

Figure D   Transverse and microscopic section of spleen

Figure E   Schematic transverse section of lymphoid tissue associated with the pharynx

1	Liver and the bile duct	16	Mesenteric ileal a.
2	Stomach	17	Antimesenteric ileal a.
3	Spleen	18	Aggregated lymph nodules (Peyer's patches)
4	Duodenum	19	Splenic a.
5	Jejunum	20	Splenic lln.
6	Ileum	21	Hilus of spleen
7	Cecum	22	Capsule
8	Colon	23	Trabeculae
9	Kidney	24	Red pulp
10	Caudal vena cava and aorta	25	White pulp
11	Gastric lln.	26	Nasopharynx
12	Hepatic lln.	27	Palate
13-15	Mesenteric lln.	28	Orophraynx
13	Jejunal lln.	29	Pharyngeal tonsil
13a	Lymphatic vessels in mesentery	30	Soft palate tonsil
14	Cecal lln.	31	Palatine tonsil
15	Colic lln.	32	Lingual tonsil

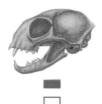

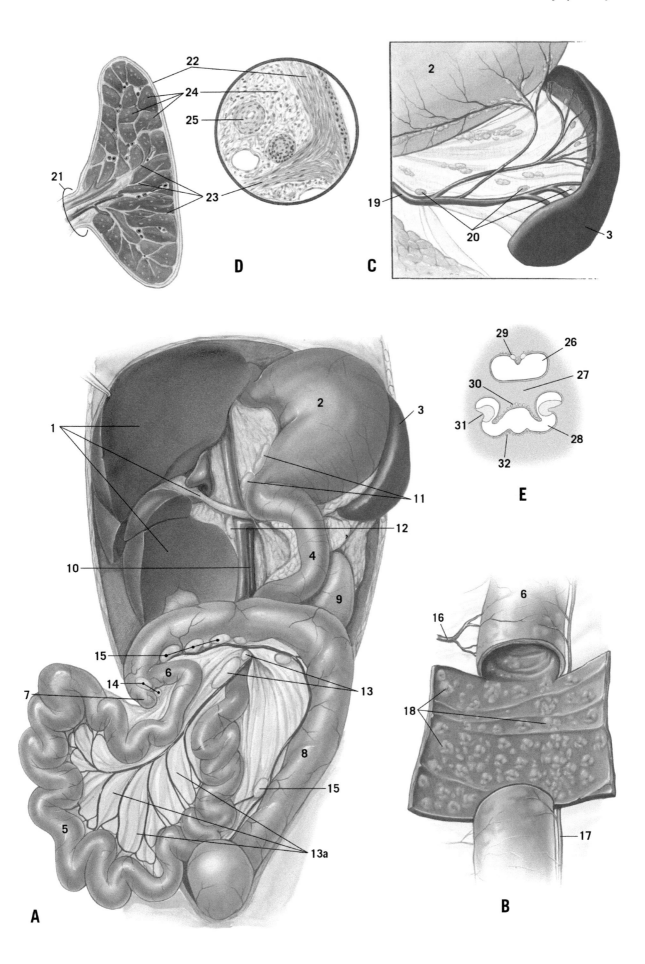

Selected References

1. Birchard SJ, Bradley RL. In: Sherding, RG (Ed): *The Cat: Diseases and Clinical Management.* 2nd Ed. New York, Churchill Livingstone Inc. 1994; 1093.

2. Crouch JE. *Text-Atlas of Cat Anatomy.* Philadelphia, Lea and Febiger, 1969; 261.

3. Hoover EA, et al. Thymectomy in preweanling kittens: Technique and immunological consequences. *Am J Vet Res* 1978; 39:99.

4. Howard KE, et al. Methodology for isolation and phenotypic characterization of feline small intestinal leukocytes. J Immunol Methods. 2005 Jul;302(1-2):36-53.

5. Lindsay FEF. Chylothorax in the domestic cat--a review. *J Small Anim Pract* 1974; 15: 241.

6. Ratzlaff MH. The superficial lymphatic system of the cat. *Lymphology* 1970; 3: 151.

7. Sherding RG. In: Birchard SJ, Sherding RG. (Eds). Saunders Manual of Small Animal Practice. 3rd Ed. St Louis, Elsevier Saunders, 2006: 115, 126.

8. Vollmerhaus B. Lymphatic system. In: Schummer A, et al. *The Circulatory System, the Skin, and the Cutaneous Organs of the Domestic Mammals.* Berlin, Verlag Paul Parey, 1981; 269.

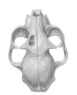

Chapter 6

Endocrine System

Antonella Borgatti Jeffreys and David J. Waters

Modified from the original chapter by David Waters

The endocrine system is a group of widely separated tissues that regulate numerous body functions through their secretions or hormones. The various endocrine organs are linked primarily by blood, by the cardiovascular system. These organs tend to be small but they can have very potent effects.

The list of endocrine organs varies from source to source. The thymus and pineal body of the brain are not included in this chapter.

Pituitary Gland

The pituitary gland (hypophysis) is located within the hypophyseal fossa of the skull, ventral to the brain stem, and consists of two lobes: (1) rostral lobe that includes most of the adenohypophysis; and (2) caudal lobe that includes the neurohypophysis. Embryologically, the adenohypophysis arises as an evagination of the oral cavity ectoderm. The neurohypophysis arises as an outgrowth of the forebrain.

The adenohypophysis is subdivided into three regions producing a variety of hormones:

1) Pars distalis: growth hormone (somatotropin), prolactin, thyrotropin (TSH), adrenocorticotropic hormone (ACTH), follicle-stimulating hormone (FSH), luteinizing hormone (LH);

2) Pars intermedia: melanocyte-stimulating hormone (MSH), ACTH;

3) Pars tuberalis: gonadotropins (LH, FSH), TSH

Most of these hormones act in turn on other endocrine organs.

The neurohypophysis is responsible for the storage and release of antidiuretic hormone (ADH), which regulates water conservation by the kidney, and oxytocin, a potent stimulus for uterine contractions and milk ejection from the mammary gland.

The blood supply to the adenohypophysis and neurohypophysis is separate. The adenohypophysis is supplied by rostral hypophyseal aa. and drained by the cavernous sinus. The neurohypophysis is supplied by branches of the rami retis and the arterial circle of the brain and drained by the cavernous sinus.

The pituitary gland is not an autonomous organ, instead is subject to precise regulation by the hypothalamus. Regulation of the adenohypophysis by the hypothalamus is facilitated by the hypophyseal portal system. Hypothalamic releasing and inhibitory factors are transported via the axons of hypothalamic neurosecretory cells to a primary blood capillary network in the proximal neurohypophysis (median eminence). The portal system transports these neurosecretory products to a secondary blood capillary network in the adenohypophysis. In response to these releasing and inhibitory factors, the adenohypophysis releases hormones that regulate the function of other endocrine glands.

The parenchyma of the neurohypophysis consists largely of axons projecting from nerve cell bodies located in the hypothalamus. ADH and oxytocin are produced in nerve cell bodies of the supraoptic and paraventricular hypothalamic nuclei. These hormones are transported along axons of the hypothalamo-neurohypophyseal tract and stored in the neurohypophysis as granules.

Pituitary neoplasms may result in, (1) compression atrophy of the pituitary gland or adjacent structures including the optic chiasm, or (2) excessive production of pituitary hormones. Pituitary (chromophobe) microadenoma with secondary bilateral adrenal hyperplasia is the most common cause of feline hyperadrenocorticism. Growth hormone-secreting pituitary adenomas have been reported. This condition is seen most frequently in middle-aged, male, mixed-breed cats. Acromegalic features are accompanied by insulin-resistant diabetes mellitus. Treatment options include medical management, radiation therapy, or surgery (hypophysectomy).

Neurogenic (central) diabetes insipidus has been reported in cats. This condition is characterized by failure of the neurohypophysis to release ADH. In most cases, the underlying lesion is unknown. Hypopituitarism and consequent dwarfism has been reported as an autosomal recessive condition.

Thyroid and Parathyroid Glands

The thyroid gland consists of two lobes (without an isthmus) located on the ventrolateral surface of the trachea just caudal to the larynx. The thyroid glands of normal cats are usually not palpable. Two parathyroid glands are associated with each thyroid gland. The external parathyroid gland is located at the cranial pole of the thyroid gland external to the thyroid capsule. The internal parathyroid gland is located within the thyroid capsule (intracapsular) and usually lies within the parenchyma of the thyroid gland. The cranial thyroid a. is the major source of blood supply for the thyroid and parathyroid glands. The caudal thyroid a. is not present in most cats.

Embryologically, the thyroid glands arise from the endoderm of the first pharyngeal pouch; the parathyroid glands arise from the third and fourth pharyngeal pouches. Variable migration of embryonic tissue explains the presence of ectopic thyroid and/or parathyroid tissue in some cats. A connective tissue capsule surrounds the thyroid parenchyma, which consists mainly of thyroid follicles. The follicles contain thyroglobulin (colloid), the iodine-rich glycoprotein precursor of thyroxine (T4) and triiodothyronine (T3). Parafollicular cells (C cells) are most frequently found between follicles. Parafollicular cells are of neural crest origin and produce calcitonin, which regulates blood calcium concentration.

Hyperthyroidism is the most common endocrine disorder of middle-aged and older cats. Clinical signs include polyuria, polydipsia, polyphagia, weight loss, and voluminous stools. Histopathologic diagnosis is usually adenomatous hyperplasia, although thyroid carcinoma has been reported. If thyroidectomy is performed, it is often performed bilaterally to ensure removal of all hyperfunctional thyroid tissue. A "normal" appearing contralateral thyroid gland is not necessarily an indication for unilateral thyroidectomy, since truly normal (non-hyperfunctional) thyroid glands are often atrophied with this condition.

Congenital hypothyroidism has been reported in cats. Clinical signs of thyroid hormone deficiency develop during the second month of life; an autoimmune etiology is suspected in some cases. Iatrogenic hypothyroidism occurs in cats that have undergone bilateral thyroidectomy or thyroid ablation with ^{131}Iodine for the treatment of hyperthyroidism.

The parathyroid parenchyma is surrounded by a thin capsule. The chief or principal cells of the parathyroid gland produce parathyroid hormone, which plays an integral role in calcium and phosphorus homeostasis. Inactive principal cells (light-staining with hematoxylin and eosin) usually predominate. Glycogen inclusion bodies are frequently found in feline principal cells. A second cell type, the oxyphil, is rare in carnivores.

Primary (idiopathic) hypoparathyroidism and primary hyperthyroidism are rare conditions of cats. Iatrogenic hypoparathyroidism with associated hypocalcemia is a serious potential complication of bilateral thyroidectomy. At surgery, preservation of external parathyroid tissue and its blood supply must be achieved. Preservation of the cranial one half of the thyroid capsule (modified intracapsular thyroidectomy) facilitates this objective.

Endocrine Pancreas

The pancreas is a lobulated organ consisting of a right limb, left limb, and body associated with the mesoduodenum and greater omentum. The blood supply to the pancreas is provided by the cranial and caudal pancreaticoduodenal aa. and pancreatic branches of the splenic a. The pancreas has both endocrine and exocrine functions. The exocrine portion of the pancreas is drained by the pancreatic duct and the variable accessory pancreatic duct (see Chapter 8 also). Embryologically, both the pancreatic islets and exocrine pancreas arise from gut endoderm.

Islet cells account for approximately 2% of the pancreatic mass and are responsible for this organ's endocrine function. They are unevenly distributed throughout the pancreas. Based on their morphologic and functional characteristics, islet cells are categorized into different subpopulations:
1) alpha cells: glucagon
2) beta cells: insulin
3) delta cells: somatostatin, gastrin, vasoactive intestinal peptide

Delta cells may play an important role in the local control of alpha and beta cell activity. Islet cell subpopulations exhibit considerable specificity with regard to their vulnerability to certain chemical agents. Cobalt chloride and alloxan are associated with selective destruction of alpha and beta cells, respectively.

Pancreatitis is the most common feline pancreatic disorder. Pancreatitis and pancreatic neoplasia represent the major indications for partial pancreatectomy. Surgical removal of up to 80% of the pancreas would not be expected to have significant endocrine consequences, since there is considerable islet cell reserve in normal individuals. However, despite this reserve, transient diabetes mellitus has been reported in other carnivores following partial pancreatectomy for insulin secreting islet cell neoplasms. The pancreas is considered vulnerable to a variety of mechanical (*e.g.,* surgical manipulation) and metabolic (*e.g.,* hypoxia) insults. Pancreatitis is not considered an important etiologic factor in feline diabetes mellitus.

Diabetes mellitus, a deficiency of insulin action, is an important endocrine disease of cats. Affected cats are usually insulinopenic (*i.e.,* low plasma insulin levels) and clinical signs include polyuria, polydipsia, polyphagia, and weight loss. Cats with diabetes mellitus may suffer from a distal polyneuropathy and assume a plantigrade stance. Degenerative lesions of alpha and beta cells, and amyloid deposition within islet cells are frequently seen in cats with diabetes mellitus. Insular amyloid deposition has also been reported in normal cats.

Adrenal Glands

The adrenal glands are paired, flattened, ovoid organs located in the retroperitoneal space immediately cranial to each kidney. The right and left adrenal glands lie in close proximity to the caudal vena cava and aorta respectively. The phrenicoabdominal a. and v. course on the surface of the adrenal glands (artery - dorsal surface; vein - ventral surface). Calcification of the adrenal gland is present in up to 30% of normal adults. Therefore, radiographic evidence of adrenal gland calcification should not necessarily be interpreted as pathologic. Accessory adrenal tissue (parovarian nodules) has been reported in cats.

Embryologically, the adrenal glands arise from mesoderm (adrenal cortex) and neural crest (adrenal medulla). Histologically, a thin capsule, consisting of dense connective tissue and smooth muscle fibers, surrounds the cortex and gives rise to trabeculae that variably penetrate the adrenal parenchyma. The adrenal cortex is highly organized into distinct zones:
1) zona arcuata (glomerulosa):   mineralocorticoids (e.g.aldosterone)
2) zona fasciculata: glucocorticoids
3) zona reticularis: glucocorticoids, sex hormones

A fourth zone (zona intermedia) is sometimes described. Mineralocorticoid production by the zona arcuata is regulated by plasma sodium, potassium, and angiotensin II concentrations, not the adenohypophysis. Therefore, hypophysectomy has no effect on the function or structure of this portion of the adrenal cortex. The production of glucocorticoids by the two internal cortical zones (zona fasciculata and zona reticularis) is under the control of ACTH (adenohypophysis) and corticotropin-releasing hormone (CRH) from the hypothalamus.

Adrenal medullary production of catecholamines is mediated by acetylcholine release from stimulated preganglionic sympathetic nerve fibers. The epinephrine and norepinephrine-producing cells of the adrenal medulla may be identified histologically by the presence of a dark brown reaction product following exposure to chromium salts (chromaffin reaction). Accessory chromaffin positive cells (paraganglia cells) may also be found remote from the adrenal glands in close proximity to the abdominal aorta. Extramedullary pheochromocytoma (paraganglionoma) is the result of neoplastic transformation of these paraganglia cells.

The relationship of the adrenal glands with other anatomic structures visualized via ventral midline celiotomy or retroperitoneal (paracostal) approach is illustrated. Adrenalectomy performed via midline celiotomy enables the surgeon to concurrently perform a thorough exploration of the peritoneal cavity; this approach also facilitates bilateral adrenalectomy. Adrenalectomy via retroperitoneal approach has been advocated to improve exposure to the adrenal gland and avoid iatrogenic, retraction-induced pancreatic trauma. Indications for unilateral adrenalectomy include neoplasms of the adrenal cortex (adenoma, carcinoma) or medulla (pheochromocytoma). Bilateral adrenalectomy may be indicated for cats with pituitary-dependent hyperadrenocorticism.

Feline hyperadrenocorticism is a rare, but recognized, clinical entity. Most cats have adrenal cortical hyperplasia secondary to pituitary microadenoma. Females appear to be at increased risk, and concurrent diabetes mellitus is frequently reported. Treatment of affected cats (unlike dogs) is usually bilateral adrenalectomy due to the ineffectiveness or unsuitability of drugs commonly used in the medical management of hyperadrenocorticism.

Primary hypoadrenocorticism has been reported in cats. Histopathologic examination of adrenal glands from affected cats reveals bilateral atrophy/destruction of all cortical zones without evidence of cause. Adrenal glands of cats with large, non-functional pituitary neoplasms often exhibit profound atrophy of the zona fasciculata and zona reticularis as a result of low circulating levels of ACTH. Unlike dogs, cats receiving exogenous corticosteroids seldom demonstrate clinical signs referable to adrenocortical suppression (secondary hypoadrenocorticism).

Ovary

In addition to the production of oocytes, the ovary is responsible for estrogen and progesterone production. Theca interna and granulosa cells surrounding developing follicles are the major sources of estrogen. Estrogen is responsible for the behavior and vaginal cytology changes associated with estrus, and also facilitates transport of spermatozoa within the female reproductive tract. Because estrogen has a profound effect on the vascularity of the uterus, an increase in uterine weight can be used as a reliable bioassay to assess the relative estrogen activity of estrogenic compounds. Granulosa lutein cells (corpora lutea) produce progesterone. Progesterone plays a critical role in preparing the reproductive tract for implantation of the fertilized ova and maintenance of pregnancy. In late gestation, placental progesterone production is sufficient to maintain pregnancy.

Ovarian hormone production is controlled by gonadotropins and gonadotropin releasing factors from the adenohypophysis and hypothalamus. Follicular maturation and estrogen secretion are stimulated by FSH and LH. Estrogen inhibits the release of FSH - releasing factor, but exerts positive feedback on LH - releasing factor secretion. Thus, estrogens play a critical role in facilitating the pre-ovulatory LH surge. LH plays an important role in the induction of ovulation, formation of the corpus luteum, and progesterone secretion. Cats in estrus maintain high circulating LH concentrations; ovulation is induced by vaginal stimulation (induced ovulation).

The first estrous cycle is usually seen at five to nine months of age. Ovulation without fertilization is followed by pseudopregnancy, a period characterized by elevated serum progesterone levels that usually lasts about 40 days. Unlike dogs, affected cats do not usually exhibit behavior changes or mammary gland enlargement. Ovarian neoplasms are rare.

Testis

The testis has both endocrine and exocrine functions. The exocrine portion of the testis consists of seminiferous tubules (tubuli contorti) that produce spermatozoa. The endocrine portion consists of interstitial (Leydig) and sustentacular (sertoli) cells. Testosterone production by the testis is regulated by the hypothalamic - pituitary - gonadal axis. Secretion of luteotropin releasing factor from the hypothalamus results in production of LH (also called interstitial cell stimulating hormone). LH stimulates testosterone production by interstitial cells and the effect of LH is potentiated by prolactin. Testosterone is responsible for secondary sex characteristics and exerts an anabolic effect on nonreproductive tissues, such as muscle, that possess 5-alpha reductase activity. Elevated serum testosterone concentrations exert negative feedback on LH secretion.

FSH and LH are essential for the development of the seminiferous tubules. In response to FSH, sustentacular cells produce: androgen binding protein, which favors high local concentrations of testosterone critical for spermatogenesis; and inhibin, a hormone that inhibits FSH release from the adenohypophysis. Sustentacular cells also contribute to a blood - testis barrier that reduces the likelihood of an autoimmune response directed toward spermatozoan antigens.

Descent of the testes into the scrotum occurs in the perinatal period. It is believed that androgens from the fetal testis facilitate testicular descent. Males are usually fertile at six to eight months of age. Retained (cryptorchid) testes do not usually produce viable spermatozoa, although their capacity to produce androgens may remain intact. Testicular neoplasms are rare.

Plate 6-1

Relative location of various endocrine organs

Figure A   Hypophysis (pituitary gland) and ventral forebrain, median section

Figure B   Thyroid and external parathyroid glands in cranial neck rotated to expose medial surface. Inset: parathyroid (left) and thyroid glands at low magnification.

Figure C   Low power magnification of pancreas section

Figure D   Relationship of adrenal glands to neighboring structures with left paracostal surgical approach

Figure E   Adrenal gland and gross section of gland

Hypophysis (pituitary gland)
1-3   Adenohypophysis
1   Pars distalis
2   Hypophyseal cleft (of Rathke's pouch)
3   Pars intermedia
4-6   Neurohypophysis
4   Pars nervosa
5   Infundibular recess
6   Infundibulum
7   Mamillary body
8   Third ventricle
9   Interthalamic adhesion
10   Optic chiasm

Thyroid and Parathyroid glands
11   External parathyroid gland
12   Thyroid gland
13   Esophagus
14   Carotid sheath
15   Cranial thyroid a.
16   Larynx
17   Principal cells of parathyroid gland
18   Follicular cells of thyroid gland
19   Colloid
20   Parafollicular cells of thyroid gland

Pancreas
21   Islet cells (endocrine function) of pancreas
22-24 Exocrine pancreas
22   Intercalated duct
23   Connective tissue septum
24   Acinar cells

Gonads
25   Testes (see chapter 9 also)
26   Ovary (see chapter 9 also)

Adrenal gland
27   Kidney
28   Renal a.,v.
29   Caudal vena cava
30   Aorta
31   Phrenicoabdominal a.
32   Phrenicoabdominal v.
33   Adrenal gland
34   13th Rib
35   Adrenal cortex
36   Adrenal medulla

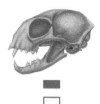

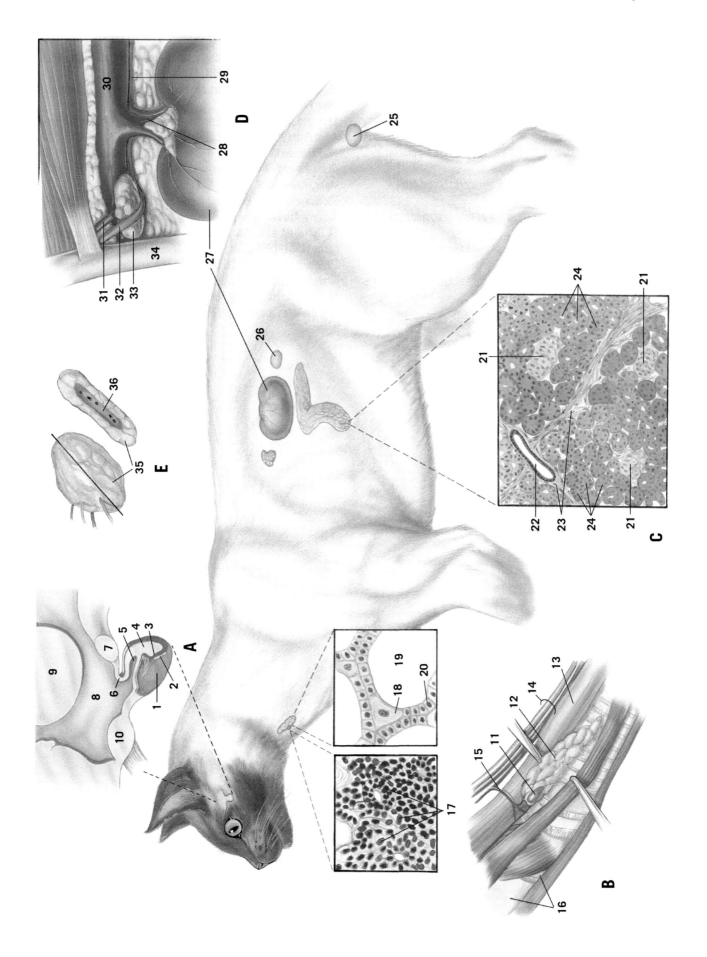

Selected References

1. Banks WJ. *Applied Veterinary Histology.* 3rd Ed. St Louis, Mosby Year Book, 1993; 408.

2. Birchard SJ. In: Bojrab MJ (ed): *Current Techniques in Small Animal Surgery,* 4th Ed. Baltimore, Williams & Wilkins, 1998; 542.

3. Bruyette DS. Feline endocrinology update. *Vet Clin North Am: Small Anim Pract* 2001; 31: 1063.

4. Cormack DH. *Ham's Histology,* 9th Ed. Philadelphia, JB Lippincott 1987; 591

5. Dellmann HD, Brown EM. *Textbook of Veterinary Histology,* 4th Ed. Philadelphia, Lea & Febiger, 1993; 270

6. Dyce KM, Sack WO, Wensing CJG. *Textbook of Veterinary Anatomy.* Philadelphia, Saunders, 2002; 210.

7. Johnston DE. Adrenalectomy via retroperitoneal approach in dogs. *J Am Vet Med Assoc* 1977; 170:1092.

8. Jones BR, et al. Preliminary studies on congenital hypothyroidism in a family of Abyssinian cats. *Vet Rec* 1992; 131:145.

9. Kramek BA, et al. Neuropathy associated with diabetes mellitus in the cat. *J Am Vet Med Assoc* 1984; 184:42.

10. Lofstedt RM. The estrous cycle of the domestic cat. *Compend Contin Educ Pract Vet* 1982;4:52.

11. Lurye JC, Behrend EN. Endocrine tumors. *Vet Clin North Amer: Small Anim Pract* 2001; 31:1083.

12. Peterson ME, Randolph JF, Mooney, CT. In: Sherding RG (ed): *The Cat: Diseases and Clinical Management.* 2nd Ed. New York, Churchill Livingstone, 1994; 1403.

13. Scavelli TD. In: Bojrab MJ (ed): *Current Techniques in Small Animal Surgery,* 4th Ed. Baltimore, Williams & Wilkins, 1998; 539.

14. Turrel JM, et al. Thyroid carcinoma causing hyperthyroidism in cats: 14 cases (1981-1986). *J Am Vet Med Assoc* 1988; 193:359.

15. Welches CD, et al. Occurrence of problems after three techniques of bilateral thyroidectomy in cats. *Vet Surg* 1989; 18:392.

16. Yano BL, Hayden DW, Johnson KH. Feline insular amyloid: association with diabetes mellitus. *Vet Pathol* 1981; 18:621.

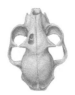

Chapter 7

Respiratory System

▌Bonnie J. Smith

Modified from the original chapter by Gwendolyn Light

Function of the respiratory system includes (1) filtering, warming, and humidifying incoming air, (2) gas exchange, and (3) thermoregulation in panting to dissipate heat. The respiratory passageway consists of the nose and nares (nostrils), nasal cavity, pharynx, larynx, trachea, bronchi, and lungs. The nose and nares admit air to the body, the nasal cavity both ameliorates the incoming air and detects scent particles in the air, the pharynx, trachea and bronchi deliver air to the lungs, the larynx functions in vocalization, and the lungs perform gas exchange. All portions of the respiratory tract contribute to panting.

Head and Neck

Nose and Nares (Nostrils)

The nose is the short relatively narrow portion of the airway extending from the exterior to the more capacious space of the nasal cavity. The nose consists of cutaneous, cartilaginous, and bony structures. The planum nasale (nasal plane or external nose) is the hairless plate of modified skin visible on the external body surface. This structure houses the nares, or nostrils. The feline planum nasale is relatively small and distinctly triangular. The skin of the planum nasale is thickened and tough, presenting numerous small, raised, circular nodules on its rostral surface. The pattern of these nodules is distinct on each individual, and a "nose print" can be used to positively identify individual cats just as fingerprints can be used to identify individual people. The planum nasale also presents the philtrum, a vertical groove bisecting the inferior half of the planum nasale into equal halves. The philtrum continues inferiorly through the median plane throughout the length of the upper lip.

The nares or nostrils are symmetrically placed at the lateral margins of the planum nasale. Cartilage supports the lateral walls of each nostril, permitting passive constant maintenance of the nasal aperture. Small muscles attaching to the nasal cartilages permit a small degree of voluntary flaring of the nostrils, as when closely examining scent or when breathing is labored through exertion or illness. Each nostril leads into a small chamber referred to as the nasal vestibule. Internally, the two nasal vestibules are divided from each other on the midline by the nasal septum. The nasal vestibule extends from the nares to the space of the nasal cavity.

Nasal Cavity

The nasal cavity consists of symmetrical right and left halves divided from each other by the vertically oriented nasal septum. A hyaline cartilage plate forms the vast majority of the nasal septum, being continued only in the caudal-most regions of the nasal cavity by a bony portion. The lateral walls and roof of the nasal cavity are formed by contributions from numerous bones of the face, but largely by the maxilla. The floor of the nasal cavity (which is also the roof of the oral cavity) is bony as well, being formed mainly from horizontal projections of the incisive, maxillary, and palatine bones. The trough-shaped part of the vomer lies on the floor of the nasal cavity, with its shallow "V" receiving and supporting the

cartilaginous portion of the nasal septum. Caudally, the dorsal region of the nasal cavity terminates at a bony partition dividing it from the cranial vault, whereas caudoventrally the nasal cavity is continuous with the nasopharynx.

Cleft palates result from developmental failure of the facial prominences to fuse, due to faulty migration of neural crest cells. In various forms of cleft palate, the medial nasal prominences do not fuse or the palatine processes of the maxillary prominences fail to fuse. Untreated, cleft palate may be lethal. In the absence of complete division of the oral and nasal cavity, ingesta may gain access to the airway and be drawn into the lungs. Death results from aspiration pneumonia. Breed-specific physical features of the head and face may also cause difficulties. Selecting for anomalies in craniofacial development resulting in shortening of the face in brachycephalic breeds such as Persians may result in difficulty breathing and inability to sustain exercise in some individuals. Craniofacial malformation of Burmese cats is a complex defect that includes cleft palate, agenesis of the planum nasale and/or nostrils, and other facial defects.

Just inside the nostrils, the short, narrow, rostral-most portion of the nasal cavity is referred to as the nasal vestibule. The space here is small and empty. The nasolacrimal duct, which drains tears from the lacrimal sac, opens into the vestibule. The middle portion of the nasal cavity is its largest region, and is sometimes referred to as its "respiratory region." This area is more spacious in all dimensions, extending from the nasal vestibule caudally through the face and ending at the choanae, the bony-edged openings at the end of the hard palate. The choanae mark the transition from the nasal cavity to the nasopharynx. Blind pockets, the paranasal sinuses (frontal and sphenoid sinuses, maxillary recess), lead from the nasal cavity by small openings into more spacious cavities within the frontal and maxillary bones. (See also the discussion of the skull in Chapter 3.)

The incisive duct is a narrow tubular passage between the rostral parts of the nasal and oral cavities. (The oral opening of the duct lays on the incisive papilla, just caudal the upper incisor teeth.) Each incisive duct also receives the duct of the ipsilateral vomeronasal organ, an elongate, tube like structure extending along the floor of the nasal cavity. These passages end blindly near the roots of the early cheek teeth. The vomeronasal organ functions largely in detection and interpretation of urinary pheromones.

The space within the nasal cavity houses the conchae or turbinates, which are intricate and delicate scroll work of bone. Each concha is anchored to the outer bony wall of the nasal cavity, and projects medially into the space of the nasal cavity. The paper-thin bone of each concha is devised into extensive scrolls that turn progressively inward. The dorsal nasal concha is the largest and longest, projecting from the dorsolateral wall of the nasal cavity toward the nasal septum. The ventral nasal concha is small, extending from the level of the second or third premolar to the canine tooth. The large, irregular middle nasal concha is a rostrally-directed extension of the ethmoid concha (see below). Together, the scrolls of the conchae cause a tremendous increase in surface area within the nasal cavity. The nasal conchae divide the nasal cavity into three spaces or meati. The dorsal nasal meatus is a small, blind-ended space between the dorsolateral wall of the nasal cavity and the dorsal concha. The middle nasal meatus is moderately sized and also blind-ended, lying between the dorsal and ventral conchae. The ventral nasal meatus is a relatively large space between the ventral concha and the floor of the nasal cavity. Importantly, the ventral nasal meatus does not end blindly, and freely communicates through the choanae with the nasopharynx. The common nasal meatus is a narrow, vertical space immediately lateral to the nasal septum, which communicates with the other three meati. Since only the ventral nasal meatus communicates directly with the nasopharynx and eventually the space common to the laryngeal and esophageal openings (the laryngopharynx), passage of instruments such as a nasogastric tube or broncho-scope obligatorily uses the ventral meatus.

The dorsal, middle, and ventral conchae are covered by respi-ratory epithelium (pseudostratified ciliated columnar). The epithelium is well provided with serous glands and numerous goblet cells. The submucosa is extremely vascular. The extensive mucosal surface thus presented provides ample opportunity to expose incoming air to warming and humidifying action, as well as the "sweeping" action of the cilia.

The dorsal, caudal-most region of the nasal cavity houses a specialized set of conchae, the ethmoidal conchae, which are an elaboration of the ethmoid bone. The ethmoid conchae are continuous caudally with the cribriform plate, the many perfora-tions of which lead directly into the cranial vault. The epithelium covering this set of conchae is olfactory, and the axons leading from the cells coalesce to form the rootlets of the olfactory nerve, which pass through the foramina in the cribriform plate to enter into the olfactory peduncles of the brain.

Pharynx

The pharynx is a soft tissue-walled tubular region leading from the caudal end of the nasal and oral cavities to the cranial end of the larynx and esophagus. Unlike the nasal cavity, the nasopharynx is not divided into right and left halves by a septum. The walls of the pharynx are muscular, and the inner wall is lined by mucosa. The several pharyngeal and palatal muscles address the changes necessary to the pharynx to permit swallowing. When the pharynx is largely relaxed, their disposition facilitates airflow directly from the nasopharynx to the laryngeal opening. The pharynx comprises three subdivisions, these being the naso-, oro-, and laryngo-pharynx. Rostrally, the soft palate divides the pharynx into two portions. As the soft palate continues caudally from the caudal end of the hard palate, it demarcates the nasopharynx dorsal to the soft palate from the oropharynx ventral to the soft palate. The position and extent of the naso- and oropharynx can be quite accurately estimated as the regions dorsal and ventral to the soft palate, respectively. More technically, the oropharynx extends from the palatoglossal arches (mucosal folds arching between the base of the tongue and the soft palate) to the base of the epiglottis. Similarly, the nasopharynx is described as extending from the choanae to the intrapharyngeal opening (the region of confluence

among the nasopharynx, oropharynx, and laryngopharynx). The nasopharynx houses the pharyngeal opening of the auditory tube, the entrance to the soft tissue tube leading to the middle ear cavity. While polyps in the nasal cavity are unusual, nasopha-ryngeal polyps are more common. Such polyps can be relatively easily visualized using the endoscope, and surgical removal is often straightforward. The laryngopharynx is the most caudal pharyngeal region, and may be loosely defined as the space dorsal to the larynx. More specifically, the laryngopharynx extends from the intrapharyngeal opening to the cranial end of the esophagus (i.e., the pharyngoesophageal limen). In communicating with both the naso- and oropharynx cranially, the laryngopharynx plays a dual role. The laryngopharynx receives air from the nasopharynx and conducts it ventrally toward the larynx, and also receives the food bolus or fluid from the oropharynx and conducts it relatively dorsally to the esophagus. Thus, in the short distance common to air and ingesta, their pathways cross each other. This crossover necessitates that the trachea and lungs be protected during deglutition, a function largely met by the movement of the epiglottis during swallowing.

During normal nasal breathing, the soft palate is relaxed and inclines ventrally, resting on the lingual base. The rostralmost tip of the epiglottis extends just into the caudal end of the nasopharynx, resting on or near the soft palate. Thus, the oropharynx is isolated from the nasopharynx, and the air passage leads directly from the nasopharynx to the laryngeal opening. In oral breathing (panting), the soft palate is raised while the epiglottis remains open, thus creating a patent airway from the oropharynx to the laryngeal opening.

Larynx

The larynx is a cartilaginous and muscular structure that joins the pharynx and trachea. The structure of the larynx is complex, owing to its functioning not only in conducting air into and out of the trachea, but also in vocalization. Three unpaired cartilages (the epiglottic, thyroid, and cricoid) and one pair of cartilages (the arytenoids) form the skeleton of the larynx. Of these, the entire epiglottic cartilage and the vocal process of the arytenoid cartilage are elastic, while the others are hyaline. The spoon-shaped epiglottic cartilage is most rostral of the laryngeal cartilages. The cartilage together with its mucosal covering composes the epiglottis. The relaxed epiglottis contributes to the smooth passage of air from the nasopharynx into the larynx. During swallowing, the epiglottis moves caudally to cover the laryngeal opening (the aditus laryngis) and protect the lower airway. The epiglottis is related to the lingual base in such a way that drawing the tongue forward while placing pressure on the lingual base also draws the epiglottis rostrally. This brings the epiglottis clearly into view, and is thereby performed during intubation to facilitate placement of the endotracheal tube through the larynx, and thus into the airway rather than the esophagus. However, cats in particular are prone to laryngospasm, or tight reflexive closure of the laryngeal opening, following any mechanical stimulation of the larynx. One missed attempt at intubation can render the procedure temporarily impossible. Application of aerosol topical anesthetic may help reduce the occurrence or severity of mechanically induced laryngospasm.

The boat-shaped thyroid cartilage is intermediate in the rostral-to-caudal sequence of laryngeal cartilages. The thyroid cartilage is placed so that the open side of the "boat" faces dorsally. The lateral surfaces of the thyroid cartilage enclose portions of the cricoid and arytenoid cartilages. The ventral surface is deeply notched with a V-shaped cleft placed with the open end of the "V" pointing caudally. Rostrally, the thyroid cartilage articulates with the thyrohyoid bones of the hyoid apparatus by means of its rostral cornu (horn). Caudally, its caudal horn articulates with the most caudal laryngeal cartilage, the cricoid cartilage. This terminal laryngeal cartilage, the cricoid, has the shape of a signet ring, being markedly wider dorsally than ventrally. The cricoid cartilage articulates cranially with the thyroid and arytenoid cartilages of the larynx, and is separated fully from the first tracheal ring by membrane.

The paired arytenoid cartilages are irregular in shape, but as a generalization may be likened to an equilateral triangle. The feline arytenoids lack the corniculate and cuneiform processes seen in other domestic carnivores. The arytenoid cartilages articulate with the thyroid and cricoid cartilages. The muscular and vocal processes of the arytenoid cartilage receive the thyroarytenoideus muscle from its extensive origin along the ventral surface of the larynx.

The numerous small muscles of the larynx are all striated. These muscles may be functionally grouped into two classes. The extrinsic laryngeal muscles are only two, the thyrohyoideus and sternothyroideus. These muscles pass between the larynx and the hyoid apparatus and sternum, respectively, and thus move the larynx as a whole. They are particularly related to gross laryngeal movements during swallowing. The five intrinsic laryngeal muscles both originate and insert upon the larynx itself. In passing among the laryngeal cartilages, these muscles serve to move the cartilages relative to each other, and function mainly in vocalization, phonation, and closure of the glottis. These muscles, together with the ligaments and articulations of the larynx, are illustrated. The m. cricoarytenoideus dorsalis warrants special note, in that it alone opens the glottis.

The laryngeal cavity is lined mainly by a noncornified stratified squamous epithelium. This relatively durable and rapidly-renewable epithelium resists the wearing forces borne by this very active region of the respiratory tract. The inner walls of the feline laryngeal cavity lack laryngeal ventricles. Nonetheless, paired laterally-placed vestibular folds are recognizable. These folds are solely mucosal, without muscular or ligamentous support. More medially, the paired vocal folds indicate the position of the vocal ligament and thyroarytenoideus muscle where they are covered by laryngeal mucosa. The glottis is a physical structure; formed by the vocal folds laterally, and by the arytenoid cartilages and their mucosal covering dorsally. The space defined by these structures is called the glottic cleft or rima glottidis. The glottis divides the laryngeal cavity into the laryngeal vestibule rostral to it, and the infraglottic cavity caudal to it. The dimensions of the glottis may be changed voluntarily as when vocalizing or holding the breath, or involuntarily as a protective reflex. The latter phenomenon is particularly well-developed in the cat, and is the source of the potential difficulties encountered during intubation mentioned earlier.

Laryngeal innervation provided by two separate branches of the vagus nerve CN X. The cranial laryngeal nerve is sensory to the cranial mucosal regions, and also motor to the cricothyroideus. The caudal laryngeal nerve (which is actually the termination of the recurrent laryngeal nerve) is sensory to the caudal mucosal regions, as well as motor to all intrinsic laryngeal muscles except the cricothyroideus.

The mechanism of purring in cats has been debated for years. Explanations encompass suggestions as diverse as vibration of the diaphragm, vibration of the cranial vena cava, and voluntary sub-vocal vibration of the vocal folds. Given the distinct vibrations palpable in the throat, the latter seems most likely.

Trachea

The trachea extends from the cricoid laryngeal cartilage in the neck to the tracheal bifurcation into the principal bronchi within the thoracic cavity dorsal to the heart. The trachea is thus described as having cervical and thoracic regions. The full length of the trachea is composed of about 40 hyaline cartilage rings. The exact number varies among individuals, usually ranging between 38 and 43. Tracheal rings are incomplete dorsally, where the space between them bridged by the trachealis muscle (smooth muscle). Connection between the rings is accomplished by annular ligaments.

Cervical Trachea

In the cranial cervical region just caudal to the pharynx, the trachea is positioned ventral to the esophagus, reflecting the relation of the larynx to the esophageal origin. Slightly caudally, about at the level of C2 or C3, the trachea shifts to attain a mostly midline position. Here the esophagus lies to the left of the trachea. The trachea maintains this general position throughout most of the neck, though it may shift to some degree during postural changes of the head and neck. The thyroid and parathyroid glands lie on the lateral tracheal surfaces just caudal to the larynx. The carotid sheath (containing the common carotid artery, vagosympathetic trunk, and internal jugular vein) courses generally along the dorsal tracheal surface cranially, shifting more laterally in the caudal cervical regions. The tracheal lymphatic trunk and the caudal laryngeal nerve also course along the trachea, slightly lateral and ventral to the carotid sheath. The ventral and lateral surfaces of the cervical trachea are in contact with the "strap" muscles of the neck. The mm. sternohyoideus are particularly closely applied to the ventral tracheal surface. Late in the neck, the esophagus shifts fully to the left of the trachea so that at and passing through the thoracic inlet, the trachea lies in direct contact with the hypaxial muscles.

Understanding of the relationship of the cervical trachea to its related structures is essential when entering the trachea through the neck as in performing a tracheostomy. To access the tracheal lumen, a ventral midline skin incision is made in the cranial cervical region. The sternohyoid muscles are identified, separated along the median plane, and reflected laterally. The exposed tracheal surface is incised transversely through the annular ligaments, being particularly careful to avoid damage to the tracheal rings, as they heal very poorly. At this point, a transtracheal wash could be performed, or a tracheostomy tube placed in the tracheal lumen and anchored to the cervical skin.

Plate 7-1

Figure A   Upper respiratory region, median section of head, nasal septum removed
Figure B   Skeleton of larynx with hyoid apparatus on the right side, ventral view
              (arytenoid cartilages not visible)
Figure C   Intrinsic musculature of larynx, lateral view with window in thyroid cartilage
Figure D   Structures typically viewed when placing an endotracheal tube
Figure E   Nose and superior lip, rostral view

1-3	Regions of nasal cavity	
1	Vestibule	
2	Respiratory region with conchae	
3	Olfactory region with conchae	

1-3   Regions of nasal cavity
   1   Vestibule
   2   Respiratory region with conchae
   3   Olfactory region with conchae
4   Frontal sinus
5   Ethmoid bone
6   Vomer
7   Sphenoid sinus
8   Hard palate
9   Soft palate
10-12 Pharynx
   10 Nasopharynx
   11 Oropharynx
   12 Laryngopharynx
13   Nasopharyngeal opening of auditory tube
14   Palatopharyngeal arch
15   Epiglottis
16   Basihyoid bone
17   Trachea
18   Esophagus
19   M. longus capitis
20   Mandubular symphysis

16, 21-25   Hyoid apparatus
   21 Thyrohyoid bone
   22 Ceratohyoid bone
   23 Epihyoid bone
   24 Stylohyoid bone
   25 Tympanohyoid cartilage
26   Thyroid cartilage (window cut in C)
27   Cricothyroid ligament
28   Cricoid cartilage
29   Tracheal cartilages
30   Annular ligaments
31   Arytenoid cartilage
32   Rostral cornu
33   Caudal cornu
35   M. arytenoideus transversus
36   M. arytenoideus dorsalis
37   M. thyroarytenoideus
38   M. cricoarytenoideus lateralis
39   M. cricothyroideus
40   Vocal cord
41   Planum nasale
42   Philtrum
43   Naris

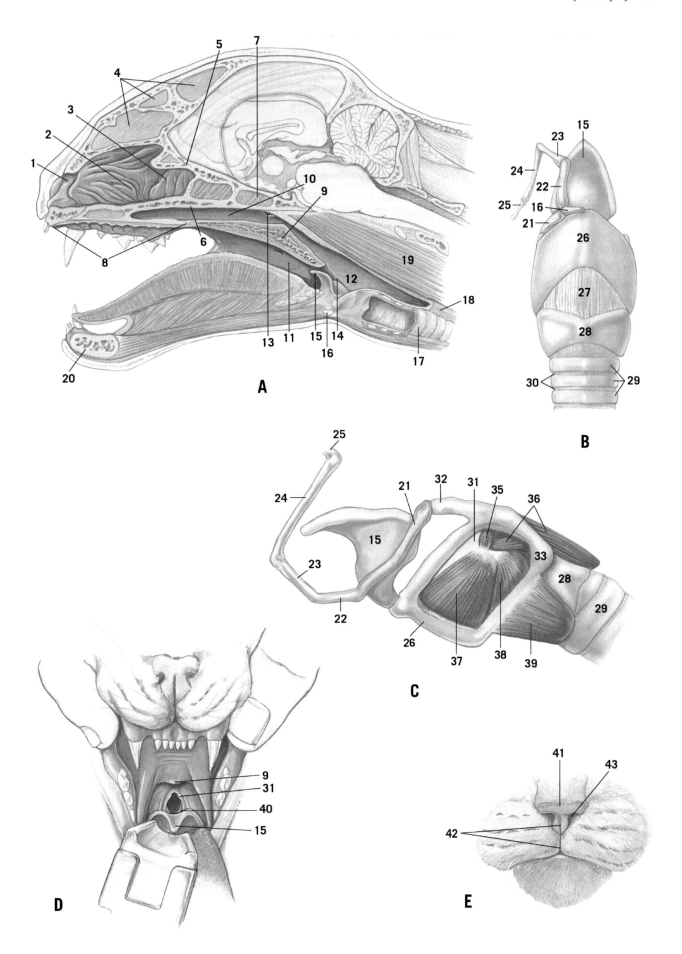

Thoracic Cavity

The thoracic cavity houses the thoracic trachea, the pleura and pleural cavities, the lungs, and the mediastium. The thoracic inlet, the thoracic walls, and the thoracic outlet, each of which includes both bony and soft tissue elements, define the thoracic cavity. The narrow thoracic inlet is bounded by the first thoracic vertebra, the first pair of ribs, and the manubrium of the sternum. The thoracic wall is formed dorsally by the vertebral bodies and hypaxial musculature, laterally and partly ventrally by the ribs and costal cartilages with their associated muscles, and ventrally by the sternum and the transversis thoracis muscle. The wide thoracic outlet is oblique, being formed by the last thoracic vertebra and rib, the costal arch, and the xiphoid process. The thoracic outlet is closed by the diaphragm, which thus forms caudal wall of the thoracic cavity and separates it from the abdominal cavity.

The diaphragm is a dome of striated muscle and tendon attaching circumferentially around the thoracic outlet. The diaphragm is convex cranially, curving into bony thorax, allowing the abdominal cavity and its organs to occupy a significant part of the bony thorax. This feature must be remembered when auscultating the lungs, so as not to incorrectly infer a pathological condition when gut sounds are heard under the caudal costal regions. The center of the diaphragm is tendinous rather than muscular. The central tendon of the diaphragm is quite large, having a shape reminiscent of a Valentine heart. This central tendon forms the apex of the curve of the diaphragm, extending as far cranially as the lower part of the sixth rib on full expiration. Individual regions of the muscular portion of the diaphragm can be described according to their attachments along the body wall. The lumbar region of the diaphragm is thick and robust, originating as paired crura (sing.: crus), columns of muscle supported by stout tendons arising from the ventral aspects of the bodies of the first three or four lumbar vertebrae. The right crus is considerably larger than the left. Both crura fan out to join the central tendon along its more dorsal regions. The thinner costal part of the diaphragm originates as segmental slips of muscle arising from the medial surfaces of the ribs and costal cartilages. These fibers also course toward and blend with the central tendon. The sternal region arises from the sternum and its relatively short fibers course fairly directly dorsally to blend with the central tendon as well.

The diaphragm presents three holes to allow specific structures to pass between the thoracic and abdominal cavities. The aortic hiatus is most dorsal, and lies between the lumbar vertebrae and the crural tendons. This opening transmits not only the aorta, but also the azygous vein, thoracic lymphatic duct, and sympathetic trunks. The esophageal hiatus lies slightly more ventrally within the right crus, transmitting the esophagus and both vagal trunks. The caval foramen perforates the central tendon on the right side of midline in the dorsal third of the tendon. This caudal vena cava passes cranially through this opening.

Diaphragmatic hernias may develop either as a congenital defect or following trauma. As a result of passage of varying amounts of the abdominal viscera through the defect, crowding of the lungs can result in dyspnea, or gastrointestinal signs may result from trapping or twisting of intestine herniated into the thoracic cavity. Often, such defects can be successfully repaired by approaching the diaphragm from its caudal surface.

Pleura

The pleurae line the thoracic wall and contact all contents of the thoracic cavity. The paired pleura are serous membranes whose final disposition is best understood if considered developmentally. The right and left pleural sacs each line one half of thoracic cavity with a single layer. Before the lungs develop, much of the thoracic cavity is empty and considerable potential space is present between the medial and lateral sides of each pleural membrane. This is the pleural cavity. The schematic illustration clearly shows that the pleural cavity contains no organs, and further that the pleural cavities are contained within the thoracic cavity. As the lungs develop from the midline, they expand into the space of the thoracic cavity, displacing the pleura as they go. The pleural lining remains intact, and the lungs (or any other organs, for that matter) never enter the pleural space. The pleural cavities are reduced to a small potential space between the lungs and the thoracic walls. Though the pleural cavities never contain organs, the membrane secretes a small amount of serous fluid into the cavity. The presence of this fluid is of paramount importance, since it is slick in nature and allows the easy sliding of the lungs within the thoracic cavity as they change dimension during ventilation. Pathologic reduction of pleural fluid causes markedly painful ventilation. While the pleural spaces are normally merely slit-like, some disease states or trauma may cause pathological accumulation of various substances within the space. In such instances, the accumulating substance can partially or almost completely fill the pleural space and expand it at the expense of the lungs. Breathing becomes difficult, and blood oxygen levels may drop markedly. Free air (pneumothorax), blood (hemothorax), pus (pyothorax), or chyle (chylothorax) are among the most common offending substances.

The mediastinum is partially defined by the medial-most regions of the right and left pleural sacs where they approach each other near the midline (mediastinal pleurae). The mediastinum is defined as these regions of pleurae together with all tissues and structures between them. Some regions of the mediastinum contain large structures such as the heart, great vessels, thymus, trachea, and esophagus. Here the two layers of mediastinal pleura do not contact each other. However, in other regions little tissue intervenes between the pleurae and they lie in direct contact. Irregularly placed, small perforations in the mediastinal pleura allow communication between the two pleural sacs.

The pleura may be subdivided into regions based upon what structure is covered by that segment of pleura. Pleura directly apposed to the lungs is called visceral or pulmonary pleura. Pleura directly applied to some part of the wall of the thoracic cavity is called parietal pleura. The parietal pleura can be further specified as costal parietal pleura where it lines the ribs and intercostals, diaphragmatic pleura on the diaphragm, and mediastinal where it lines the mediastinum. The pericardial mediastinal pleura, covering the pericardium, is a sub region of mediastinal pleura often considered separately from the others. Each of these regions is directly continuous with the others since pleura originates as a single sheet of tissue lining half the thoracic cavity. In certain areas, small free folds of pleura are formed as visceral pleura reflects to form parietal pleura. The most prominent of these are the pulmonary ligaments at the reflection of visceral to mediastinal pleura, and the plica venae cavae, a fold of pleura surrounding the caudal vena cava. The plica venae cavae, together with the pleural covering the mediastinum, pericardium, and diaphragm, forms a potential space termed the mediastinal recess. The accessory lobe of the right lung occupies the recess.

The line of pleural reflection is the line along which the costal pleura reflects onto the diaphragm. Dorsally, this line begins at about the last rib; the line curves ventrally and cranially in a cranially-concave line to the eighth costal cartilage. The lungs do not expand to the point of reaching the line of pleural reflection. Their caudal edge, the basal border of the lung, more or less parallels the line of pleural reflection a short distance cranial to it. The basal border of the lung begins dorsally at about the eleventh intervertebral space, and curves cranioventrally to the costochondral junction of the sixth rib. The two layers of pleura thus lie in contact with each other as a short gap between the basal border of the lung and the line of pleural reflection. This region is termed the costodiaphragmatic recess, for the two regions of pleura forming it. The cranial-to-caudal dimension of the costodiaphragmatic recess varies with stage of respiration, becoming smaller on inspiration and larger on expiration. As with all serous membranes in the body, normally a thin film of serous fluid lies between these two pleural layers. Thus, the costodiaphragmatic recess offers a convenient region in which to access the pleural cavity and its contents. Since the recess freely communicates with the other regions of the pleural cavity, any substance in it is representative of the pleural contents as a whole. Further, since no organ lies in immediate proximity, this region is a convenient site to obtain representative samples of pleural fluid or other contents without jeopardizing the heart or lungs. This procedure, thoracocentesis, is best performed in the middle of the eighth intercostals space, just dorsal to the costochondral junction.

Respiratory Muscles

The muscles of the thoracic wall together with the diaphragm achieve the changes in dimension of the thoracic cavity necessary for ventilation. Enlarging the thoracic cavity lowers the pressure within, allowing inspiration. Conversely, decreasing the size of the cavity causes exhalation. Since inspiration is the more difficult of the two actions, most of the mural thoracic musculature and the diaphragm are function during inspiration. Elevation of the ribs and caudal movement (contraction) of the diaphragm are inspiratory movements, while sinking of the ribs and cranial movement of the diaphragm are expiratory movements. Though the diaphragm is by far the greatest contributor to ventilation, its contribution is not essential. Diaphragmatic paralysis does render breathing more difficult, but ventilation adequate to support life long-term is possible using only the muscles of the thoracic wall.

Thoracic Trachea

The thoracic trachea begins as the most dorsal visceral structure entering the thoracic cavity, where it is directly apposed to the m. longus colli. The thoracic trachea lies in the mediastinum. The trachea gradually inclines ventrally from its entrance to the thorax, and attains a position ventral to the esophagus at the level of the aortic arch. In departing from its parallel course with the vertebral column, a space develops between the trachea and the vertebrae that is readily apparent in lateral radiographs. Changes in this normal triangular shape of this space suggest some anomaly in the trachea or surrounding structures. The trachea terminates near the heart base, where it divides into the two principal (main stem or primary) bronchi.

Principal Bronchi

The right and left principal bronchi arise from the trachea and diverge toward the lungs. The bronchi enter the medial surfaces of the lungs, adjacent to the major vessels. Upon entering the lungs, each primary bronchus undergoes progressive division and re-division into progressively smaller airways. First among these are lobar bronchi, destined to enter each primary lobe of a given lung. Next segmental bronchi arise that in turn arborize in to smaller bronchioles. Histologically, bronchioles lack cartilage. These bronchioles continue to divide into smaller and smaller passages, which terminate in alveolar ducts to alveolar saccules. The alveolar saccules comprise multiple alveoli, which are the sites of gas exchange. Adults of the lungworm, *Aelurstrongylus abstrusus*, reside in small airways of the terminal bronchioles and alveolar ducts, as well as in the vascular pathways of the small pulmonary arteries.

Lungs

The lungs are the largest organs of the thoracic cavity. The pulmonary root or hilus lies on the medial surface of each lung, and is the collection of airways (bronchi), vessels, and nerves that pass from the mediastinum into or out of the lungs. Each lung is divided into externally-visible lobes based upon internal branching of the bronchi. Deep superficial grooves on the external surface of the lungs are suggestive (though not entirely directly reflective) of these divisions. These interlobar fissures divide the right and lungs into grossly-visible lobes. The larger right lung comprises four lobes: the cranial, middle, caudal, and accessory lobes. All but the latter are visible from the lateral surface. The accessory lobe (lying within the mediastinal recess) approximates the median plane, and surrounds a portion of the caudal vena cava. The smaller left lung has only two lobes, the cranial and caudal. However, the cranial lobe is divided into cranial and caudal parts. The fissure between these lobes is quite deep, and gives the strong impression that the two parts could be separate lobes. However, both these portions are supplied by the same the lobar bronchus; hence, they are considered parts of one lobe rather than separate lobes. Along the ventral border of each lung, the separation between two lung lobes creates the cardiac notch. In these small regions, the pericardium directly contacts the thoracic wall, making the heart or pericardial cavity accessible to needle puncture without also piercing the lung. The relatively poorly-developed left cardiac notch lies between the caudal part of the left cranial lobe and the left caudal lobe. On the right, the cardiac notch lies between the right cranial and middle lobes.

Much of the thoracic wall under which the lungs lie is itself covered by epaxial musculature or muscles of the thoracic limb. Thus, the portion of the body wall through which the lungs may be most directly auscultated is quite small. This triangular region, the auscultation triangle, is bordered on each side by the m. triceps brachii cranially, dorsally by the lateral edge of the epaxial muscles, and caudally by a curving line from the sixth costo-chondral junction to the eleventh intercostals space. (Note that the basal border of the lung extends more caudally than the caudal boundary of the auscultation triangle, because the caudal most regions of the lung are too thin to permit accurate detection of air sounds within them.)

Innervation to the lungs is entirely autonomic. Parasympathetic tone constricts airways, while sympathetic tone may dilate or constrict the airways dependent upon which receptors are involved.

Vascular supply to the lungs comprises two separate flows and functions. One, the nutritive flow, is designed to bring oxygen and nutrients to the pulmonary parenchyma while removing metabolic wastes from it. The bronchial vessels accomplish this function. In contrast, the functional supply, accomplishes delivery of deoxygenated blood to the alveoli for the purposes of as exchange. Branches of the pulmonary artery serve this purpose. The location of the functional (deoxygenated) pulmonary vessels with respect to the bronchi is illustrated. This classic relationship is used diagnosing of several cardiac anomalies that result in discrepancies causing discrepancies in distribution between the two sets of vessels.

A small number of adult parasites can occupy the pulmonary tissues (rather than bronchi). The adult lung fluke, *Paragonimus kellicotti*, establishes permanent cystic cavities in alveolar tissue. Other species that cause pulmonary parenchymal disease include *Toxoplasma* spp. and the heartworm, *Dirofilaria immitis.* Heartworm disease was once thought of as mainly a canine concern, and both treatment and prophylactic regimens are well-established in dogs. However, feline heartworm disease is now recognized as occurring with significant and increasing frequency. Severe and life-threatening thromboemboli may develop as a result of *D immitis* infection, as well as possibly from treatment of the disease. Prophylaxis is thus the most prudent course.

Plate 7-2

Figure A   Schematic illustration of relationship of pleura, pleural cavity, and some
structures of the thoracic cavity through development, transverse section.
Right hand illustration only shows heart and pericardium in place

Figure B   Location of lungs, auscultation triangle, and line of pleural reflection, left
lateral and right lateral view. Shaded area denotes the auscultation triangle;
red dotted line denotes the location of the median portion of the diaphragm;
blue dotted line denotes line of pleural reflection

1 Thoracic vertebra	**10** Parietal pericardium
2 Thoracic wall; bone, cartilage, and/or muscle	**11** Visceral pericardium
3 Sternum	**12** Pericardial cavity
4 Mediastinum	**13** Heart
5-7 Pleura (diaphragmatic pleura not shown)	**14** Rib 6
5 Costal (parietal) pleura	**15** Rib 10
6 Mediastinal (parietal) pleura	**16** Diaphragm
7 Pulmonary (visceral) pleura	**17** Epaxial muscle
8 Pleural cavity	**18** Basal border of the lung
9 Lung, developing or adult	**19** Potential pleurocentesis (thoracocentesis) site
	20 Cardiac notch

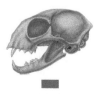

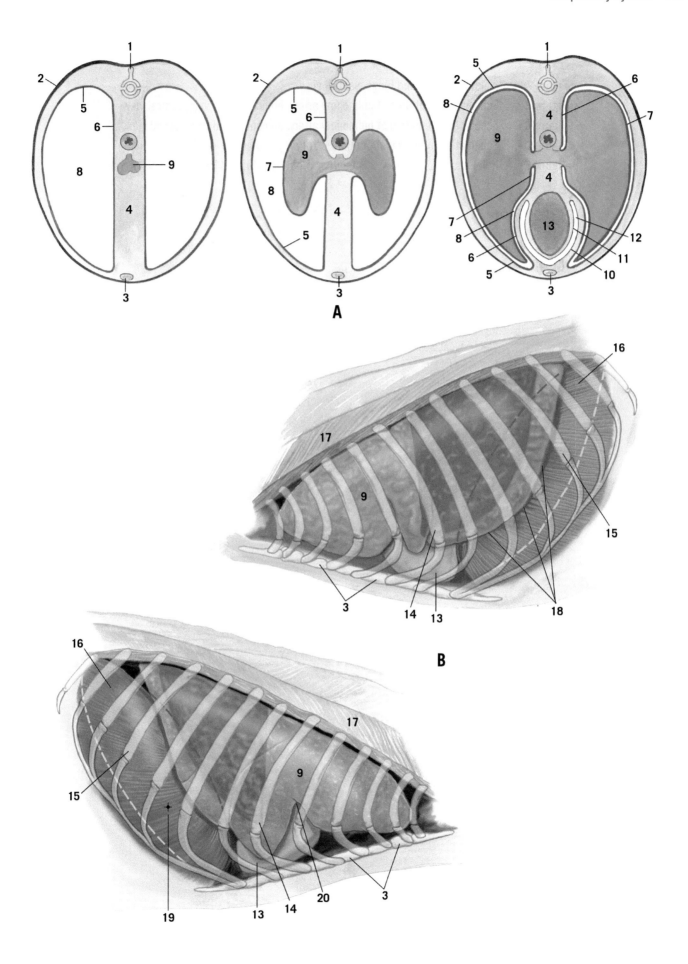

Plate 7-3

Figure A   Isolated bronchi and lungs, ventral view
Figure B   Schematic orientation of pulmonary artery, bronchus, and vein, ventral view
Figure C   Schematic orientation of pulmonary artery, bronchus, and vein, lateral view
Figure D   Schematic illustration of termination of air passageway
Figure E   Relationship of cervical esophagus, carotid sheath, and trachea, craniolateral view.

1	Trachea	10	Pulmonary a
2	Principal bronchus	11	Pulmonary v
3-4	Left lung	12	Respiratory bronchiole
3	Left cranial lobe	13	Alveolar ducts
4	Left caudal lobe	14	Alveolar sac
5-8	Right lung	15	Alveoli
5	Right cranial lobe	16	Esophagus
6	Right middle lobe	17	Carotid sheath; common carotid a, internal jugular v, vagosympathetic trunk
7	Right caudal lobe		
8	Accessory lobe		
9	Lobar bronchus	18	Recurrent laryngeal n

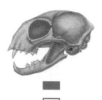

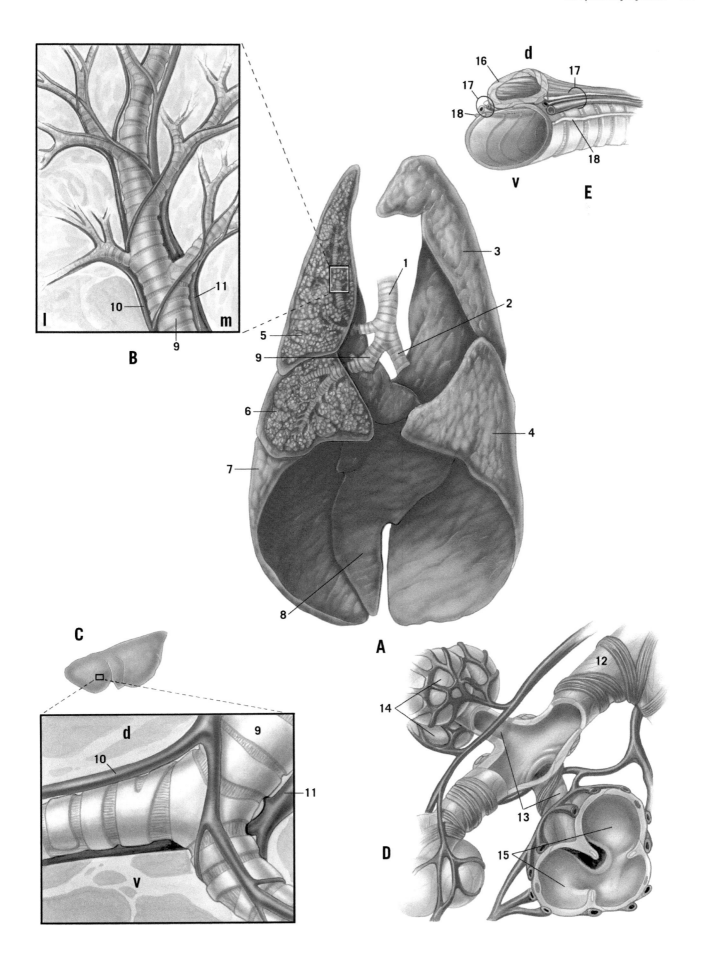

B

l   m

11
10
9

5
1
9

6

7

8

A

3

2

4

d
16
17
17
18
18

v

E

C

d

10
9
11

v

D

14

12

13

15

Selected References

1. August JR, Bahr A. In: August JR (Ed): *Consultations in Feline Internal Medicine,* Volume 5. St. Louis, Elsevier Saunders. 2006; 347.

2. Dyce KM, Sack WO, Wensing CJG. *Textbook of Veterinary Anatomy.* 3rd Ed. Philadelphia, WB Saunders, 2002; 148, 403.

3. Kerins AM, Breathnach R. In: Chandler EA, Gaskell CJ, Gaskell RM (Eds). *Feline Medicine and Therapeutics.* 3rd Ed. Oxford, Blackwell Publishing, Ltd. 2004; 325.

4. Levy JK, Ford RB. In: Sherding RG (Ed). *The Cat: Diseases and Clinical Management.* 2nd Ed. St. Louis, Elsevier Saunders, 1994; 947.

5. Muilenburg RK, Fry TR. In: Harari J (Ed). *Veterinary Clinics of North America, Small Animal Practice: Topics in Feline Surgery.* Philadelphia, WB Saunders. 2002; 839.

6. Schummer A, Nickel R, Sack WO. *The Viscera of the Domestic Mammals.* 2nd revised ed. New York, Springer-Verlag. 1979; 211, 247.

7. Venker-van Haagen AJ. In: Ettinger ST, Feldman EC (Eds). *Textbook of Veterinary Internal Medicine,* 6th ed. St. Louis, Elsevier Saunders, 2005; 1186.

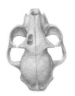

Chapter 8

Digestive System

■ Jill A. Barnes

Modified from the original chapter by James Smallwood

The digestive system consists of those body structures and organs that function in the prehension, transport, and breakdown of food, in the absorption and temporary storage of absorbed nutrients, and in the discharge and elimination of alimentary waste products from the body. The major components of the system include the mouth and pharynx, the alimentary canal, the liver, and the pancreas. As a predatory carnivore, the digestive system of the cat is relatively uncomplicated, yet highly adapted for capturing and digesting the bodies of smaller mammals and birds, which represent its primary prey in the wild.

Mouth and Pharynx
Teeth
Typical of the carnivore, the teeth of the cat are appropriately modified for grasping, puncturing, and tearing (cutting) rather than true mastication. With the exception of "crunching" dry food, cats do little if any actual chewing. A relatively large diastema, or carrying space, is present immediately caudal to the canine teeth. There are no first premolars and no lower (inferior) first or second premolars; the molars consist of a single tooth on each side, upper and lower. Due to this reduction in premolars and molars, the cat has the fewest teeth of any common domestic mammal with a permanent dental formula of:

2 (Incisors3/3, Canines 1/1, Premolar 3/2, Molar 1/1) = 30.

The only permanent teeth that do not have deciduous predecessors are the four molars so that the deciduous dental formula is:

2 (I 3/3, C 1/1, P 3/2) = 26.

Kittens typically begin to eruption of their deciduous teeth during their third postnatal week, and their permanent teeth are all in place by about six months of age.

The only tooth with three roots is upper (superior) P4. When the mouth is closed, the upper sectorial tooth (P4) slides across the vestibular surface of the lower sectorial tooth (M1), producing an effective scissor-like cutting action.

Root abscesses associated with upper P4 may produce a draining tract ventral to the eye or may erode into the orbit and rupture into the conjunctival sac. Some of the small incisor teeth may be loose or lost in older cats. Anodontia, a complete absence of teeth, has been reported in the cat. Periodontal disease is the most common condition affecting the mouth of the cat.

Oral Cavity
The oral cavity is bounded rostrally and laterally by the lips and cheeks, and extends caudally to join the oropharynx at the level of the caudal border of the hard palate. When the mouth is closed the oral cavity is divided by the teeth into the oral cavity proper and the oral vestibule. The latter is the space peripheral to the teeth, bounded by the lips and cheeks, and into which liquid medication can be administered. In addition to diffuse salivary (labial) glands, the lips contain large sebaceous and apocrine glands. The secretion of these circumoral glands is used in grooming and is frequently rubbed off on other objects, apparently as a scent marker substance. The upper lips (and nose) are divided by a median groove, the philtrum. Labial granuloma (eosinophilic granuloma) is a chronic lesion of undetermined etiology that affects the lip of the cat, usually near the midline of the upper lip.

Additional salivary tissue (buccal glands) is present in the cheeks, especially at the angle of the mouth. The cheeks are primarily supported by the m. buccinator, which functions to discharge material in the oral vestibule back into the oral cavity proper.

The oral cavity is bounded dorsally by the hard palate, which is formed by processes of the incisive, maxillary, and palatine bones, covered by a tough mucous membrane. The hard palate is characterized by about seven palatine ridges, separated by transverse rows of highly cornified papillae. Cleft palate (palatoschisis) is occasionally seen as a congenital defect in newborn kittens.

Just caudal to the central incisor teeth is a small eminence, the incisive papilla, along side of which are the small openings of the right and left incisive ducts that lead to the nasal cavity and vomeronasal organ.

The sublingual caruncles, which contain the openings of the mandibular and major sublingual ducts, are located in the floor of the oral cavity, to either side the rostral end of the lingual frenulum.

Tongue
When the mouth is closed, the tongue occupies most of the space within the oral cavity. Although not used for food prehension, the highly mobile apex of the tongue functions in licking, grooming, and serves as a ladle to lap liquids into the floor of the oral cavity when drinking.

The dorsum of the tongue is characterized by highly cornified, caudally directed filiform papillae, which function as a stiff brush for grooming. The carpet of filiform papillae on the rostral two thirds of the dorsum of the tongue is dotted by the small, circular fungiform papillae. Fungiform papillae are concentrated near the edges of the tongue and have large taste buds associated with them.

General sensory innervation to the rostral two thirds of the tongue is via the lingual n. (from mandibular n. of cranial nerve V), while the taste buds associated with the fungiform papillae receive special sensory innervation from cranial nerve VII.

The body and root of the tongue are less mobile than the apical part. These parts function in bolus formation by pressing food against the hard palate, and in propelling the bolus through the pharynx during swallowing. At the junction of body and root, and arranged in a caudally pointed V pattern are four to six vallate papillae. Diffuse areas and solitary nodules of lymphoid tissue are present on the root of the tongue forming the lingual tonsil. General and special sensory innervation to the caudal third of the tongue is provided via the glossopharyngeal n. (cranial nerve IX).

The bulk of the tongue consists of intrinsic skeletal muscle bundles, mixed with connective and adipose tissue. The intrinsic muscles and several important extrinsic muscles (*e.g.*, genioglossus, styloglossus, and hyoglossus) are bilaterally symmetrical, and are divided by a thin septum. Each half of the tongue receives motor innervation via the hypoglossal n. (cranial nerve XII) of that side. The tongue is a richly vascular organ and will bleed profusely when lacerated. Cats subjected to heat stress can dissipate excessive body heat from the tongue by panting. The principal blood supply to each half of the tongue is via the lingual a. and v. While under general anesthesia, the lingual a. can be used to take the pulse.

Lacerations of the tongue, neoplasia, chemical and electrical burns, foreign-body penetration, and string foreign-body strangulation are some of the conditions affecting the mouth of the cat. Stomatitis and/or glossitis can also be manifestations of various systemic diseases including ulcerations related to feline rhinotracheitis virus and calicivirus infections, uremia, and immune system abnormalities.

Salivary Glands

In addition to the diffuse salivary tissue located within the walls of the oral cavity, the cat has several paired salivary glands. The consolidation of buccal glands at the angle of the mouth is sometimes described separately as the molar gland. As the name implies, the loosely encapsulated, V-shaped parotid gland cradles the base of the ear. Principal intraglandular ducts (radicles) unite near the ventral angle of the distinctly lobulated gland to form the parotid duct, which crosses the surface of the masseter muscle to reach the cheek. It then continues in the substance of the cheek to open on the parotid papilla, opposite upper P4.

Nestled in the angle between the maxillary and linguofacial vv. is the ovoid, well-encapsulated mandibular gland. The mandibular duct leaves the rostral aspect of the gland, passes between the mandible and lingual muscles, and continues along the floor of the oral cavity to reach the sublingual caruncle, upon which it opens. Closely associated with the mandibular duct, and applied to the rostral surface of the mandibular gland is the monostomatic sublingual gland, from which the major sublingual duct arises. This duct closely accompanies the mandibular duct to the sublingual caruncle. Although uncommon, ranulas and salivary mucoceles resulting from damage to the mandibular-sublingual duct system, do occasionally occur in the cat.

Scattered along the course of the major sublingual duct, in the floor of the oral cavity are many lobules of the polystomatic sublingual gland. As the name implies, numerous minor sublingual ducts arise from these lobules and empty directly into the sublingual recess of the oral cavity. The dorsal buccal glands of the cat are consolidated to form the distinct zygomatic salivary gland, which is located in the ventral part of the orbit. Its major duct opens about 3 mm caudal to upper M1 and several minor ducts open caudal to the major duct. Due to the alkaline nature of the feline mouth (pH 8-9) analgesics such as buprenorphine can be applied and absorbed transmucosally.

Pharynx

The pharynx represents an intersection between the digestive and respiratory systems. When viewed in sagittal section, it is a Y-shaped area, consisting of three parts. The nasopharynx, which lies dorsal to the soft palate, is part of the respiratory system (see Chapter 7 also). Ventral to the soft palate and continuous with the oral cavity is the oropharynx. When the tongue is drawn out of the mouth, the junction of the oral cavity and oropharynx is defined by the palatoglossal arches laterally. In the normal breathing position, the soft palate rests on the root of the tongue, and its caudal border lays rostroventral to the apex of the epiglottic cartilage. The soft palate contains diffuse salivary (palatine glands) and lymphoid tissue. The ovoid palatine tonsils are located in bilateral depressions (tonsilar fossae) in the dorsolateral walls of the oropharynx. When not inflamed, the tonsils are largely concealed by mucosal flaps (semilunar folds).

The oropharynx extends caudally to the base of the epiglottic cartilage, where it is continued by the laryngopharynx. This part of the pharynx continues the digestive tract dorsal to and lateral to each side of the laryngeal opening to join the esophagus at the level of the caudal border of the cricoid cartilage. The bilateral channels that pass around the larynx, which serve to carry liquid or semiliquid material, are called the piriform recesses.

When solid food is swallowed, it is directed dorsal to laryngeal opening into the caudal part of the laryngopharynx by the root of the tongue. As this occurs, the elastic epiglottic cartilage is folded back to cover the laryngeal opening. Except during swallowing, the laryngopharynx is closed by the pharyngeal constrictor muscles (mm. hyopharyngeus, thryopharyngeus, cricopharyngeus), which may be assisted in this function by engorgement of the pharyngeal venous plexus located in the wall of the laryngopharynx. During swallowing, the root of the tongue acts like a plunger to push the bolus quickly into the laryngopharynx. The pharyngeal constrictor muscles must relax to receive and capture the bolus, and then promptly contract in a cranial to caudal sequence to capture the bolus and propel it caudally into the esophagus. The junction of the laryngopharynx with the esophagus is subtly marked by an annular mucosal fold, the pharyngoesophageal limen, which forms a threshold at the origin of the esophagus.

Plate 8-1

Figure A   Location of major salivary glands, lateral view

Figure B   Location of teeth, lateral view, not all incisors and roots visible

Figure C   Tongue with location of various papillae, dorsal view. Inset: cornified filiform papillae

Figure D   Oral and pharyngeal regions associated with the digestive system, sagittal section, medial view

Figure E   Positive contrast esophagram, lateral view. Radiograph provided courtesy of Diagnostic Imaging (Radiology) Service, Veterinary Teaching Hospital, North Carolina State University College of Veterinary Medicine

1	Parotid salivary gland
1'	Its duct
2	Mandibular salivary gland
2'	Its duct
3	Sublingual salivary gland
3'	Its duct
4	M. masseter
5	M. digastricus
6	M. brachiocephalicus
7	M. parotidoauricularis
8	Superior incisor 2
9	Superior incisor 3
10	Superior canine
11	Superior premolar 2
12	Superior premolar 3
13	Superior premolar 4
14	Superior molar 1
15	Incisive bone
16	Maxilla
17	Inferior incisor 3
18	Inferior canine
19	Inferior premolar 3
20	Inferior premolar 4
21	Inferior molar 1
22	Mandible
23	Apex of tongue
24	Body of tongue
25	Root of tongue
26	Median sulcus
27	Filiform and fungiform papillae

28	Foliate papillae
29	Vallate papillae
30	Epiglottis
31	Hard palate
32	Soft palate
33	Nasal cavity
34	Palatoglossal arch
35	Oral cavity
36	Mandibular symphysis
37-39	Pharynx
37	Nasopharynx
38	Laryngopharynx
39	Oropharynx
40	Nasopharyngeal opening of auditory tube
41	Palatopharyngeal arch
42	Semilunar fold of palatine tonsil
43	Basihyoid bone
44	M. Geniohyoideus
45	M. Genioglossus
46	Esophagus
46'	Esophagus with "herringbone" pattern of mucosa
47	Trachea
48	Scapulae
49	T12 Vertebra
50	Stomach
51	Liver
52	Diaphragm
53	Heart
54	Sternum

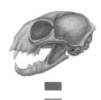

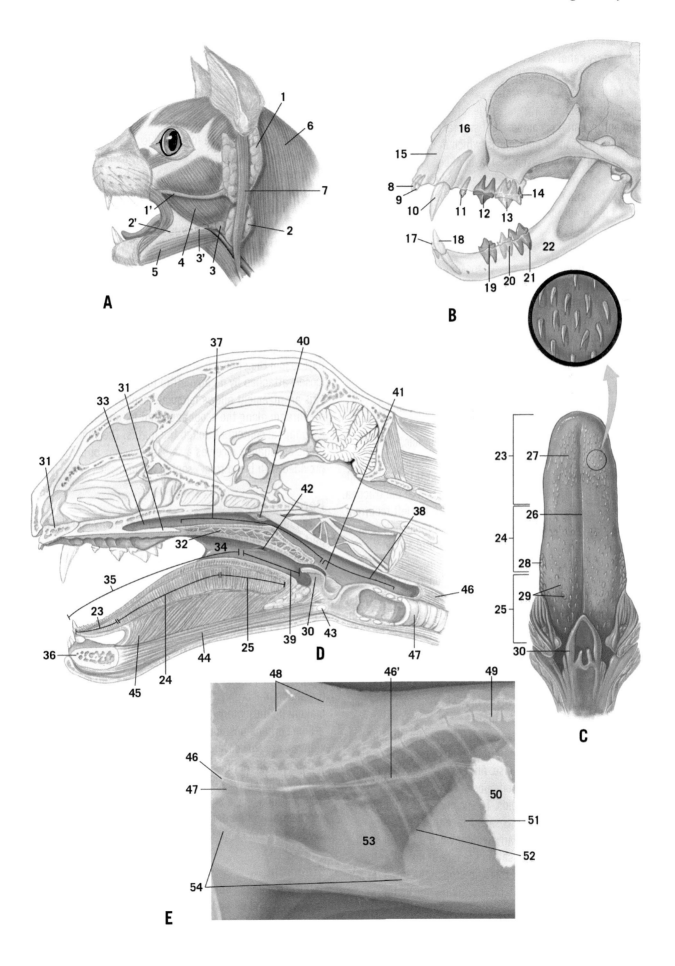

Alimentary Canal

The alimentary canal consists of a musculomembranous tube that extends from the laryngopharynx to the anus. The proximal to distal components of this digestive tube are the esophagus, stomach, small intestine, large intestine, and anal canal. The wall of the alimentary canal is composed of several layers: (1) mucosa; (2) submucosa; (3) tunica muscularis, which may be divided into several layers; and (4) an adventitial layer of connective tissue. Because the liver and pancreas discharge products into the alimentary canal and play a vital role in digestion, these organs are included in this discussion of the digestive system.

Esophagus

The esophagus begins at the pharyngoesophageal limen, dorsal to the caudal border of the cricoid cartilage, where it is surrounded by fibers of the m. cricopharyngeus. Except when distended by a bolus or other intraluminal body, the esophagus is closed and flattened. The mucosa, which contains no glands, is characterized by distinct longitudinal folds. Mucous glands are present in the submucosa only in the area of the pharyngoesophageal limen. Cranial to the base of the heart, the tunica muscularis consists of striated muscle, while caudal to the heart, this layer consists of smooth muscle.

The esophagus can be divided into cervical, thoracic, and abdominal parts. The cervical part begins dorsal to the trachea, but in the caudal part of the neck typically slides off to the left side of the trachea to enter the thoracic inlet. In addition to the trachea, the cervical esophagus is closely associated with the left recurrent laryngeal n., and left carotid sheath. This part of the esophagus receives blood from branches of the common carotid aa. and innervation through branches of the vagus nn. and sympathetic trunks. The cervical esophagus is normally flattened, with one surface against the trachea and other peripheral to it. The thoracic part of the esophagus inclines dorsally in the cranial mediastinum to return to its position dorsal to the trachea. It passes to the right side of the aortic arch, crosses the dorsal aspect of the tracheal bifurcation, and continues through the caudal mediastinum to the esophageal hiatus. Near the level of the heart it becomes associated with branches of the vagus nn., which accompany the esophagus through the esophageal hiatus.

Coinciding with the change from striated to smooth muscle in the muscular coat, there is an abrupt change in the mucosal pattern at the level of the heart base. Although the distinct longitudinal folds continue, there is superimposed on them, a pattern of distinct transverse mucosal folds. The combined longitudinal and transverse folds create a mucosal surface that resembles overlapping roof tiles. This is clearly evident when a barium paste esophagram is performed in the cat. In the lateral radiograph, the barium coating of the caudal thoracic esophagus takes on a characteristic "herringbone" pattern, resembling the vertebral column of a fish. It should be emphasized that this is the normal esophagram pattern for the cat, and should not be confused with an esophageal foreign-body. The principal blood supply to the caudal part of the esophagus is from branches of the bronchoesophageal aa. Because the thoracic esophagus is located between the two pleural sacs, this part receives an additional complete or partial serosal covering provided by the reflection of mediastinal pleura upon it.

Obstructive esophageal foreign bodies are uncommon in the cat, however, nonobstructive foreign objects such as sewing-needles, fish-hooks, and string are occasionally found in the esophagus. Obstruction of the esophagus near the base of the heart may result from abnormal development of the major vessels arising from the embryologic aortic arches, which can produce vascular rings that constrict the esophagus. The most common of these occurs when the definitive aortic arch arises from the right fourth embryonic arch instead of the left arch. Both congenital and acquired hypomotility of the esophagus (megaesophagus) has been reported in the cat. Congenital hypomotility may be hereditary and is most often seen in Siamese and Siamese-related breeds.

The esophagus passes through the right crus of the diaphragm at the esophageal hiatus and is continued as a short abdominal part to join the stomach at the cardia. The esophagus is only loosely attached by its adventitia to the borders of the hiatus. This arrangement allows for some respiratory excursion of the diaphragm along the esophagus and for unrestricted passage of esophageal contents through the hiatus. The short abdominal part of the esophagus receives a serosal covering of peritoneum and is provided with blood from esophageal branches of the left gastric a.

Peritoneum

The internal surface of the abdominal cavity and the cranial part of the pelvic cavity is lined by a serous membrane called peritoneum. This lining is continued from the wall of the cavities onto the surface of the digestive organs and some urogenital organs. The portion of peritoneum lining the abdominal and pelvic wall is referred to as parietal peritoneum; that lining the surface of appropriate organs is visceral peritoneum. Double layers of peritoneum extending (connecting) between parietal and visceral peritoneum can be referred to as mesentery, omentum, or ligaments. All blood vessels, lymphatics, and nerves supplying the abdominal organs travel between the two layers of peritoneum making up mesentery, omentum, and ligaments.

Some organs positioned against the body wall such as the kidneys, are only covered by peritoneum on one surface.

Because all peritoneal surfaces are ultimately continuous with each other, the peritoneum encloses a peritoneal cavity that contains only a small amount of serous fluid. Because the peritoneum and peritoneal cavity extends partly into the pelvic cavity, the term is not synonymous with abdominal cavity.

Stomach

The esophagus enters the stomach at the cardia (cardiac opening). When viewed in the ventrodorsal perspective, the stomach of the cat is distinctly J-shaped, consisting of a fundus, body, and pyloric region. This segment of the embryonic gut is enlarged and rotated so that its visceral surface is directed caudodorsally (against intestines), and its parietal surface faces cranioventrally (against liver). Differential embryonic growth results in two distinct curvatures. The greater curvature is directed primarily toward the left and caudoventrally, whereas the lesser curvature faces, for the most part, toward the right and craniodorsally. As the stomach fills, the greater curvature of the gastric body moves caudoventrally, whereas the lesser curvature remains relatively fixed in position.

As demonstrated in ventrodorsal (or dorsoventral) radiographs of upper gastrointestinal contrast studies, the moderately full stomach of the cat lies entirely within the left half of the abdominal cavity, with the pylorus located near the median plane. The fundus is the dome-like part of the stomach that projects dorsal to the cardia. The body comprises the major part of the organ from the level of the cardia to the angular notch of the lesser curvature. Distal to this notch, the pyloric antrum tapers to the narrower pyloric canal, which terminates at the pylorus.

The gastric wall consists of the mucosa, a well developed submucosal layer, a laminated tunica muscularis, which varies in thickness over different parts of the stomach, and a serosal covering of visceral peritoneum. At the cardia, there is an abrupt change in mucosal epithelium from the stratified squamous epithelium of the esophagus to the simple columnar epithelium of the more distal part of the alimentary canal. Thus the entire stomach of the cat is glandular, and the mucosal surface is characterized by the presence of gastric folds or rugae. These irregular folds are oriented predominantly in a longitudinal direction and are more prominent when the stomach is empty. As a protection from the gastric acid and enzymes, the mucosal surface is normally coated with a thin layer of mucus secreted by the epithelial cells.

The gastric mucosa contains many glands, which are concentrated by type in distinct regions of the stomach. The cardiac gland region, which contains seromucous glands, forms a narrow, annular zone immediately distal to the cardiac opening. Lining the fundus and most of the body is the thicker, darker mucosa of the region of the proper gastric glands. The tubular glands in this region contain the acid-producing parietal cells and the enzyme releasing chief cells. The entire pyloric region and a narrow strip along the lesser curvature, which extends proximally to the cardiac region, are covered by a lighter, thinner mucosa forming the pyloric gland region. This area contains branched mucous-producing glands. The mucosa rests on a loose submucosal layer of connective tissue, which adds tensile strength to the wall and allows the muscular coat to slide over the mucosa as the stomach contracts and relaxes.

The arrangement of the smooth muscle fibers forming the tunica muscularis follows the general GI pattern of outer longitudinal and inner circular layers, with the addition of an intervening third layer of internal oblique fibers over the fundus and greater curvature of the body. At the cardia, the internal oblique fibers thicken to form the cardiac loop, the limbs of which continue distally along the lesser curvature, forming the boundaries of the gastric groove. Although well defined along the curvatures, the outer longitudinal

fibers fan out obliquely across the parietal and visceral surfaces, forming the external oblique fibers. The inner circular layer of fibers, which is not present in the fundus, is best developed in the pyloric region, where it is markedly thickened at the pylorus to form the pyloric sphincter.

The serosa of the stomach is formed by visceral peritoneum, which closely invests and strengthens the tunica muscularis. Along the greater curvature, the visceral peritoneum reflects from the stomach as a two-ply fold of greater omentum (embryonic dorsal mesogastrium). The part of the greater omentum that attaches the stomach to the spleen forms the gastrosplenic ligament, while the most proximal part that attaches directly to the diaphragm forms the gastrophrenic ligament. Similarly, the visceral peritoneum reflects along the lesser curvature as a two-ply fold of lesser omentum (embryonic ventral mesogastrium), which attaches the stomach and proximal duodenum to the liver.

Blood supply to the stomach is via the three major branches of the celiac a. (see Chapter 4 also). The principal arteries of the stomach course along the greater and lesser curvatures and give off branches to the gastric wall at regular intervals. Venous blood from the stomach is collected by the gastroduodenal and splenic vv., which carry it to the hepatic portal v. for circulation through the liver.

Autonomic innervation of the stomach is via branches of the vagal trunks, and through sympathetic nerves from the celiac and cranial mesenteric plexi.

Acute gastritis is a common disease in the cat. Although in many cases the exact cause is never identified, trichobezoars (hairballs) are frequently incriminated in the cat, especially in long-haired breeds.

Intestines

Typical of the carnivore, the intestines of the cat are not highly modified and constitute a relatively simple tubular continuation of the alimentary canal from pylorus to anus. The intestines are divided into the small intestine, the large intestine, and the anal canal. The intestines are attached to the dorsal body wall by the mesentery. During embryologic development, the intestines rotated approximately 270° around a vertical axis in a counter-clockwise (when viewed from ventral) direction. As a result of this embryologic gut rotation, the mesentery was twisted around the cranial mesenteric artery forming the root of the mesentery, the colon was pulled across cranial to the mesenteric root, and the duodenum was pulled around caudal to the mesenteric root. The arteries, nerves, and lymphatics are distributed to the bowel between the two layers of connecting peritoneum that form the mesentery.

The intestinal wall consists of a mucosa, submucosa, tunica muscularis, and except for the terminal part of the rectum and anal canal, a serosa formed by visceral peritoneum. The intestinal mucosa is lined by simple columnar epithelial cells mixed with a variable population of mucus-producing goblet cells, which become more prevalent in the large bowel. Many transient folds of variable height are characteristic of the mucosal surface of the intestines. Intestinal glands are present in the mucosa throughout

Plate 8-2

Figure A   Stomach and proximal duodenum, omentum removed, sectioned to reveal lumen, ventral view

Figure B   Duodenum at entrance of bile and pancreatic ducts, dorsal view

Figure C   Schematic illustration of layers of intestine

Figure D   Schematic diagram of the relationship of peritoneum, peritoneal cavity, and some structures of the abdominal cavity through development.

1 Esophagus	21 Lymphatic nodules
2 Diaphragm	22-23 Tunica muscularis
3-11 Stomach	22 Inner circular layer
3 Gastric folds	23 Outer longitudinal layer
4 Lesser curvative	24 Jejunum
5 Greater curvature	25 Vertebra
6 Cardia	26 Abdominal body wall
7 Fundus	27 Parietal peritoneum
8 Body	28 Visceral peritoneum
9 Pyloric antrum	29 Peritoneal cavity
10 Pyloric canal	29' Omental bursa
11 Pyloric sphincter	30 Dorsal mesogastrium, becomes greater omentum
12 Descending duodenum	30' Superficial leaf, greater omentum
13 Pancreas	30" Deep leaf, greater omentum
14 Bile duct	31 Ventral mesogastrium, becomes lesser omentum and falciform ligament
15 Pancreatic duct	31' Lesser omentum
16 Major duodenal papilla	32 Spleen
17 Accessory pancreatic duct (inconstant)	33 Pancreas
18 Minor duodenal papilla (inconstant)	34 Stomach
19 Mucosa	35 Liver
20 Submucosa	

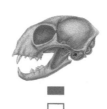

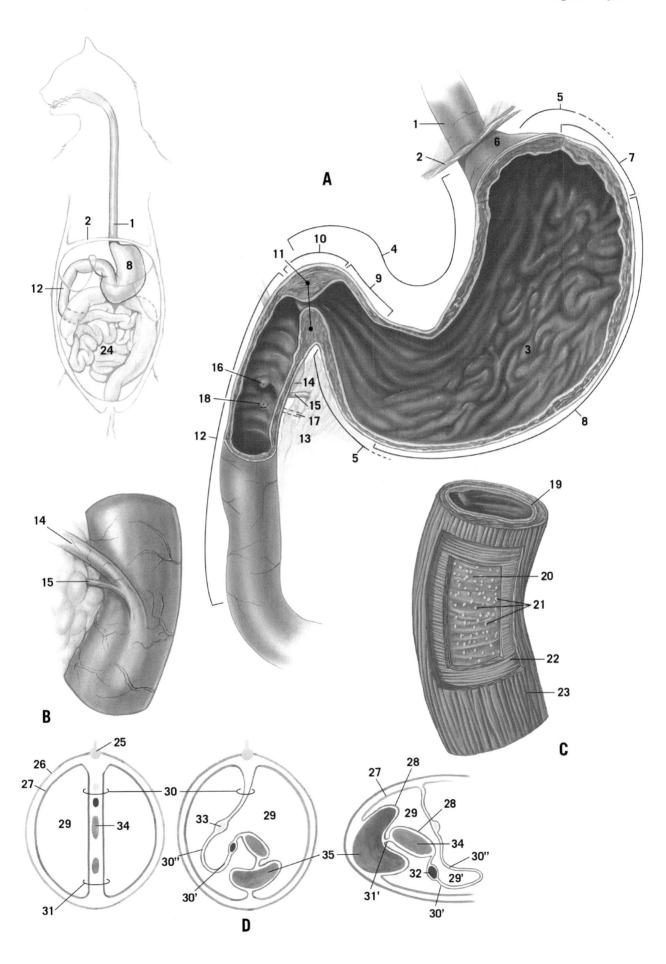

A

B

C

D

the intestines. In addition to solitary nodules, the cat has a few grossly evident patches of aggregated lymph nodules located in the bowel wall, mostly along the antimesenteric aspect of the small intestine. The submucosa, which contains nerves and a major vascular network, adds considerable tensile strength to the bowel wall and provides the principal holding layer when the gut is sutured. Also, because of its loose arrangement, the submucosa allows for the tunica muscularis to contract largely independent of the mucosa, thereby creating the transient mucosal folds and effecting the normal peristaltic movement of ingesta through the bowel. The tunica muscularis consists of a thin outer longitudinal layer and a thicker inner circular layer.

Small Intestine

The small intestine consists of the duodenum, jejunum, and ileum. It extends from the pylorus to the cecocolic junction and receives the product of gastric digestion (chyme) from the stomach.

In addition to transient folds, the mucosal surface of the small intestine is characterized by the presence of a carpet-like covering of intestinal villi, which greatly increase the absorptive surface area of the bowel.

Blood supply to the small intestine is by branches of the cranial mesenteric a. Venous return from the small intestine is collected primarily by the cranial mesenteric v., a major tributary of the hepatic portal v. (see Chapter 4). Lymph, which also serves in the transport of absorbed of fat (chyle) from the small intestine, passes through mesenteric lymph nodes, and subsequently through the visceral trunk to the cisterna chyli (see Chapter 5).

The most proximal small intestine forms the duodenum, which is relatively fixed in position by its short mesentery, the mesoduo-denum. From the pylorus, the short cranial part of the duodenum courses cranially, turns sharply to the right, and then turns caudally at the cranial duodenal flexure to be continued along the right side of the abdomen as the descending duodenum. The most proximal duodenum contains submucosal duodenal glands. Just distal to the cranial duodenal flexure, the bile duct and pancreatic duct obliquely penetrate the mesenteric border of the descending duodenum. From the point of initial penetration, the ducts continue distally within the wall for a short distance to reach the mucosal surface at the major duodenal papilla, upon which they open. The minor duodenal papilla is only present in those cats in which the accessory pancreatic duct persists, which has been reported to be approximately 20%. If present, the minor papilla is located about 2 cm distal to the major duodenal papilla, in the mesenteric wall of the duodenum.

The descending duodenum passes caudally to about the level of the 5th lumbar vertebra, where it turns to the left and then cranially at the caudal duodenal flexure, and is continued as the ascending duodenum. The ascending duodenum passes cranially to the duodenojejunal flexure, which marks the junction of these two parts of the small intestine. Near the root of the mesentery, and just distal to this flexure, the mesentery lengthens to form the mesojejunum. The jejunum is by far the longest part of the small intestine, and because of its relatively long mesentery, is free to move into whatever unoccupied space is available within the abdomen. Except in the pregnant queen, jejunal loops typically fill most of the middle part of the abdominal cavity, between stomach and liver cranially, and around the urinary bladder caudally. During middle to late gestation, the jejunum is displaced craniodorsally by the gravid uterus and is compressed into whatever space is made available by accommodation of the stretched abdominal walls.

The short, terminal portion of the small intestine is designated the ileum. The junction of jejunum and ileum is not marked by any gross or microscopic line of distinction. When the small intestine is pulled away from the cecum, however, the ileocecal fold will be stretched so that it can be traced to its attachment along the antimesenteric border of the small bowel. The point where the proximal edge of the ileocecal fold joins the small intestine can be considered as the junction of jejunum and ileum. Because the cecum of the cat is small, the ileocecal fold is short, and thus the ileum represents only the terminal few cm of small intestine. As the ileum approaches the cecum, it is directed cranially, where it passes medial to the cecum to join the large intestine at the cecocolic junction. The ileum projects into the lumen of the large bowel to empty on the ileal papilla.

The most common clinical manifestation of intestinal disease in the cat is diarrhea. Among the many causes of diarrhea are dietary problems, parasitism, and systemic disorders, especially infectious diseases. Enteric pathogens of cats include numerous viral, bacterial, mycotic, and rickettsial organisms. Intestinal parasites that affect the cat include helminths (ascarides, hookworms, tapeworms) and protozoa (coccidia, toxoplasma, giardia). Heavy infestations of ascarides most frequently affect young kittens, in which many adult worms may inhabit the small intestine. Large numbers of adult worms interfere with peristalsis and can result in stasis or even mechanical obstruction of the bowel.

Other forms of intestinal obstruction include those caused by foreign-body, intussusception, volvulus, incarceration of the bowel in a hernia, adhesions or stricture, intra-abdominal abscess or granuloma, and intestinal neoplasia. The most common intestinal neoplasms of the cat are lymphosarcoma and adenocarcinoma.

Large Intestine

The large intestine consists of the cecum, colon, rectum, and anal canal. Blood supply to the large intestine by via branches of the cranial mesenteric, caudal mesenteric, and internal pudendal aa. Except for that from the rectum, venous blood from the large intestine is collected primarily by the caudal mesenteric v., a tributary to the hepatic portal v., and lymphatic drainage passes through mesenteric lln. to reach the cisterna chyli.

The cecum of the cat is a short, comma shaped diverticulum that forms the most proximal division of the large bowel. Despite its small size, an unusually large accumulation of lymph nodules is found in the cecum of the cat. At the level of the ileal papilla, the cecum is continuous with the colon at the cecocolic junction.

The colon of the cat is relatively short. The initial part is directed cranially along the right side of the abdomen as the ascending colon, which, at about the level of the second lumbar vertebra, turns to the left at the right colic flexure. The transverse colon continues from right to left, immediately cranial to the root of the mesentery, and then turns caudally at the left colic flexure. The descending colon continues caudally along the left dorsal abdominal wall, and then curves medially to continue as the rectum at the pelvic inlet.

The rectum passes caudally through the dorsal part of the pelvic cavity to be continued by the anal canal. The cranial part of the rectum has a serosal covering of visceral peritoneum, and is attached to the dorsal wall of the pelvic cavity by the mesocolon; however, the rectum extends beyond the line of peritoneal reflection so that its more caudal part is retroperitoneal and does not have a serosal covering. The rectum is provided with autonomic inner- vation from nerves of the pelvic plexi, which are located alongside the peritoneal portion of the rectum and the hypogastric nn., which course caudally from the caudal mesenteric plexus. The outer longitudinal muscle layer of the rectum condenses dorsally to form a distinct band of fibers, the m. rectococcygeus, which continues dorsal to the anal canal and attaches to the ventral surface of the first few caudal vertebrae. When the cat raises its tail for defecation, the m. rectococcygeus tenses to provide a supportive stay for contraction of the rectum against the fecal material.

The anal canal is the short, terminal part of the alimentary canal that surrounds the anus, which is the caudal opening of the digestive system. In contrast to the rest of the large intestine, the anal canal is lined by stratified squamous epithelium, and the junction of the two types of epithelia is marked by the anorectal line. Even though distinct longitudinal folds or columns are poorly defined in the cat, the area immediately caudal to the anorectal line is referred to as the columnar zone. This zone ends at the junction of the intestinal mucosa and the skin of the anus, which forms the anocutaneous line (intermediate zone). The terminal part of the anal canal, which is lined by skin, is referred to as the cutaneous zone. Located bilaterally in the walls of the cutaneous zone are the two orifices of the paranal sinuses (anal sacs). The foul-smelling secretion that collects in these sinuses and is expelled from their orifices is produced by the glands of the paranal sinuses, which are located within the walls of the sacs (see Chapter 2).

The inner circular layer of the tunica muscularis of the anal canal is thickened to form the internal anal sphincter m. In addition, a striated muscle sphincter encircles the anal canal, forming the external anal sphincter m. innervated via the caudal rectal n.

The terminal part of the rectum and the anal canal are flanked bilaterally by the mm. levator ani and coccygeus. These paired striated muscles and their associated fascial connections form the pelvic diaphragm. This important diaphragm functions to close the pelvic cavity caudally around the alimentary canal, and thus prevent herniation of abdominal and pelvic viscera during the abdominal press of defecation.

Colitis, colonic neoplasia, and megacolon are uncommon diseases in the cat.

Plate 8-3

Figure A   Section of jejunum; Inset: schematic illustration of intestinal villi
Figure B   Junction of small and large intestine, ventral view
Figure C   Distal rectum and anal canal, dorsal view
Figure D   Anus with location of anal sac, caudal view

1	Jejunum	12	Transverse colon
2	Mucosa, submucosa, tunica muscu-laris, and visceral peritoneum	13	Descending colon
3	Jejunal a., v.	14	Rectum
4	Mesojejunum	15	Caudal reflection of peritoneum
5	Ileum	16	Anal canal
6	Ileal papilla	17	Anorectal line
7	Cecum	18	Columnar zone
8	Ascending colon	19	Cutaneous zone
9	Cecal In	20	Internal anal sphincter m.
10	Ileocecal fold	21	Paranal sinus (anal sac)
11	Ileocolic a., v.	**21'**	Its duct
		22	External anal sphincter m.

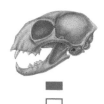

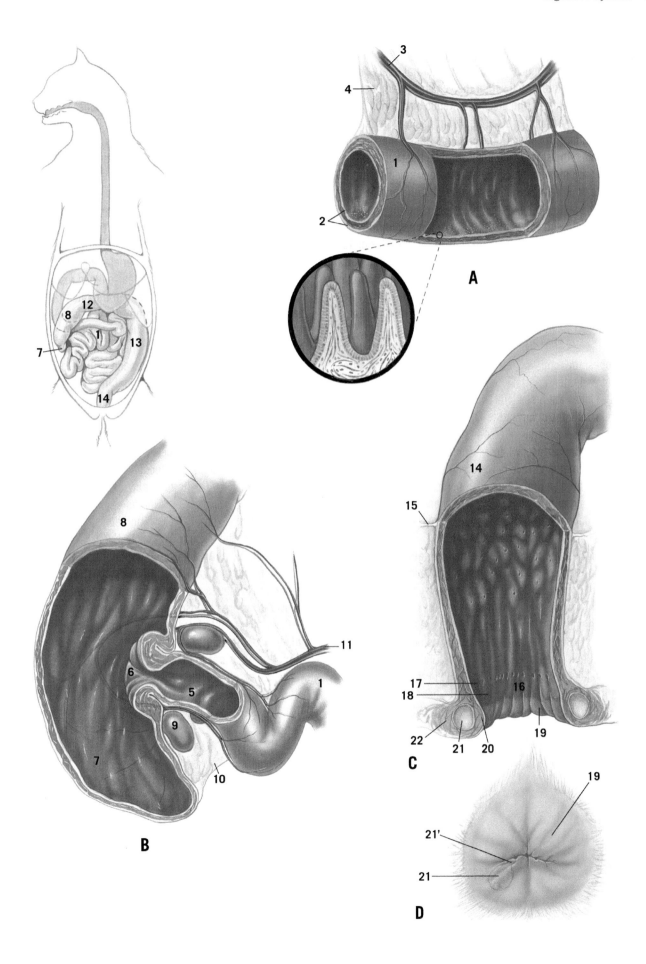

A

B

C

D

Liver and Gallbladder

The glandular tissue of the liver develops embryologically as an outgrowth of glandular mucosa from the primordial duodenum. Being strategically interposed within the venous system, between the gastrointestinal tract and general systemic circulation, the liver serves as a complex blood filter that has hundreds of metabolic functions. Its major duties include the synthesis of most plasma proteins, the storage of carbohydrates, the synthesis, degradation, and mobilization of lipids, the conversion of the end-products of protein catabolism to urea and uric acid, and the removal of waste products from the blood resulting from the breakdown of red blood cells. By extracting many harmful substances from the portal blood and converting these toxins to less harmful or innocuous compounds, the liver plays an important role in detoxification. A major function of the liver is the formation and elimination of bile, which serves to buffer the pH of the intestinal fluid, and aids in the emulsification and absorption of fats. During fetal life, the liver also functions in hematopoiesis.

The liver of the cat is divided into right, left, quadrate, and caudate lobes; the right and left lobes are subdivided by fissures into medial and lateral parts. Occasionally, the quadrate and right medial lobes are fused. The liver is located almost entirely within the intrathoracic part of the abdominal cavity. Because its convex surface is intimately related to the diaphragm, it is termed the diaphragmatic surface, while its concave visceral surface is related to the parietal surface of the stomach and other organs. The liver is oriented so that its rounded border is directed dorsally, and its sharp border projects caudolaterally and caudoventrally. The short abdominal part of the esophagus crosses the dorsal border of the liver at the esophageal notch.

The notch for the round ligament of the liver (embryonic umbilical vein) denotes the division between the left and quadrate lobes. The round ligament is located in the free edge of a peritoneal fold, the falciform ligament, which attaches the round ligament to the diaphragm. The thin falciform ligament of the cat (unlike that of the dog) does not serve as a major fat storage depot. The left medial lobe is much smaller than the left lateral lobe. The quadrate lobe lies ventral to the porta of the liver and between the round ligament and the gallbladder. The hepatic porta is the concentrated area on the visceral surface where the hepatic portal

v. and branches of the hepatic a. enter, and the bile duct leaves the organ. Dorsal to the hepatic porta is the caudate lobe, which has caudate and papillary processes. As the name implies, the caudate process projects caudally and is closely related to the right kidney. The cranial extremity of the kidney is caressed by the renal impression of the caudate process. Projecting into the lesser curvature of the stomach is the papillary process of the caudate lobe, which is concealed by the lesser omentum. The caudal vena cava is embedded in the dorsal border of the liver as it crosses the caudate lobe. Also embedded in the liver between the quadrate and right lobes is the gallbladder. The right medial lobe is larger than the right lateral lobe.

The gallbladder occupies a deep fossa within the liver, which allows it to be seen from both the parietal and visceral surfaces of the organ. The gallbladder is a pear-shaped reservoir for the accumulation and temporary storage of the bile that is produced by the liver. Occasionally, there may be complete or partial duplication of the gallbladder. From its ventrally located fundus and body, the gallbladder tapers to a neck, which joins the dorsally directed cystic duct. As the cystic duct approaches the hepatic porta, it is joined by hepatic ducts from individual liver lobes, some of which may have already joined to form a common hepatic duct. The united cystic and hepatic ducts form the bile duct, which passes within the hepatoduodenal ligament (part of lesser omentum) to the proximal part of the descending duodenum, opening on the major duodenal papilla (see duodenum).

In addition to the falciform ligament, the liver is closely attached to the diaphragm by the short coronary ligament, which encircles the area of the esophageal notch and embedded caudal vena cava. At each end of the coronary ligament, the peritoneal fold lengthens slightly so that, when the liver and diaphragm are separated, right and left triangular ligaments can be demonstrated. The falciform ligament also blends with the coronary ligament ventrally. Most of the liver is covered by visceral peritoneum; however, the coronary ligament divides into two limbs that circumscribe a small area nuda, where the liver is attached directly to the diaphragm. It is within this area that the hepatic vv. leave the parietal surface of the liver to enter the caudal vena cava. The functional blood supply of the liver enters via the hepatic portal v., while the nutritional supply is provided by branches of the hepatic a. (from the celiac a.). Blood from these two sources mixes within the sinusoidal blood capillaries of the liver, and is then collected by branches of the hepatic vv., which deliver it to the caudal vena cava.

Because of its dynamic role in hundreds of metabolic processes, the liver is subject to injury by a multitude of infectious, metabolic, and toxic diseases. Noninfectious, inflammatory hepatic diseases account for the majority of liver disorders diagnosed in clinical practice. Many of these are related to toxins or to drug-induced liver injury. Congenital portosystemic shunts, which allow portal blood to bypass the liver and enter systemic circulation directly, are seen occasionally in the cat and are often manifested clinically by neurologic signs. The liver is also a frequent site of both primary and metastatic neoplasms. In cases of diaphragmatic hernia, the liver is usually involved, particularly in peritoneopericardial hernia in the cat.

Pancreas

The pancreas develops embryologically as two buds from the duodenum, and, like the liver, the glandular tissue of the pancreas represents an extension of the glandular mucosa of the duodenum. Subsequent cellular differentiation results in the pancreas assuming both exocrine and endocrine functions. In terms of the digestive system, it is the exocrine function that is of primary interest. (For endocrine functions, see Chapter 6).

Pancreatic secretion (juice), which is excreted into the duodenum, contains sodium bicarbonate to neutralize the hydrochloric acid of gastric origin, and important enzymes, necessary for the digestion of carbohydrates, fats, and proteins. Acidification of the small intestinal contents caused by the lack of pancreatic bicarbonate can lead to serious impairment of small bowel function. In the absence of pancreatic enzymes, absorbable nutrients would not be available to the animal, resulting in malnutrition and starvation. Intestinal hormones (e.g., cholecystokinin-pancreozymin and secretin) play a major role in the regulation of pancreatic secretion.

The pancreas of the cat is a pale, lobulated organ, which consists of a body and right and left lobes. The body is that part of the pancreas nestled in the bend of the cranial part of the duodenum, and from which the two lobes diverge. The body and right lobe, located between the layers of the mesoduodenum, are closely associated with the duodenum. The right lobe extends caudally along the mesenteric border of the duodenum to the level of the caudal flexure. The thicker left lobe extends between the layers of the deep wall of the greater omentum, where it is related primarily to the stomach.

The dorsal pancreatic bud grows into the dorsal mesentery, whereas the ventral pancreatic bud develops in association with the liver in the ventral mesentery. The pancreatic tissue arising from the two buds grows together forming the body of the pancreas, and the initially separate duct systems coalesce with one another. If the connection of the dorsal pancreatic bud persists postnatally, it is designated the accessory pancreatic duct, and if that of the ventral bud, which is closely associated with the bile duct remains patent, it forms the pancreatic duct. As noted above, the pancreatic duct of the cat is constant, but the accessory pancreatic duct persists only about 20% of the time. If the latter degenerates prenatally, there is no need for a minor duodenal papilla, and none will be present.

The pancreas receives blood from branches of the celiac and cranial mesenteric aa. Venous blood from the pancreas is collected by several tributaries to the hepatic portal v. Parasympathetic nerves from the vagus n. stimulate increased secretion of the pancreatic enzymes, whereas sympathetic stimulation through branches of the celiac and cranial mesenteric plexi result in diminished secretory activity.

Pancreatic acinar cells contain packets of digestive enzymes known as zymogen granules. If the enzymes become activated within the pancreas, autodigestion occurs, causing severe inflammation of the gland. And, because of the close proximity of the pancreas to other organs (e.g., duodenum, liver, jejunum, stomach, and colon), pancreatitis can cause inflammation of these organs as well. Toxoplasmosis and feline infectious peritonitis are infectious diseases that involve the pancreas of the cat. Chronic pancreatitis in the cat is persistent, producing smoldering inflammation and vague signs of illness. When pancreatic acinar cell function is severely impaired, a syndrome of nutrient maldigestion and malnutrition ensues. Primary neoplasms that affect the feline pancreas include adenoma and adenocarcinoma.

Plate 8-4

Figure A   Liver and gallbladder, lesser omentum removed, caudal (visceral) view (left)
and cranial (parietal) view

Figure B   Pancreas, ventral view

Figure C   Gallbladder and bile duct, dorsal view

1	Left lateral lobe	13	Coronary lig
2	Left medial lobe	**13a**	Left triangular ligament
3	Quadrate lobe	**13b**	Right triangular ligament
4	Right medial lobe	14	Falciform lig
5	Right lateral lobe	15	Round lig of liver
6-8	Caudate lobe	16	Left (gastric) lobe of pancreas
6	Caudate process	17	Right (duodenal) lobe of pancreas
7	Renal impression	18	Body of pancreas
8	Papillary process	19	Exocrine duct system
9	Gall bladder	20	Pancreatic duct
10	Hepatic portal vein	21	Accessory pancreatic duct (inconstant)
11	Caudal vena cava	22	Bile duct
12	Hepatic vv.	23	Hepatic ducts
		24	Cystic duct

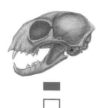

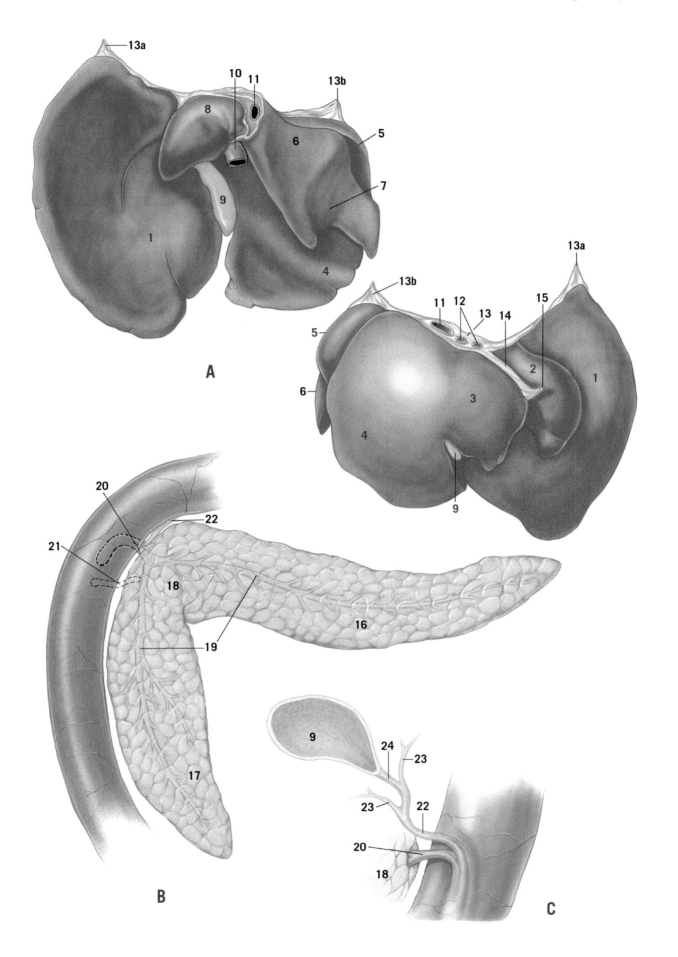

Selected References

1. Caney SMA, Gruffydd-Jones, TJ. In: Ettinger SJ, Feldman EC (Eds). *Textbook of Veterinary Internal Medicine: Diseases of the Dog and Cat.* 6th Ed. St. Louis, Mo., Elsevier Saunders, 2005;1448.

2. Center SA: In: Grant, GW, Strombeck, DR (Eds). Strombeck's Small Animal Gastroenterology, 3rd Ed. Philadelphia, WB Saunders Co, 1996, p 860.

3. Crouch JE. *Text-Atlas of Cat Anatomy.* Philadelphia, Lea & Febiger, 1969;143.

4. De Lahunta A, Habel RE. *Applied Veterinary Anatomy.* Philadelphia, WB Saunders, 1986:15.

5. Elzay RP, Hughes RD. Anodontia in a cat. *J Am Vet Med Assoc* 1969;154:667.

6. Hall EJ, German AJ. In: Ettinger SJ, Feldman EC. Eds. *Textbook of Veterinary Internal Medicine: Diseases of the Dog and Cat.* St. Louis, Mo., Elsevier Saunders, 2005;1332.

7. Jergens AE. In: Ettinger SJ, Feldman EC (Eds). *Textbook of Veterinary Internal Medicine: Diseases of the Dog and Cat.* 6th Ed. St. Louis, Mo., Elsevier Saunders, 2005;1298.

8. Mathews, KG, Bunch SK. In: Ettinger SJ, Feldman EC (Eds). *Textbook of Veterinary Internal Medicine: Diseases of the Dog and Cat.* 6th Ed. St. Louis, Mo., Elsevier Saunders 2005, 1453.

9. Nickel R, Schummer A, Seiferle E, Sack WO. *The Viscera of the Domestic Mammals.* 2nd revised Ed. New York, Springer-Verlag, 1979.

10. O'Brien TR. Radiographic Diagnosis of Abdominal Disorders in the Dog and Cat. Philadelphia, WB Saunders, 1978;211.

11. Schebitz H, Wilkens H. *Atlas of Radiographic Anatomy of the Cat.* Parey Verlag 2004.

12. Smallwood JE, Morris EL. Radiographic Aids, The Esophagram, Series 10 (Spring 1977). The Quaker Oats Company, Chicago, Illinois.

13. Smith, MM. In: Ettinger SJ, Feldman EC (Eds). *Textbook of Veterinary Internal Medicine: Diseases of the Dog and Cat.* 6th Ed. St. Louis, Mo., Elsevier Saunders 2005;1290.

14. Todoroff RJ, Pavletic MM. In: Holzworth J, ed. Diseases of the Cat. Philadelphia: W. B. Saunders, 1987;68.

15. Washabau RJ, Holt DE. In: Ettinger SJ, Feldman EC. Eds. *Textbook of Veterinary Internal Medicine: Diseases of the Dog and Cat.* St. Louis, Mo., Elsevier Saunders, 2005;1378.

16. Wilkinson GT. In: Wilkinson GT (Ed). *Diseases of the Cat and their Management.* Melbourne: Blackwell Scientific Publications. 1984;463.

17. Williams DA., Steiner JM. In: Ettinger SJ, Feldman EC. Eds. *Textbook of Veterinary Internal Medicine: Diseases of the Dog and Cat.* St. Louis, Mo., Elsevier Saunders, 2005;1489.

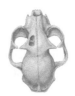

Chapter 9

The Urogenital System

Bonnie J. Smith

The urogenital system includes the organs that produce, transport, and store liquid waste, together with the female or male reproductive organs. These two systems are often considered as one unit because some parts, such as the vestibule in the female (queen) and the penis in the male (tom), are shared by both systems. This is a reflection of a common embryologic origin.

Urinary Organs

The urinary system includes the kidneys, ureters, urinary bladder, and urethra. The kidneys function in continuous filtration of the blood and production of urine (including the attendant electrolyte and pH balancing), while the ureters transport urine to the urinary bladder. The urinary bladder temporarily stores the urine, and at appropriate times expels it into the urethra, which transports it to the vestibule of the queen or the exterior of the tom.

Kidney and Ureter

The feline kidney is proportionately larger than that of the dog, and has the typical smooth "bean" shape usually associated with this organ. The kidney presents a cranial and caudal pole, a dorsal and ventral surface, a longer and convex lateral border, and a shorter and concave medial border. The medial border is indented at its midpoint as the hilus, an area often likened to the "eye" of a bean. The hilus is the area where vascular, nervous, and excretory structures enter or leave the kidney. Both kidneys lie with their dorsal surfaces largely flat against the dorsal abdominal wall just ventral to the transverse processes of the lumbar vertebrae. Feline kidneys are situated relatively farther caudally in the body cavity than in dogs. The right kidney typically extends from the first to the fourth lumbar vertebrae, while the left kidney typically extends from the second to the fifth lumbar vertebrae.

The kidneys are covered by peritoneum only on their ventral surfaces (see also Chapter 8). Thus, renal hemorrhage or rupture of the ureter may result in localized collection of fluid near the dorsal body wall rather than diffusion of the fluid among the abdominal organs. The attachments of the feline kidneys to the body wall are relatively loose, rendering the kidneys somewhat mobile and therefore relatively easy to palpate. The left kidney may be somewhat pendulous, rendering it particularly accessible to palpation. This feature results in its occasionally being mistaken for an abnormal mass. The loose attachments of the kidneys also render them fairly easy to grasp through the body wall and firmly immobilize in preparation for percutaneous renal biopsy.

The kidney is invested by a tough fibrous capsule. The feline renal capsule is characterized by a feature unique among domestic mammals: the readily visible capsular vv. Typically, three or four veins are present on the dorsal as well as ventral surfaces of the kidney. The tributaries of each vein begin near the convex lateral border, one each near the cranial pole, midpoint, and caudal pole. The fine tributaries of the veins form an arborizing pattern over the external surface of the capsule. The veins converged toward the

hilus, where they drain into the renal v. The presence of these large capsular vv. on the surface of the kidney places the cat at some increased risk of hemorrhage after percutaneous renal biopsy.

On sectioning, the capsule should peel readily from the surface of the organ; adhesions indicate renal pathology. When sectioned mid-sagittally, the hilus is associated with the renal sinus, which is a space containing fat, the initial branches of the renal a., the terminal tributaries of the renal v., the renal nn., and the renal pelvis (the expanded proximal end of the ureter). Several (approximately 4 or 5) extensions from the renal pelvis, termed pelvic recesses, extend laterally into the renal tissue. The pelvic recesses receive urine from the collecting tubules and transport it to the renal pelvis.

The sectioned kidney reveals the relatively thin outer layer of cortex. The fresh cortex appears faintly granular due to the plethora of glomeruli present in this region. In addition to the glomeruli and associated vessels, the renal cortex houses the renal capsules, proximal convoluted tubules, and distal convoluted tubules of the nephrons The deeper and thicker medulla demonstrates a darker outer layer (closer to the cortex), and a paler inner region (closest to the hilus). The medulla houses the nephric loops (of Henle) and collecting ducts of the nephrons. When sectioned longitudinally, the fresh medulla presents a faintly striated appearance, owing to the presence of the myriad elongate, hairpin nephric loops and collecting ducts. Near the hilus, the subdivision of the medulla into pyramidal subdivisions (renal pyramids) becomes evident. The pyramids converge into the renal papillae, which drain into the renal pelvis. On the median plane, the renal papillae fuse to form a renal crest that projects into the renal pelvis. The paler medullary region nearest the hilus forms a ridge, the renal crest, which projects into the renal pelvis.

The renal aa. are large, reflecting the fact that together the kidneys receive 25 percent of the cardiac output. The renal a. branches on entering the hilus and quickly divides again to form the interlobar aa. The interlobar aa. ascend toward the cortex, traveling between the renal pyramids. At the corticomedullary junction, the arcuate aa. branch from the interlobar arteries at approximately a right angle and arch over the surface of the renal pyramid. Small interlobular aa. ascend from the arcuate aa. into the substance of the cortex and give rise to the afferent arterioles of the glomeruli. The fate of the efferent arterioles leaving the glomerular capillary tuft depends on the level of the parent glomerulus within the cortex. Efferent arterioles from more superficial and mid-cortical glomeruli divide into the peritubular capillary network, the complex net of capillaries surrounding the cortical labyrinth of the convoluted tubules. Efferent arterioles of the deeper cortex near the corticomedullary junction descend into the medulla as the hairpin curves of the vasa recta, which run parallel to the nephric loops. Additional blood supply to the medulla arrives through some vasa recta arising directly from the arcuate aa.

The ureters are muscular tubes conducting urine from the kidney to the urinary bladder via peristaltic contractions. Each ureter leaves the kidney at the hilus and courses retroperitoneally along the dorsal body wall toward the urinary bladder. On nearing the urinary bladder, each ureter inclines slightly ventrally to access the rounded upper part of the bladder. The ureters enter the dorsal surface of the bladder at an oblique angle, tunneling through the muscular bladder wall a short distance before entering the lumen. This slanted entrance into the bladder results in pressure being put along the length of the ureter within the bladder wall as the filling bladder stretches, assisting in prevention of reflux of urine from the bladder into the ureter and potentially the kidney.

The Urinary Bladder

The location of the urinary bladder varies with its degree of distension. The full bladder extends over the brim of the pelvis and lies on the ventral abdominal wall as far cranially as the umbilicus, with only the omental apron between it and the parietal peritoneum. When empty, the bladder contracts greatly and lies much farther caudally, near the pelvis. The feline bladder, however, never recedes as far caudally as does the bladder in other domestic species, and always lies at least partially within the abdomen. This abdominal positioning facilitates cystocentesis (i.e., collection of urine performed by inserting a needle directly through the abdominal wall and into the bladder). The abdominal positioning also results in most of the bladder being covered by peritoneum.

The apex of the bladder is its relatively rounded cranial end. During fetal life, the apex communicates with the allantoic cavity by means of a connection termed the urachus. Occasionally remnants of the urachus persist into postnatal life, forming a diverticulum at the apex of the bladder. Because the wall of this urachal diverticulum is not well muscled and may not empty properly, the blind pocket may form a site for recurrent bacterial infections, and may require surgical correction. The apex of the bladder is continued by the body, which is the largest and most distensible part of the organ. Caudally, the body narrows to the neck, which funnels into the proximal (preprostatic) portion of the urethra. The neck of the feline bladder is notably longer and narrower than in other species, and the distinction between the end of the neck and the beginning of the urethra is sometimes described as difficult to discern. The ureters typically enter near the neck of the bladder. The entrance of the ureters and the exit of the urethra together define a triangular area at the caudal aspect of the bladder termed the vesicular trigone.

The arrangement of the bladder's smooth muscle fibers in the region of the neck is such that, as the bladder fills and expands, the muscle fibers in the neck constrict the neck of the bladder and occlude the outflow tract. As the bladder contracts, the orientation of these fibers changes so that the neck relaxes and urine can flow into the urethra. Muscle in this area is sometimes referred to as the "internal urethral sphincter."

The urethra leaves the bladder at the neck and courses caudally along the midline. The intrapelvic portion of the urethra is surrounded by the thick urethralis muscle. At the level of the pubis, a narrow band of skeletal muscle surrounds the urethra as the voluntarily controlled ("external") urethral sphincter. The female urethra is short, straight, and relatively wide, and passes directly to the vestibule. The (external) urethral sphincter surrounds approximately the midpoint of the short female urethra. The male urethra follows a long, curving course that begins with the pelvic portion within the pelvic cavity. This portion of the urethra overlies the pelvic symphysis and extends as far as the pelvic outlet. The ("external") urethral sphincter of males is located in this area. The luminal diameter of the pelvic urethra is much wider than in the later parts, a factor important in considering the most likely site for urethral obstruction by urinary crystals or stones. At the pelvic outlet, the male urethra narrows significantly, leaves the pelvic cavity, and enters into the base of the penis as the penile urethra. The penile urethra courses through the full length of the organ and opens to the exterior on the distal tip of the penile glans at an opening termed the urinary meatus. The length, curve, and narrowness of the male urethra render urinary catheterization of toms much more difficult than in queens. The procedure is further complicated by the difficulty of prolapsing the small, short, conical penis from the prepuce and retaining it in an externalized position without compressing the narrow penile urethra.

Young adult cats of both sexes are prone to feline urologic syndrome (FUS), a disease characterized by dysuria (painful or difficult urination) with or without hematuria (blood in the urine). However, the incidence has decreased significantly over the last 2 decades with advances in feline nutrition. Partial or complete obstruction of the urethra by urinary crystals or sediments may occur, and is far more common in toms than queens due to the length and narrowness of the penile urethra. Castrated males may be more frequently affected than intact males, although disagreement exists on this matter. Excessive grooming of the perineal region is also frequently noted. Affected cats of both sexes make frequent attempts at urination accompanied by straining and/or signs of discomfort or pain (stranguria). Obstructed cats develop signs of uremia and progressive distension of the urinary bladder. Catheterization of such patients is requisite, despite the difficulties involved.

Perineal urethrostomy may be indicated in toms with severe, recurrent episodes of FUS accompanied by urethral obstruction. In this procedure, castration is first performed if the cat is intact. Subsequently, the majority of the penis is removed. The urethra is opened just distal to the bulbourethral glands at the level of the ischial arch, which is the region where the wider pelvic urethra begins to narrow down to the narrow penile urethra. The urethra is sutured to the skin of the perineal area, thus creating a short, straight, relatively wide urethra essential similar to that of the queen that is much less vulnerable to obstruction.

Plate 9-1

Figure A   Urinary organs with digestive organs removed and urinary bladder opened, ventral view

Figure B   Schematic illustration of a nephron and associated vessels

Figure C   Kidney, transverse, median and sagittal sections

1	Diaphragm
2	Caudal vena cava
3	Abdominal aorta
4	Adrenal gland
5	Kidney with capsular veins
6	Renal a, v
7	Ureter
8	M. transversus abdominis
9	M. psoas major
10	Testicular a, v
11	Ductus deferens
12	Orifice of ureter
13	Vesicular trigone
14-18	Nephron
14	Glomerular (bowman's) capsule
15	Proximal convoluted tubule
16	Descending part of nephric loop (loop of henle)

17	Ascending part of nephric loop (loop of henle)
18	Distal convoluted tubule
19	Collecting duct
20	Afferent arteriole
21	Glomerulus
22	Efferent arteriole
23	Peritubular network
24	Vasa recta
25	Renal capsule
26	Renal cortex
27	Renal medulla
28	Renal crest
29	Renal pyramid
30	Interlobar a, v
31	Arcuate vessels
32	Renal pelvis
33	Renal sinus

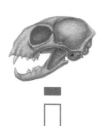

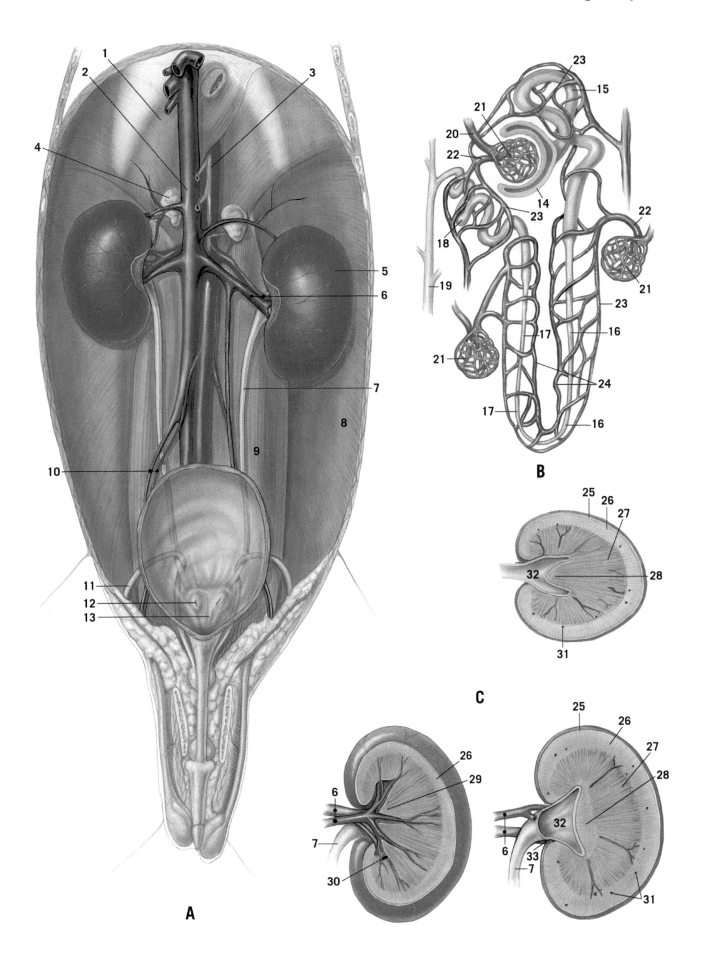

A

B

C

Plate 9-2

Figure A   Urinary bladder showing distended and contracted positions in relation to the pelvis, ventral view, as drawn from contrast radiograph

Figure B   Urinary organs drawn from excretory urogram, lateral view

Figure C   Junction of ureter and urinary bladder, sagittal section

Figure D   Schematic illustration of male urinary organs; inset: enlargement of penile urethra with urinary calculi

  1   Urinary bladder
  2   Neck of bladder
  3   Kidney
  4   Ureter
  5   Urethra
     5'   Penile urethra
  6   Ureterovesicular junction
  7   Penis
  8   Urinary calculi in urethral lumen
  9   Ductus deferens
10   Testis, covered by visceral vaginal tunic

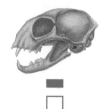

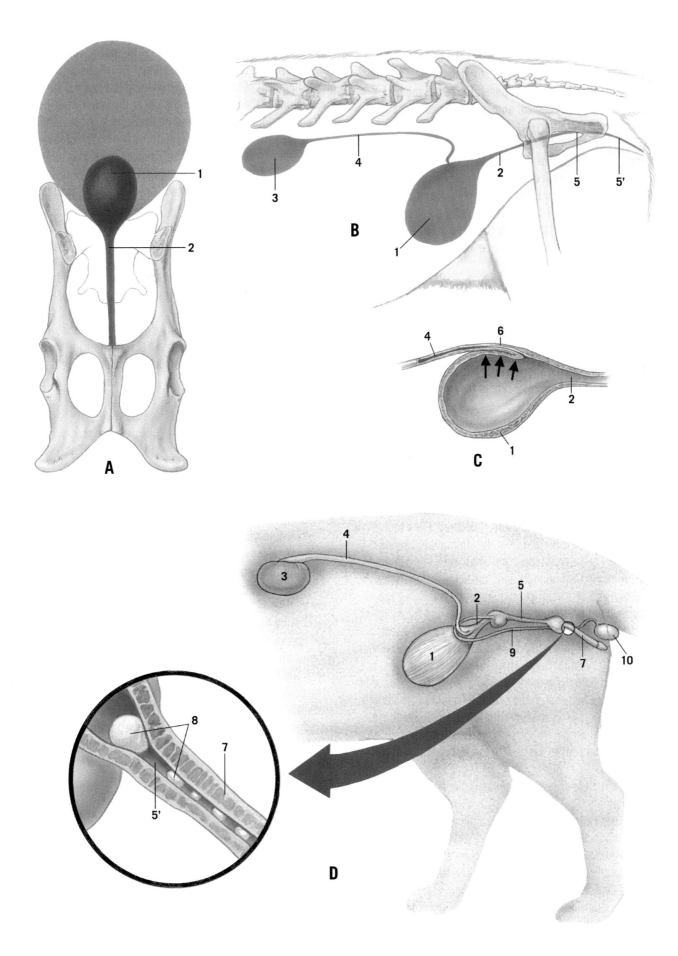

Male Genital Organs

The male genital organs of the cat include the testes, epididymis, ductus deferens, accessory sex glands (prostate and bulbourethral glands), urethra, and penis. The testes produce sperm (the cellular part of semen) and sex hormones (see also Chapter 6). Some maturation of sperm takes place within the testes, and further maturation as well as transport of the sperm takes place in the epididymis. At ejaculation, the terminal part of the epididymis expels the sperm into the ductus deferens, which carries sperm to the pelvic urethra. At that point, most of the fluid portion of the semen is added to the ejaculate by the prostate and bulbourethral glands. The urethra (both the pelvic and penile portions) transports the semen to the exterior.

Scrotum, Testes, Epididymis, and Ductus Deferens

The testes are contained within a cutaneous pouch termed the scrotum. Several aspects of the feline scrotum are unusual among domestic mammals. The feline scrotum is not pendulous, but lies high on the caudal surface of the thighs, just ventral to the anus. Among domestic mammals, only the boar has a similar placement of the scrotum. Further, the scrotal skin of the tom is densely covered with fine hair.

The wall of the scrotum consists of skin, smooth muscle (tunica dartos) and the external spermatic fascia. The internal cavity of the scrotum is divided into two separate compartments, right and left. The actual contents of each scrotal compartment that can be relatively easily separated from it are the m. cremaster, the spermatic cord, the vaginal tunics, the epididymis, and the testis. The m. cremaster is rather poorly developed in the tom, but as in other species is derived from the internal abdominal oblique muscle. The vaginal tunics, an evagination of peritoneum into the scrotum via the inguinal canal, are serous membranes that are recognized as a more external parietal layer lining the internal surface of the internal spermatic fascia, and the more internal visceral layer covering the external surface of the testis. The potential space between the parietal and visceral vaginal tunic is the cavity of the vaginal tunic, which normally contains a small amount of serous fluid. As with all serous cavities, the presence of the potential space and associated serous fluid allows for smooth movement of the organs associated with the space. In this case, the serous layers allow the testes to be moved slightly further away from or closer to the body to assist with thermoregulation of the organ.

The overall structure of the feline testis is similar to that of most domestic mammals. The testis is generally oblong and is covered by a thick fibrous capsule, the tunica albuginea. The feline testes are oriented obliquely within the scrotum.

The epididymis is a lengthy tubular structure situated mainly along the dorsolateral surface of the testis. The length of the tube is belied by its external appearance, since it is extremely tortuous and actually much longer than the size of the organ as grossly visible to the eye. The epididymis consists of a head, which receives the efferent ductules at the cranial end of the testis;

a body, which lies along the dorsolateral surface of the testis; and a tail that lies at the caudal end of the testis. The tail of the epididymis is anchored to the caudal end of the testis by the proper ligament of the testis, as well as to the internal surface of the scrotum by the ligament of the tail of the epididymis. Like the testis, the epididymis is oriented obliquely within the scrotum, so that the head of the adjacent epididymis is directed cranioventrally and the epididymal tail is directed caudodorsally. This orientation may be remembered by considering that the epididymis lies "tail to tail," with the tail of the epididymis oriented toward the tail of the tom.

The ductus deferens is a muscular tube that delivers sperm to the pelvic urethra. The ductus deferens leaves the tail of the epididymis, and is at first quite sinuous as it courses cranially along the epididymal border. The ductus deferens straightens once it passes the cranial edge of the testis, at which point it enters into the spermatic cord.

The spermatic cord is the rope-like collection of structures passing one way or another between the scrotum and the abdominal cavity via the inguinal canal. Accompanying the ductus deferens within the cord is the tiny artery of the ductus deferens, testicular vessels, lymphatics, and nerves. The testicular artery and artery of the ductus deferens travel out of the abdomen toward the testis, while the testicular vein, lymphatics, and sensory nerves travel into the abdomen from the scrotum. The testicular artery is notably coiled along its course within the spermatic cord, and the testicular vein forms a thick network of veins termed the pampiniform plexus, which is woven around the testicular artery. This arrangement serves to somewhat reduce the temperature of the blood arriving at the testis, since heat tends to move from the warmer arterial blood into the cooler venous blood within the pampiniform plexus. This effect is of course advantageous to the testis, which requires a temperature lower than core body temperature in order to successfully produce viable sperm. Conversely, by accepting heat from the arterial blood, the cooler venous blood leaving the testis is warmed slightly before it returns to the systemic circulation, reducing the need to expend metabolic energy to re-warm that blood to core body temperature.

The contents of the spermatic cord are invested with serous membranes continuous with the visceral vaginal tunic surrounding the testis. The mesoductus deferens is a separate fold surrounding only the ductus deferens; the remainder of the contents of the spermatic cord is enclosed collectively by a fold termed the mesorchium.

On reaching the interior of the abdominal cavity, the ductus deferens turns caudally toward the pelvis, loops around the ureter near the bladder, passes through the substance of the prostate gland, and enters the dorsal part of the pelvic urethra on a small eminence termed the colliculus seminalis.

Accessory Genital Glands

The tom possesses two accessory genital glands, the prostate and bulbourethral glands. In the definitive form, the prostate gland appears to be a single gland, and is intimately associated with the urethra just caudal to the neck of the urinary bladder. The bilobed, rounded prostate gland covers the dorsal and lateral surfaces of the urethra. The small, paired bulbourethral glands lie at the caudal end of the pelvic urethra on its dorsal surface, at the level of the ischial arch. Visualization of these glands is rendered a bit difficult due to their being covered by the bulbospongiosus muscle (see below). The location of the bulbourethral glands can offer an important mark during perineal urethrostomy by marking the terminal end of the pelvic urethra and the site at which to suture the urethral mucosa to the skin. However, they are less useful as a landmark in castrated male since they atrophy in the absence of the tropic influence of testosterone.

Penis

The overall structure of the feline penis is similar to that of most domestic mammals. Given the overall size of the species, the portions are all present in miniature.

The penis is composed of three erectile (or cavernous) tissue bodies. That termed the corpus cavernosum penis (CCP) originates as the paired crura, which arise from the ischial arches. The CCP is invested throughout its length by a thick, white, extremely tough connective tissue layer termed the tunica albuguinea. (Note should be made that, though each testis is invested by a similar connective tissue layer also termed "tunica albuguinea," these respective connective tissue regions are each entirely separate from each other.) Each crus passes at first a bit ventrally and then caudally and medially to join its fellow on the midline. The fused region of CCP continues cranially within the penis in a position ventral to the urethra, which runs along its ventral surface in a shallow groove. From the point of origin of each crus to the point where each fuses on the midline with its fellow, each crus is covered by skeletal muscle termed the ischiocavernosus mm. Once the two crura fuse, the muscular cover is lost but the tunica albuguinea is retained. In carnivores, the erectile tissue of the CCP within the glans ossifies, and takes the form of a bone termed the os penis. In the tom, the os penis is approximately five millimeters long. The os penis possesses a small groove on its dorsal surface in which the urethra runs, thus demonstrating its derivation from the CCP.

A second erectile tissue body, the corpus spongiosum penis (CSP), originates as the bulb of the penis. The penile bulb lies at the level of the ischial arch, on the midline between the converging crura. The bulb of the penis is covered by its own layer of skeletal muscle, the bulbospongiosus. Just past the ischial arch, the CSP decreases abruptly and greatly in size, and the covering of the bulbospongiosus muscle ends. At this point, the CSP is reduced to a very narrow sleeve of tissue immediately surrounding the urethra and extending to its opening at the urinary meatus.

The third erectile tissue body is termed the corpus spongiosum glandis (CSG – not to be confused with the very similar-sounding CSP). The CSG is confined to the most distal region of the penis, the glans. The glans surrounds the os penis and urethra.

Based upon the location and characteristics of the three erectile tissue bodies, the penis may be divided into three regions. The root of the penis is the most proximal region, where the crura are separate from each other and the penile bulb lies between them. The body of the penis is the portion where the two crura have fused, and the urethra runs ventral to them surrounded by the narrow casing of CSP. The free part generally corresponds to the glans, where the CSG is elaborated into the most superficial layer of erectile tissue.

As with other portions of the male genital system, the feline penis has certain unique characteristics. The penis is quite short compared to all other domestic mammals, and retains its embryological orientation. Thus, the body and glans of the penis are directed caudally rather than cranially, and the preputial opening points directly caudally from a position ventral to the scrotum. As a result, the tom assumes the same posture as the queen to urinate, and squats to void urine. Also, the feline glans penis is relatively thin and indistinct, present as a conical region of erectile tissue surrounding the distal end of the penis. Though not possessing large amounts of erectile tissue, the glans of adult intact males possesses striking distinctive surface structures: numerous rows of projecting, proximally-directed, keratinized spines. After copulation, these spines strongly scrape the vaginal wall of the queen, an effect necessary to induce ovulation in this species. The penile spines regress almost completely after castration.

Despite the peculiar orientation of the feline penis, copulation in cats is essentially similar to that in other quadrupeds. As the erection develops, the penis changes its orientation and projects cranially between the tom's thighs, achieving a position similar to that of most quadrupeds, and the tom mounts the queen in the fashion characteristic of other domestic mammals.

Due to the caudal direction of the tom's non-erect penis, determination of the sex of kittens is rather difficult compared with sexing the offspring of other domestic mammals. Since penis as well as the scrotum is positioned high on the caudal surface of the things, one cannot simply observe the ventral belly wall for the presence of the prepuce and penis. Consequently, the perineal region must be examined for the relative separation of the anus and the preputial or vulvar opening - the anogenital distance. In male kittens, the anogenital distance is greater, since the scrotum will eventually enlarge significantly in size in the space between the anus and preputial orifice. In female kittens, the distance is much shorter. Nonetheless, sexing a single kitten can still be a challenge. Until one is very familiar with this characteristic, sexing is most easily performed when one has the entire litter in hand to facilitate comparison among individuals.

The cat is one of the simplest species in which to perform castration. Initially, the sex of the animal should be carefully confirmed (see immediately above). Due to the singular position of the tom's genitals, pet owners may have difficulty determining the gender of their pet. Presentation of young queens for castration or young toms for ovariohysterectomy is far from unheard of. To be assured that the cat is male, the presence of descended testes within the scrotum should be confirmed.

After the cat is anesthetized (often using short-acting injectable anesthetic, due to the ease and quickness of the typical procedure), the scrotum is plucked free of hair or closely shaved, and appropriately cleaned. One testis is grasped through the scrotal skin so that the skin is drawn tense. With the testis immobilized, a long incision, from the dorsal edge of the scrotum to the ventral edge, is made through the skin. The parietal vaginal tunic may or may not be incised. The testis is exteriorized from the scrotum, with or without its overlying tunic. Several approaches to ligation of the spermatic cord may be employed. In the simplest form, the testis is removed from its tunic as well as the scrotum, and a length of the spermatic cord also exteriorized. The spermatic cord is carefully crushed (but not divided) with hemostats to promote clotting and hemostasis, the testis removed, and the spermatic cord simply knotted on itself (an admittedly more risky technique). Alternately, following careful crushing of the cord and removal of the testis, the ductus deferens can be separated from the remainder of the contents of the spermatic cord (a procedure facilitated by the separate investiture of these two sets of structure

by separate serous layers), and the two resulting portions square-knotted on each other. The most meticulous approach is to carefully crush the cord, remove the testis, and place a ligature in the crushed region. In all methods, the stump of the cord is examined carefully for bleeding, and if none is observed, allowed to retract into the scrotum. The entire procedure is then repeated on the other side. The scrotum is not closed, but the edges of each incision are separated from each other a final time to reduce fibrin adhesions and promote good drainage. Antibiotic therapy is unnecessary.

Cryptorchidism and monorchidism are fairly common in the cat. Retained testes are most frequently located near the inguinal canal. Occasionally they may be located higher in the body cavity, anywhere from the deep inguinal ring to as far cranially as the caudal pole of the kidneys, the level of their embryological origin. Thus, removal of such retained testes requires a different and more complex approach and anesthesia, since the procedure has at least the possibility of progressing to surgery within the abdominal cavity.

When performed before sexual maturity, castration has the added benefit of greatly reducing or possibly eliminating the aggressive and territorial behavior of males, reducing or avoiding numerous problems such as bite wounds, bite abscesses, territorial marking (scratching and "spraying") and so forth. Even intact males several years old often lose a noticeable amount of their undesirable "tom" behavior after castration. However, clients should be advised that, even in pre-pubescent toms, castration will not guarantee absence of such behaviors.

Urine spraying is a behavior problem most common in male cats, usually but not always intact toms. This "problem" is actually a normal behavior pattern associated with territorial marking. The behavior becomes a problem when the tom performs it in an area unsatisfactory to his owners, usually inside the home on furniture, walls, door frames, and so forth. The urine has a particularly objectionable smell. Sprayed objects are extremely difficult to successfully clean, and sometimes must be discarded. When spraying, the tom (or, rarely, queen) voids from a characteristic posture. Rather than squatting as when simply urinating, the cat stands with its rear directed at the object to be marked and the tail erect and sometimes slightly "fluffed". The ears are frequently directed caudally. The cat voids a small amount of urine directly caudally (recall the unique orientation of the feline penis) while vibrating the tail quickly. When finished (and again in contrast to a normal urination), no attempt is made to cover the urine.

Because urine spraying is a behavioral problem associated with territorial activity, neutering of the cat before sexual maturity greatly reduces but does not necessarily eliminate the problem. Castration of intact toms displaying this activity may eliminate the problem, or at least reduce its frequency.

Plate 9-3

Figure A   Male genital system with some muscles and prepuce removed, dorsal view
Figure B   Penis, dorsal view
Figure C   Glans penis in castrated and intact male, dorsal view
Figure D   Structures common to male genital and urinary systems with urethra opened ventrally, ventral view
Figure E   Junction of male genital and urinary systems, median section
Figure F   Left testis, lateral view and sagittal section

1	Urinary bladder	18	Corpus spongiosum penis
2	Ureter	19	Corpus cavernosum penis
3	Neck of bladder	20	Tunica albuginea penis
4	Testis within vaginal tunics and spermatic fascia	21	Corpus spongiosum glandis
		22	Os penis
	4' Testis within visceral vaginal tunic	23	Penile spines
	4" Testis	24	Exrenal urethral orifice
5	M. cremaster	25	Colliculus seminalis
6	Spermatic cord	26	Urethral crest
7	Inguinal canal	27	Crus of penis
8	Testicular a, v	28-30	Epididymis
9	Ductus deferens		28 Head
10	Prostate gland		29 Body
11	Urethra		30 Tail
12	Bulbourethral gland	31	Efferent ductules
13	M. ischiocarvernosus (covering crus of penis)	32	Rete testis
		33	Mediastinum testis
14	M. bulbospongiosus (cut in A and lower B)	34	Seminiferous tubules
15	M. retractor penis (cut in A and lower B)	35	Tunica albuginea testis (covered by layer of visceral vaginal tunic)
16	Body of penis	36	Proper ligament of the testis
17	Glans penis	37	Spermatic fascia (lined by layer of parietal vaginal tunic)
		38	Pampiniform plexus

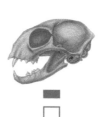

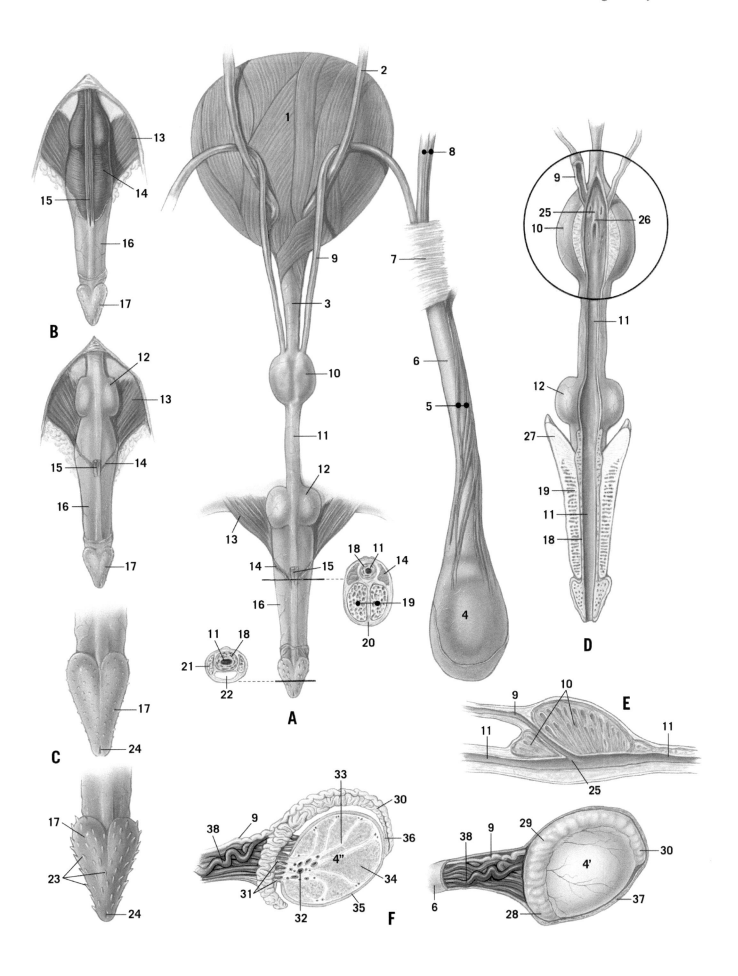

Plate 9-4

Figure A   Body posture attained during spraying

Figure B   Body postures attained during copulation

Figure C   Schematic illustration of relative changes in size and orientation of penis in nonerect (top) and fully erect (bottom) state

1   Pelvic symphysis
2   Testis in scrotum
3   Prepuce, sagittally sectioned
4   Bulbourethral glands covered by muscle
5   Body of penis
6   Glans penis

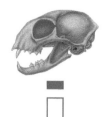

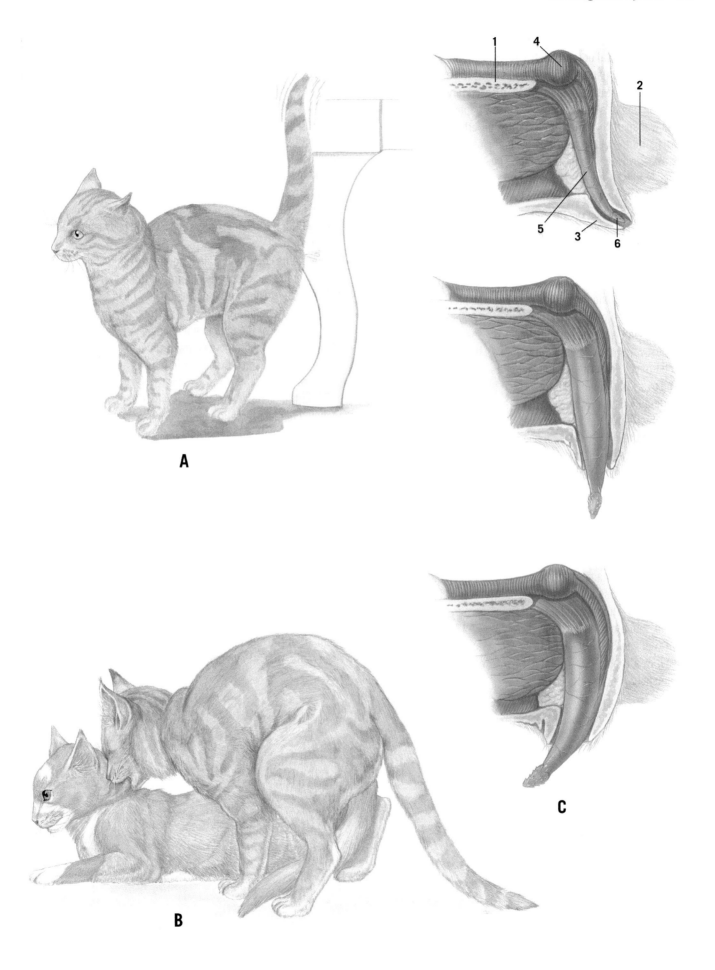

A

B

C

1 4

2

5 3 6

Female Genital Organs

The female genital or reproductive organs are the ovaries, uterine tubes, uterus, vagina, vestibule, and vulva. The ovaries are responsible for the maturation and release of secondary oocytes, as well as production of sex hormones (see also Chapter 6). The uterine tubes transport the unfertilized oocytes or fertilized ova to the uterus, and the uterus nurtures the embryos and fetuses through gestation by way of formation of the placenta.

The ovaries, uterine tubes, and uterus are supported by a fold of peritoneum termed the broad ligament of the uterus, similar to the manner in which the mesenteries suspend the intestinal tract. Though the broad ligament is largely thin and transparent similar to intestinal mesentery, portions contain significant amounts of smooth muscle, which add to its ability to support the uterus during pregnancy. However, unlike the intestinal mesentery, most of the broad ligament contains little fat. The broad ligament comprises three parts, each related to a specific region of the reproductive tract. The portion supporting the ovaries is termed the mesovarium, the mesosalpinx enfolds the uterine tube, and the largest part, the mesometrium, supports the uterus.

The ovaries of the queen are located just caudal to their corresponding kidney, at approximately the level of the third or fourth lumbar vertebra. The left ovary lies more caudally than the right, similar to the kidneys. Once a queen begins to cycle, the surface of the ovary becomes uneven due to the presence of maturing and atretic follicles or corpora lutea.

Each ovary is suspended from the body wall by the mesovarium and suspensory ligament. The mesovarium (the portion of the broad ligament related to the ovary) is thin, fine, and transparent, similar to other folds of peritoneum. In the free edge of the mesovarium runs the suspensory ligament, a dense band of tissue more similar a ligament at a joint than to peritoneal folds. The suspensory ligament runs from the cranial pole of each ovary to the dorsal body wall just caudal to the diaphragm in the area of the last rib, and provides most physical support of the ovary. A second stout (but very short) ligamentous band, the proper ligament of the ovary, attaches the caudal pole of each ovary to the tip of the uterine horn.

The uterine tube (oviduct or salpinx) takes a tortuous course between the ovary and the proximal uterine horn. The ovarian end of the uterine tube is expanded into the funnel-shaped, diaphanous infundibulum, which envelops the medial surface of the ovary and functions to capture the oocytes at ovulation. The mesosalpinx, the portion of the broad ligament supporting the uterine tube, is a lateral extension of (and thus continuous with) the mesovarium. Together, the mesosalpinx on the lateral side and the mesovarium on the medial side of the ovary form the ovarian bursa ("purse"), which envelops the ovary. The feline mesosalpinx (unlike the canine) contains little fat, and thus the ovary is routinely visible through the mesosalpinx regardless of the body condition of the queen.

The uterus comprises paired horns, the single body, and the single cervix. The uterus lies mainly in the abdominal cavity, with only the cervix lying in the pelvic cavity. The uterine horns are quite elongate, extending from the uterine tube (at the level of the ovary) through much of the abdominal cavity nearly to the pelvic inlet. Elongate uterine horns are characteristic of species that bear their young in litters, since the multiple fetuses are gestated along the length of the horns.

Toward the caudal end of their course, each uterine horn inclines medially to meet its fellow on the midline, where the two separate horns fuse together to form the single uterine body. The uterine body of the queen is quite short, being approximately one-fifth the length of the horns. Rather than serving as a site of gestation, the main function of the uterine body is to provide the initial portion of the route to the exterior for both uterine horns.

The portion of the broad ligament supporting the uterine horns and body is termed the mesometrium. A secondary fold of mesentery extends from the lateral surface of the mesometrium and projects from it at approximately a right angle. The round ligament of the uterus runs in the free edge of this fold, beginning at the tip of the uterine horn and ending shortly distal to the superficial inguinal ring. The round ligament of the uterus is the remnant of the presumptive gubernaculum, which, had the embryo been male, would have guided the testis to the scrotum.

The uterine body meets caudally with the uterine cervix, a short, extremely muscular structure that connects the uterus and vagina. The cervix serves as a sphincter and stout guardian in isolating the interior of the uterus from the external environment (and thereby assisting in keeping the uterine lumen sterile) at all times other than estrus and parturition.

The exact location of the uterus varies according to three factors: whether a non-pregnant queen has previously produced a litter, the current gravid or non-gravid state, and the stage of gestation when present. Despite experiencing tremendous excursions within the abdominal cavity during pregnancy, the uterus of queens in good condition can return to nearly the location it occupied before the first pregnancy. In the non-gravid queen, the uterine horns and body are suspended from the dorsal body wall relatively high in the body cavity by the mesometrium, and resting on the coils of the jejunum in approximately the dorsal half of the abdomen. Once pregnancy occurs, the enlarging uterus slowly sinks ventrally in the abdomen, gradually displacing the intestines. The smooth muscle within the mesometrium allows marked stretching to occur while still providing support for the greatly enlarged organ. As gestation progresses, the uterus advances cranially as well. At term, only the two walls of the greater omentum are interposed between the uterus and the ventral body wall, and the uterus may extend as far cranially as the diaphragm.

During pregnancy, both the uterus and its vascular supply enlarge greatly. The size and tortuosity of the ovarian and uterine vessels at term are many times that observed at any other time, even during estrus. In early pregnancy, enlargement of the uterus occurs mainly at the sites of embryonic implantation, resulting in a beaded or "sausage" appearance of the uterine horns. The uterus enlarges more uniformly as pregnancy progresses, and the constrictions along the uterine horns between fetuses become less distinct and are eventually lost.

The vagina, a thin-walled, muscular tube, extends caudally from the cervix toward the exterior. Its function is to receive the penis during copulation so that semen can be deposited near the cervix, and also to conduct the contents of the uterus toward the exterior of the body.

The vagina ends at the vestibule, which begins where the urethra enters the distal urogenital tract. Thus, the vestibule serves both the reproductive and urinary systems. The vestibule is also a tubular region, and extends from the entrance of the urethra to the vulva. The walls of the queen's vestibule contain diffuse bits of cavernous tissue, but these are not organized into a discrete vestibular bulb as is seen in the bitch. Paired major vestibular glands are present, which produce mucus to facilitate both copulation and parturition. The vestibule ends at the vulva, which is the terminal end of the female urogenital tract.

The vulva of the queen is composed of paired labia, thickened swellings that meet dorsally in a rounded commissure and ventrally in a more pointed commissure. The queen's vulva is densely covered with fine hair. The ventral commissure encloses the clitoris, a small erectile tissue body homologous to the penis. The small size of the clitoris in all species together with the overall small size of cats results in the feline clitoris being particularly small. Nonetheless, despite its small size, the clitoris of the queen has identifiable components similar to those of the penis, including paired crura, a body, and a glans.

Ovariohysterectomy is the most commonly performed abdominal surgery in queens. The organs are approached through the ventral midline of the caudal abdomen. The uterine horn may be located by gently displacing the jejunum and using an oophorectomy (spay) hook or finger to "hook" the uterine horn. Gentle traction on the uterine horn will exteriorize the horn and allow it to be traced cranially to the ovary and its vessels. The ovarian vessels are identified, clamped, ligated, and transected. The uterine horn is then traced caudally to its junction with the uterine body, and the opposite uterine horn is followed cranially from the uterine body to reveal the second ovary. This ovary is removed in a manner identical to the first. The mesometrium is divided as the two uterine horns are elevated to expose the uterine body. During this procedure, the ureters should be positively identified and avoided. The uterine vessels and uterine body and vessels are ligated, and transected, and the uterine horns and body are removed. In a routine ovariohysterectomy, the cervix remains behind.

Plate 9-5

Figure A   Female genital and urinary organs, ventral view
Figure B   Schematic illustration of ovary and uterine tube, partly sectioned
Figure C   Isolated female genital organs; inset: dorsal section of uterine body, ventral view
Figure D   Vestibule with dorsal wall opened, dorsal view

1	Kidney	16	Corpus albicans
2	Ureter		(**14-16** Not present simultaneously at mature stages)
3	Urinary bladder		
4	Suspensory ligament	17	Proper ligament of the ovary
5	Ovary	18	Fimbria
6	Uterine tube (oviduct)	19	Round ligament of the uterus
7	Uterine horn	20	Body of uterus
8	Broad ligament (mesometrium part)	21	Velum uteri
9	Vagina	22	Cervix
10	Vestibule	23	External uterine ostium
11	Vulva	24	Fornix of vagina
12	Rectum, cut	25	Urethra
13	Pelvic symphysis, split and retracted	26	External urethral orifice
14	Follicles in various stages of maturity	27	Remnants of mesonephric ducts
15	Corpus luteum	28	Duct of major vestibular glands
		29	M. constrictor vestibuli
		30	Fossa clitoridis
		31	M. constrictor vulvae

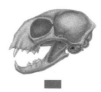

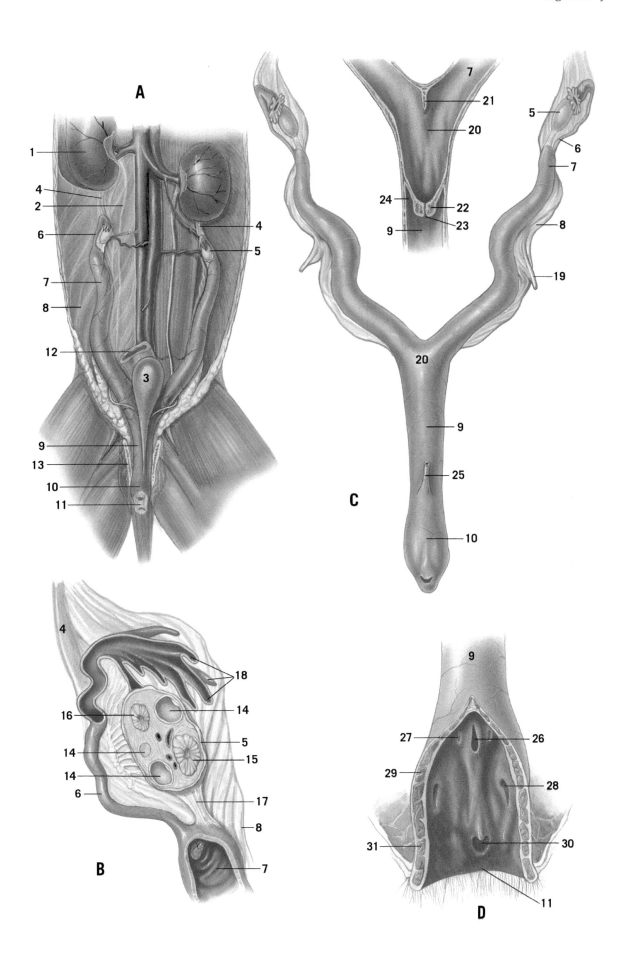

Plate 9-6

Figure A   Gravid uterus, in situ, ventral view
Figure B   Fetus with embryonic membranes transected and reflected
Figure C   Female and male external genitalia of kittens, caudal view

1	Liver	7	Fetus
2	Greater omentum, transected and removed	8	Umbilical cord
		9	Amnionic membrane
3	Intestines	10	Allantoic membrane
4	Late gestational uterus	11	Chorionic membrane
5	Zonary placenta	12	Anus
6	Urinary bladder	13	Vulva
		14	Prepuce

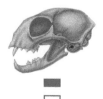

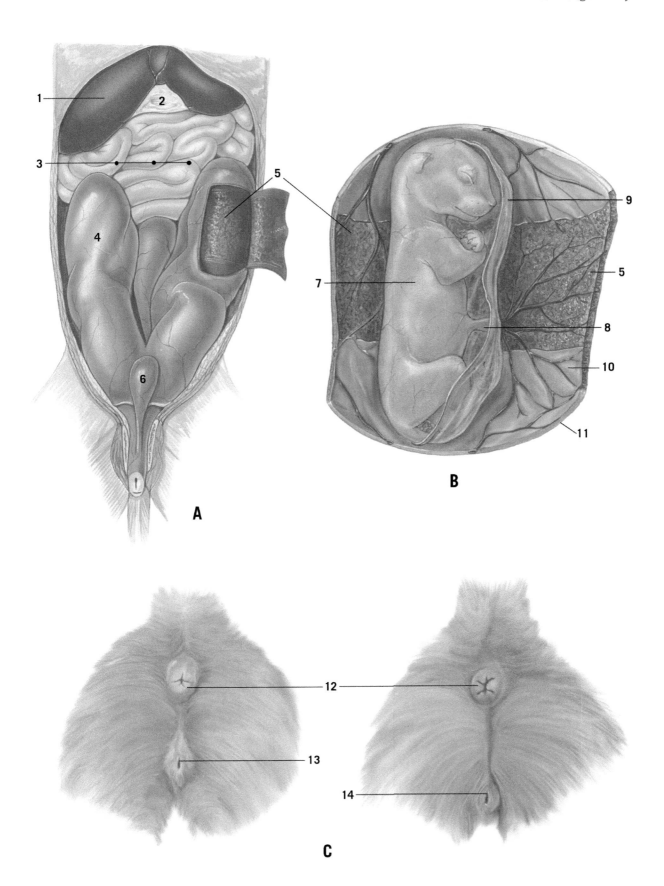

Selected References

1. Barsanti JA, Finco DR, Brown SA. In: Sherding RG (Ed). *The Cat: Diseases and Clinical Management.* 2nd ed. New York, Churchill Livingstone, 1994; 1769.

2. Bartges JW. In: August JR (Ed). *Consultations in Feline Internal Medicine,* Vol. 5. St. Louis, Elsevier Saunders. 2006; 441.

3. Bojrab MJ, Constantinescu GH. In Bojrab MJ (Ed): *Current Techniques in Small Animal Surgery.* 4th ed. Baltimore, Williams and Wilkins, 1998; 468.

4. Dyce KM, Sack WO, Wensing CJG. *Textbook of Veterinary Anatomy Textbook of Veterinary Anatomy.* 3rd Ed. Philadelphia, WB Saunders, 2002; 166, 430, 437.

5. Flanders JA, Harvey HJ. In: Sherding RG (Ed). *The Cat: Diseases and Clinical Management.* 2nd Ed. New York, Churchill Livingstone, 1994; 1825.

6. Gaskell CJ. In: Chandler EA, Gaskell CJ, Gaskell RM (Eds). *Feline Medicine and Therapeutics.* 3rd Ed. Oxford, Blackwell Publishing, Ltd. 2004; 313.

7. Hostutler RA, Chew DJ, DiBartola SP. In: Richards JR (Ed): *Veterinary Clinics of North America: Small Animal Practice: Advances in Feline Medicine.* Philadelphia, Saunders. 2005; 147.

8. Schummer A, Nickel R, Sack WO. *The Viscera of the Domestic Mammals.* 2nd revised Ed. New York, Springer-Verlag. 1979; 282.

9. Smith CW. Perineal urethrostomy. In: Harari J (Ed). *Veterinary Clinics of North America, Small Animal Practice: Topics in Feline Surgery.* Philadelphia, WB Saunders. 2002; 917.

10. Watson A. Vaginal ring and round ligament of the uterus in the female cat. Anat. Histol, Embrgol. 2009; 319

11. Westropp JL, Buffington J, Chew DJ. In: Ettinger ST, Feldman EC (Eds). *Textbook of Veterinary Internal Medicine,* 6th ed. St. Louis, Elsevier Saunders. 2004; 1828.

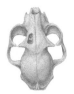

Chapter 10

Nervous System

Lola C. Hudson

Because the cat has been used widely for neurologic research over decades, there is more detailed information in the scientific literature about the feline nervous system than any other domestic species and frequently this feline information is extrapolated to other veterinary species. The anatomy and physiology of the nervous system is complex, but an understanding is critical to clinical neurology. Neurologic signs are related more to *where* a lesion is located rather that to *what* a lesion is.

Neuroanatomic Systems

The nervous system is frequently divided for ease of understanding into the central nervous system (CNS), the peripheral nervous system (PNS), and the autonomic nervous system (ANS). But, there is considerable anatomic and physiologic overlap between these systems. This overlap should always be remembered when dealing with neuroanatomy. As an example, a motor neuron may have its nerve cell body in the spinal cord (CNS) but its axon will leave the CNS via a ventral root and spinal nerve (PNS); thus, parts of a single neuron are in both systems.

Central Nervous System

The CNS is classically defined as the brain and spinal cord. These structures develop from the neurepithelium of the embryonic neural plate, neural groove, and neural tube. Malformations of these embryonic structures can result in death of a fetus, or conditions like spina bifida or syringomyelia in kittens.

Initially, the nerve cell bodies (gray matter) are surrounded by the processes (white matter) of the nerve cell bodies. This relationship of gray and white matter is maintained in the adult spinal cord, but secondary migration of cell groups and growth in the embryonic brain also results in areas where gray matter surrounds white matter (cerebral and cerebellar cortex), and where gray and white matter are intermixed (reticular formation of brain stem). Functionally related clusters of nerve cell bodies within the CNS are referred to as "nuclei" while functionally related bundles of nerve processes may be called "tract," "fasciculus," "lemniscus," "stria," "peduncle," or other terms.

Meninges

In addition to the bony protection provided by the skull and vertebrae, the brain and spinal cord are covered by 3 layers of connective tissue - the meninges. Meningiomas are the most common intracranial neoplasm found in cats. There is a predilection for older (10+ years), male cats. The outermost layer is called the dura mater and it is the thickest, most opaque layer. In the skull, this layer is closely applied to the periosteum of the cranial vault so that there is no epidural space between bone and dura mater. At the various foramina where cranial nerves leave the skull, the dura mater becomes continuous with the epineurium with the exception of cranial nerves I, II, and VIII. Also, there are 3 locations where double folds of dura mater exist. One, the falx cerebri, is located in the longitudinal fissure between the 2 cerebral hemispheres. Another, the tentorium cerebelli, is located in the transverse fissure between the cerebrum and cerebellum, and surrounds the midbrain. The tentorium cerebelli may completely ossify in the mature cat. A third fold, the diaphragma sellae, bridges the sella turcica in the base of the cranial vault, and contains a small foramen through which the pituitary stalk passes. If the brain is being removed intact in a necropsy, then these double folds of dura mater must be removed first to avoid tearing the brain. These folds of dura mater can also play a very important role in injuries or diseases that cause shifting and/or swelling of the brain. The growth of a brain tumor or brain edema can result in such crowding of the cerebrum or cerebellum that these structures herniate beneath the falx cerebri or tentorium cerebelli. Such herniation can put tremendous pressure on the brain stem ventral to these structures and can possibly kill the cat.

The dura mater also surrounds the spinal cord and extends somewhat caudal to the termination of the spinal cord, ending at about the first caudal vertebra in cats. The dura mater covers the roots of the spinal nerves to the level of the intervertebral foramina, where it then becomes continuous with the epineurium. In the vertebral column, there is an epidural space between bone and dura mater that contains the semifluid epidural fat and vertebral venous sinuses.

Deep to the dura mater is the arachnoid membrane. The arachnoid membrane is held against the dura mater by the pressure of the cerebrospinal fluid (CSF) in the subarachnoid space. The arachnoid membrane follows the large contours of the CNS but, at certain locations, it does not follow the CNS contours exactly. A clinically important enlarged subarachnoid space is the cerebellomedullary cistern (cisterna magna). The cerebellomedullary cistern is accessible for withdrawal of CSF samples or introduction of contrast material for myelography. Alternatively, the subarachnoid space of the spinal cord within the lumbar vertebrae is accessible.

Deep to the arachnoid membrane and subarachnoid space is the pia mater. This membrane is tightly adhered to the surface of the CNS and follows the contours faithfully. The pia mater contains the larger arteries that supply the CNS. In the spinal cord, the pia mater has periodic lateral thickenings, called the denticulate ligaments. These ligaments help to suspend and anchor the spinal cord within the meninges.

For cranial nerves I, II, and VIII, the meninges extend the full length of these nerve trunks. Technically, these "nerves" are evaginations of the brain itself. Potentially, these provide a direct route for infections moving from the periphery to the brain.

Blood Vessels

The brain of the cat is supplied by branches from the arterial circle (circle of Willis) and branches of the basilar a. The arterial circle itself is formed from anastomoses of the basilar a. and rami retis. (Because the mature cat does not maintain the internal carotid a., other vessels - the rete mirabile maxillaris and rami retis - take over its function.) The spinal cord is supplied by 3 longitudinally oriented arteries, a ventral spinal a. and a pair of dorsal spinal aa., which receive periodic contributions from spinal arteries.

The venous drainage of the brain is by several large sinuses that travel from the dorsal areas of the brain caudally, then travel ventrally in the caudal skull, and finally, rostrally to the base of the cranial vault. There are several connections with veins external to the skull.

A pair of vertebral venous sinuses located in the epidural space drains the spinal cord. They occasionally interconnect across the midline and regularly have lateral connections to veins external to the vertebral column. (For more information about blood supply, see Chapter 4.)

Brain

The embryonic brain develops from 3 vesicles of the rostral neural tube into 5 divisions of the mature brain: telencephalon, diencephalon, mesencephalon, metencephalon, and myelencephalon (medulla oblongata).

Another commonly used term in neuroanatomy is "brain stem": this is comprised of the diencephalon, the mesencephalon, the pons (not the cerebellum), and myelencephalon.

Ventricular System

The lumen of the embryonic neural tube remains in the mature CNS as the ventricular system, which is lined with ependymal cells and filled with CSF.

The first and second ventricles, or lateral ventricles, are located in the cerebrum, one within each cerebral hemisphere of the brain. The lateral ventricles are separated from each other on the midline by the septum pellucidum. Each lateral ventricle is connected independently to the third ventricle by an interventricular foramen. The third ventricle, which is located in the diencephalon, is best seen on a median section and roughly resembles a doughnut in shape. From the caudal part of the third ventricle, the mesen-cephalic aqueduct extends through the mesencephalon. This tube is narrower at the rostral end and gradually enlarges into a fourth ventricle, which is located between the cerebellum and the pons/ rostral myelencephalon. Lateral apertures from the fourth ventricle communicate with the subarachnoid space approximately at the level of the vestibulocochlear nerve (cranial nerve VIII). The caudal end of the fourth ventricle closes into a small tube - the central canal - that is located in the caudal myelencephalon and spinal cord. The point of closure of the 4th ventricle into the central canal is called the obex.

Each of the ventricles contains a choroid plexus that produces CSF by passive filtration of blood and active secretion. There is a relatively constant production and flow of CSF through the ventricular system and into the subarachnoid space where the majority of absorption takes place. Hydrocephalus, defined as an increase in CSF volume, may result in expansion of the ventricular system at any or all levels with compromise of nervous tissue. If hydrocephalus is present in the neonate, the entire cranial vault may be grossly enlarged, and the junction of frontal and parietal bones (the bregma) may remain permanently open.

Telencephalon

The telencephalon is phylogenetically the youngest area and is composed of the cerebrum or 2 cerebral hemispheres. The telencephalon covers a large portion of the remaining brain and can be readily seen on dorsal, lateral, and ventral views. The feline cerebrum has a convoluted surface. Each elevation is called a gyrus and the groove separating adjacent gyri is called a sulcus or fissure. (Several gyri and sulci are identified in the illustrations.)

The gray matter on the surface of the cerebrum is comprised of 6-7 cell layers and is called the cerebral cortex. The relative thickness of the layers varies from region to region.

Deep to these cell layers in the core of each gyrus is an area of white matter. Collectively, these cores of white matter are the corona radiata. Even deeper in each cerebral hemisphere are the basal nuclei (gray matter) - caudate nucleus, claustrum, amygdala body, and lentiform (putamen plus pallidum) nucleus. The basal nuclei are associated with motor function and behavior.

The telencephalon has also been subdivided into various functional lobes. The location of these lobes roughly corresponds to the area of cerebrum underlying the skull bone of the same name. Although any given function is not totally confined to a designated lobe, lesions in a lobe may be manifested clinically as disruptions of these designated roles. The frontal lobe contains part of the motor cortex involved with voluntary movement and contains areas associated with psychomotor skills. The parietal lobe is associated also with the motor cortex and the somesthetic interpretation center (conscious perception and localization of proprioception, pain, touch, and temperature). The occipital lobe functions in visual interpretation. The temporal lobe is associated with auditory function, behavior, and memory. The piriform lobe is found on the ventral surface of the cerebrum; it is not convoluted. This area functions in olfaction.

The major connection between the left and right cerebral hemispheres is the corpus callosum, most easily seen on a median section as a long, fairly thick strip of white matter.

Ventral to the corpus callosum and septum pellucidum is the body of the fornix. The fornix is the white matter connection between the hippocampal gyrus and nearby areas and the brain stem, particularly the mamillary bodies.

The major connection between each hemisphere and the rest of the brain is the internal capsule (white matter), which cannot be seen on the surface of the intact brain.

Diencephalon

The diencephalon consists of the thalamus, which takes up most of its bulk, and the smaller areas of epithalamus, subthalamus, metathalamus, and hypothalamus.

Part of the thalamus can be seen on the dorsal surface of the brain after the cerebral hemispheres are removed. On a median section, the interthalamic adhesion can be seen as an oval of solid tissue in the center of the third ventricle. This is an area of fusion between left and right thalami. The thalamus functions as a sensory relay center, receiving general sensory impulses and trans-mitting them to the telencephalon as well as receiving cortical projections.

The epithalamus includes the striae habenularis, the habenular nuclei, and the pineal body located on the dorsal midline at the caudal diencephalon.

The metathalamus includes the lateral geniculate and medial geniculate bodies, which relay special sensory impulses for sight and hearing, respectively, to the cerebral cortex where final integration and perception occurs. The geniculate bodies grow caudally over the dorsorostral mesencephalon during development.

The subthalamus cannot be seen on the surface of the brain but is located between the thalamus and hypothalamus at the transition of diencephalon and mesencephalon.

The portion of the hypothalamus that can be seen on the ventral surface of the brain extending caudal to the optic chiasm includes the small paired mamillary bodies on the caudoventral diencephalon, and the tuber cinereum, which is the tissue surrounding the base of the pituitary stalk. The hypothalamus functions in association with the autonomic nervous system and the endocrine system (see Chapter 6 also).

The optic chiasm is the point where the left and right optic nn. meet on the ventral diencephalon and where about 65% of the feline optic fibers cross the midline. Optic tracts lead from the optic chiasm on the ventral and lateral surface of the diencephalon. Each optic tract contains fibers from both the left and right optic nn. These optic nn, chiasm, and tracts are part of the visual pathways, for both conscious vision and pupillary light reflexes (see Chapter 11 also).

The telencephalon and diencephalon together may be referred to as the forebrain or prosencephalon and are often considered as a unit when localizing neurologic lesions.

Mesencephalon

Immediately caudal to the diencephalon is the mesencephalon or midbrain. Dorsally, the rostral colliculi and caudal colliculi can be seen if the cerebral hemispheres are removed. (These 4 mounds of tissue may also be referred to as the corpora quadrigemina.)

These rostral and caudal colliculi are associated with visual and auditory functions, respectively. Each rostral colliculus is connected to the ipsilateral lateral geniculate body (both function in vision) by a short, white matter brachium. Similarly, each caudal colliculus is connected to the medial geniculate body (both with auditory function) by a brachium on the lateral surface of the mesencephalon. The commissure of the caudal colliculi (also white matter) can be seen joining these structures across the dorsal midline.

The portion of the mesencephalon dorsal to the plane of the mesencephalic aqueduct is called the tectum and includes the previously discussed corpora quadrigemina; tissue ventral to the aqueduct is the tegmentum. Within the tegmentum are the important motor nuclei, the red nucleus, the substantia nigra, and motor nuclei of CNs III and IV. The substantia nigra of the cat does not contain melanin despite its name.

The crus cerebri can be seen on the ventral surface of the mesencephalon. These white matter structures represent the continuation of *some* motor fibers that were in the internal capsule. The depression between the crura cerebri is called the interpeduncular fossa.

Metencephalon

The embryonic rhombencephalon (hindbrain) develops into the metencephalon and myelencephalon. The metencephalon consists of the cerebellum dorsally and the pons ventrally.

The cerebellum has a central portion called the vermis and two lateral hemispheres. The surface of the cerebellum is highly convoluted with folia and sulci or fissures. There are 3 cerebellar lobes separated by fissures: rostral lobe, caudal lobe, and flocculonodulus. Each lobe includes a part of vermis and lateral hemispheres. The lobes are further divided into several lobules.

The cortex on the surface of the cerebellum has 3 layers - the external molecular layer, the piriform neuron (Purkinje cell) layer, and the granular layer. The white matter of the cerebellum may be called the medulla. On a median section, this medulla has a branching appearance and is called the arbor vitae.

Deep within the cerebellum are 3 pairs of cerebellar nuclei. The axons from these cerebellar nuclei are virtually the sole conduit of impulses out of the cerebellum to the remainder of the nervous system. The cerebellum is connected to the rest of the brain by pairs of rostral, middle, and caudal cerebellar peduncles; all impulses into or out of the cerebellum must pass through a cerebellar peduncle.

The basic function of the cerebellum is to coordinate motor activity, which is primarily achieved by inhibitory synapses onto motor neurons and interneurons. The cerebellum does not initiate voluntary or involuntary movement. Cerebellar dysfunctions are frequently manifested as dysmetria, intention tremors, increased muscle tone, and loss of menace response.

Cerebellar hypoplasia is seen occasionally and can be the result of in utero panleukopenia virus infections or may be the result of certain drug treatments (like griseofulvin) of a pregnant queen.

If the cerebellum is removed to reveal the dorsal pons, this usually tears the thin roof plate of the fourth ventricle. This roof plate, which is essentially the ependymal layer plus associated meninges, is called the medullary velum. In the floor of the fourth ventricle, the median sulcus on the midline and the sulcus limitans on the ventrolateral floor can be seen.

The pons includes a central area with indefinite borders called the reticular formation, which is not visible on any external surface. The reticular formation is a mixture of white and gray matter. Within the rostral area of the reticular formation (extending into the mesencephalon) is the functional site of the ascending reticular activating system (ARAS). This functions in maintaining alertness, or awareness via the cerebrum. On the ventral surface of the pons, the prominent transverse pontine fibers can be seen. These can be followed laterally and dorsally as they become the middle cerebellar peduncle. Just dorsal (deep) to the transverse pontine fibers are the longitudinal fibers of the pons that are the caudal continuation of the crus cerebri of the mesencephalon.

Associated with pons are the important motor nuclei, the nuclei of the reticular formation, part of the vestibular nuclei (discussed below), and the motor nucleus of cranial nerve V.

Myelencephalon

The myelencephalon or medulla oblongata is the most caudal part of the brain and completes the transition to the spinal cord. The reticular formation is continued in the central part of this division. Within this portion of the reticular formation are cardiac, swallowing, respiratory, and vomiting centers.

The dorsal surface of the myelencephalon reveals the caudal part of the fourth ventricle and the obex. The narrow bundle of fibers crossing the base of each caudal cerebellar peduncle is the dorsal acoustic stria. Lateral to the fourth ventricle at the level of the dorsal acoustic stria is the area of the 4 vestibular nuclei. These are an important part of the vestibular system, which functions in maintaining equilibrium and normal posture. The rostral continuation of fasciculi in the dorsal funiculus of the spinal cord can be seen caudal to the level of the obex. Dorsolaterally, the spinal tract of cranial nerve V can be seen. Ventrally, just caudal to the transverse pontine fibers, is another, smaller, bundle of transversely oriented fibers called the trapezoid body[a], which is part of the auditory pathway. A midline ventral median fissure is present ventral to and caudal to the trapezoid body, and is continued onto the spinal cord. To each side of this fissure, the longitudinally oriented pyramids can be seen; these are the continuation of the longitudinal fibers of the pons. Caudally, the pyramids can be seen decussating (crossing the midline), and this decussation marks the border between brain and spinal cord.

Nuclei of the reticular formation, part of the vestibular nuclei, and motor nuclei of cranial nerves VI, VII, IX-XII are important motor nuclei located in the myelencephalon.

---

[a]Some authors include the trapezoid body and other structures in this same plane as part of the metencephalon. The argument arises because, in humans, the transverse pontine fibers cover the trapezoid body and the caudal edge of the transverse pontine fibers is the border between metencephalon and myelencephalon. In common domestic animals, including the cat, the transverse pontine fibers do not cover the trapezoid body.

Plate 10-1

Figure A   Brain with portion of left hemisphere removed, dorsal view
Figure B   Brain with portion of right hemisphere removed, ventral view
Figure C   Brain, lateral view
Figure D   Brain, median section, medial view
Figure E   Brain with cerebrum and cerebellum removed (brain stem), dorsal view

Telencephalon
1   Precruciate gyrus
2   Cruciate sulcus
3   Postcruciate gyrus
4   Marginal gyrus
5   Marginal sulcus
6   Ectomarginal gyrus
7   Rostral suprasylvian sulcus
8   Middle suprasylvian sulcus
9   Caudal suprasylvian sulcus
10 Ectosylvian gyrus
11 Occipital gyrus
12 Hippocampal gyrus
13 Fornix
14 Prorean sulcus
15 Lateral rhinal sulcus
16 Piriform lobe
17 Olfactory bulb
18 Lateral olfactory stria
19 Medial olfactory stria
20 Proreus gyrus
21 Coronal sulcus
22 Rostral compositus gyrus
23 Pseudosylvian fissure
24 Sylvian gyrus
25 Caudal compositus gyrus
26 Medial rhinal sulcus
27 Cingulate gyrus
28 Splenial sulcus
29 Suprasplenial sulcus
30 Lateral ventricle
31 Caudate nucleus
32 Cerebral cortex
33 Internal capsule (cut to remove cerebral hemisphere)
34 Septum pellucidum

35 Corpus callosum
36 Rostral commissure
37 Longitudinal fissure

Diencephalon
38 Optic n. (Cranial n. Ii)
39 Optic chiasm
40 Optic tract
41 Tuber cinereum'
42 Infundibulum
43 Mammillary bodies
44 3rd Ventricle
45 Pituitary gland (hypophysis)
46 Interthalamic adhesion
47 Stria habenularis
48 Pineal gland
49 Thalamus
50 Lateral geniculate body
51 Medial geniculate body

Mesencephalon
52 Oculomotor n. (Cranial n. Iii)
53 Crus cerebri
54 Mesencephalic aqueduct
55 Rostral colliculus
56 Brachium of caudal colliculus
57 Caudal colliculus
58 Trochlear n. (Cranial n. Iv)

Metencephalon cerebellum
59 Vermis
60 Lateral hemisphere
61 Culmen
62 Declive
63 Ansiform lobule
64 Paramedian lobule

65 Dorsal paraflocculus
66 Flocculus
67 Ventral paraflocculus
68 Primary fissure
69 Uvulonodularis fissure
70 Medulla(white matter)
71 Nodulus
72 Lingula pons
73 transverse pontine fibers
74 trigeminal n. (cranial n. V)
75 Cerebellar peduncles
76 4th Ventricle
77 Abducens n. (cranial n VI)

Myelencephalon
78 Facial n. (cranial n VII)
79 Vestibulocochlear n. (cranial n. VIII)
80 Glossopharyngeal n. (cranial n. IX)
81 Vagus n. (cranial n. X)
82 Accessory n. (cranial n. XI)
83 Hypoglossal n. (cranial n. XII)
84 Trapezoid body
85 Pyramids
86 Pyramidal decussation
87 Dorsal acoustic stria
88 Obex
89 Fasciculus gracilis
90 Fasciculus cuneatus
91 Spinal tract of V (of trigeminal nerve)

Spinal Cord
92 Ventral roots of 1st cervical nerve
93 Spinal cord
94 Central canal

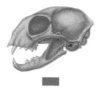

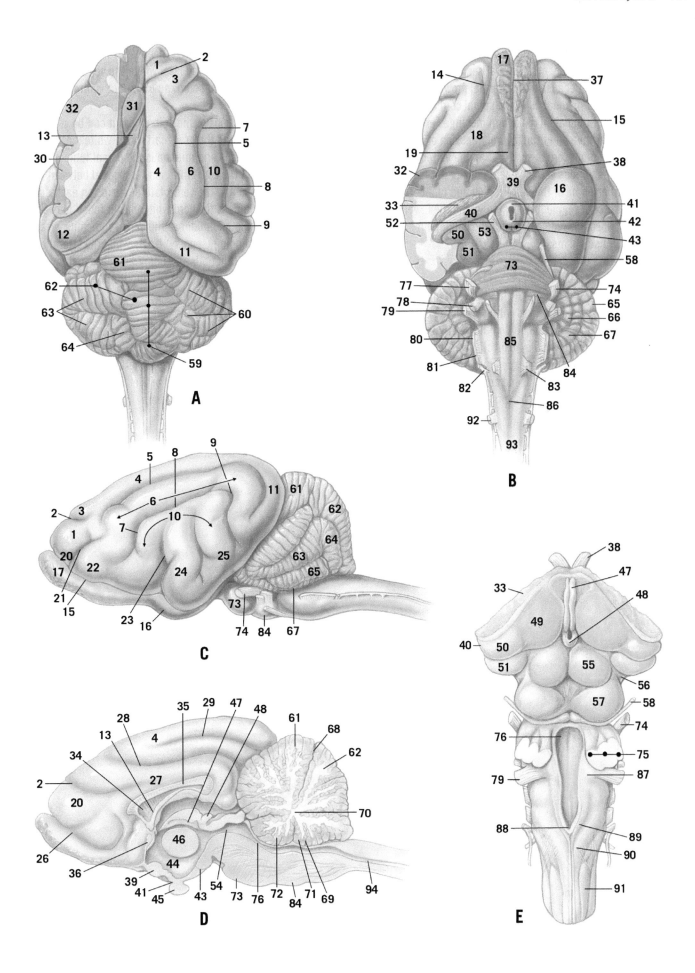

Spinal Cord

The feline spinal cord has 8 cervical segments, 13 thoracic segments, 7 lumbar segments, 3 sacral segments, and about 5 caudal segments. Because of differential growth between the vertebral column and spinal cord, the spinal cord ends at about the level of S_1[b] vertebra in cats. (The spinal meninges extend further caudally and may give an initial false impression of a longer spinal cord.) Since the spinal cord is shorter than the vertebral canal containing it, the various cord segments do not necessarily directly correspond to vertebrae of the same region and number. For example, the S_2 cord segment is located within the L_6 vertebra. This difference is especially noticeable with the caudal lumbar, sacral, and caudal cord segments.

Grossly, 2 areas of enlargement are visible: one is the cervical intumescence formed by segments C_6-T1(T_2)[c] located within vertebrae C_5-T_1 and the other is the lumbosacral intumescence formed by segments L_4-S_3 located within vertebrae L_4-L_6. These 2 areas correspond to the origin of spinal nerves that innervate the forelimb and hindlimb/genitalia, respectively. The tapering end of the spinal cord is called the conus medullaris.

The dorsal median sulcus is found on the dorsal midline of the spinal cord. At the level where the dorsal rootlets of spinal nn. join the spinal cord, a shallow groove, the dorsolateral sulcus, can be seen on each side. Ventrally, a deep ventral median fissure is present on the midline. At the level where the ventral rootlets of spinal nn. leave the spinal cord, an indistinct ventrolateral sulcus is present.

On transverse sections of the spinal cord it can be seen that the white matter surrounds the gray matter. The white matter between the dorsolateral sulcus and midline is the dorsal funiculus; the lateral funiculi are the cord white matter located between the dorsolateral sulcus and the ventrolateral sulcus on each side. The ventral funiculus is the cord white matter found between the ventrolateral sulcus and midline. The dorsal funiculus essentially contains only ascending (sensory) tracts while the lateral and ventral funiculi contain both ascending and descending (motor) tracts. These tracts connect the cord and brain or connect different areas of spinal cord.

The central gray matter of the spinal cord has roughly a butterfly or "H" configuration when seen on transverse section. The exact shape and relative amount of the gray matter varies from region to region and reflects the amount of peripheral tissue being innervated. The dorsal horn (upper part of the "H") is associated with sensory function while the ventral horn (lower part of the "H")

[b]Frequently, a shorthand method for designating vertebrae, spinal cord segments, and spinal nerves is used. It consists on a capital letter followed by a single or range of Arabic number(s). The letters indicate the region - C for cervical, T for thoracic, L for lumbar, S for sacral, Ca or Cd for caudal. The single number can represent an individual structure, as in this case, or the maximum number of structures in that region. The range of numbers indicates more than one specific structure or a variable maximum number of structures.

is associated with motor function. The dorsal and ventral horns are found in all segments of the spinal cord and develop from the embryonic alar plate and basal plate, respectively. The zona intermedia (between dorsal and ventral horns) and its lateral projection, the lateral (or intermediolateral) horn, is associated with autonomic motor function and can be recognized in the thoracic, cranial lumbar, and sacral segments. The zona intermedia develops from the basal plate.

At the center of the spinal cord sections, the small central canal can be seen. Like other areas of the ventricular system, it is lined with ependymal cells and contains CSF.

In cats, the conditions most frequently resulting in spinal cord lesions are trauma, ischemic neuromyopathy, and spinal lymphosarcoma. The lymphosarcomas occur most frequently in cats of less than 2 years-of-age and the majority of these cats are positive for feline leukemia virus.

Rabies is a lethal, viral disease of the CNS that can be contracted by and transmitted by cats. Because of wildlife reservoirs, pet cats that are not vaccinated for rabies can become infected by diseased wildlife or unvaccinated pets and then be the source of rabies to humans. Surprisingly, there are still states/provinces in North America that do not require rabies vaccination of cats even though the local wildlife harbors the disease.

Upper Motor Neurons and Lower Motor Neurons

Clinical neurology frequently refers to upper motor neurons (UMNs) and signs related to UMN dysfunction, and to lower motor neurons (LMNs) and signs related to LMN dysfunction. Each type is motor in function as the names imply. A LMN is responsible for carrying motor impulses from the CNS into the periphery to its target, often striated muscle. A UMN is responsible for carrying motor impulses from "higher" brain centers, such as the cerebral cortex and basal nuclei, to LMNs. UMNs of cats synapse indirectly onto LMNs, through interneurons (connecting neurons). All UMNs and their tracts are located within the CNS. Therefore, UMN signs are associated with CNS lesions. The nerve cell bodies of LMNs are located in motor nuclei of cranial nerves in the brain stem and in the lateral (autonomic) and ventral horns of the spinal cord segments. The axons of LMNs extend into the periphery. Therefore, LMN signs can result from either CNS or PNS lesions.

The placement of a cord segment or nerve in parenthesis following an indicated range indicates that such a segment or nerve sometimes contributes to that range.

Plate 10-2

Figure A   Magnetic resonance mid-sagittal brain scout image with orientation and location of transverse sections indicated

Figures B-N   Magnetic resonance image of transverse sections of brain. Sections correspond to lines 3-15 consecutively on the scout image A. Colors correspond to brain divisions indicated by the key.

Images provided courtesy of Diagnostic Imaging (Radiology) Service, Veterinary Teaching Hospital, North Carolina State University College of Veterinary Medicine

1	Cerebellum (dorsal metencephalon)	10	Lateral ventricle
2	Obex	11	Corpus callosum
3	4th ventricle	12	Lateral geniculate body
4	Pons (ventral metencephalon)	13	Medial geniculate body
5	Caudal colliculus	14	Thalamus
6	Mesencephalic aqueduct	15	3rd ventricle
7	Rostral colliculus	16	Interthalamic adhesion
8	Tegmentum region of mesencephalon	17	Internal capsule
9	Hippocampus	18	Caudate nucleus
		19	Optic chiasm

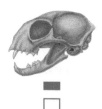

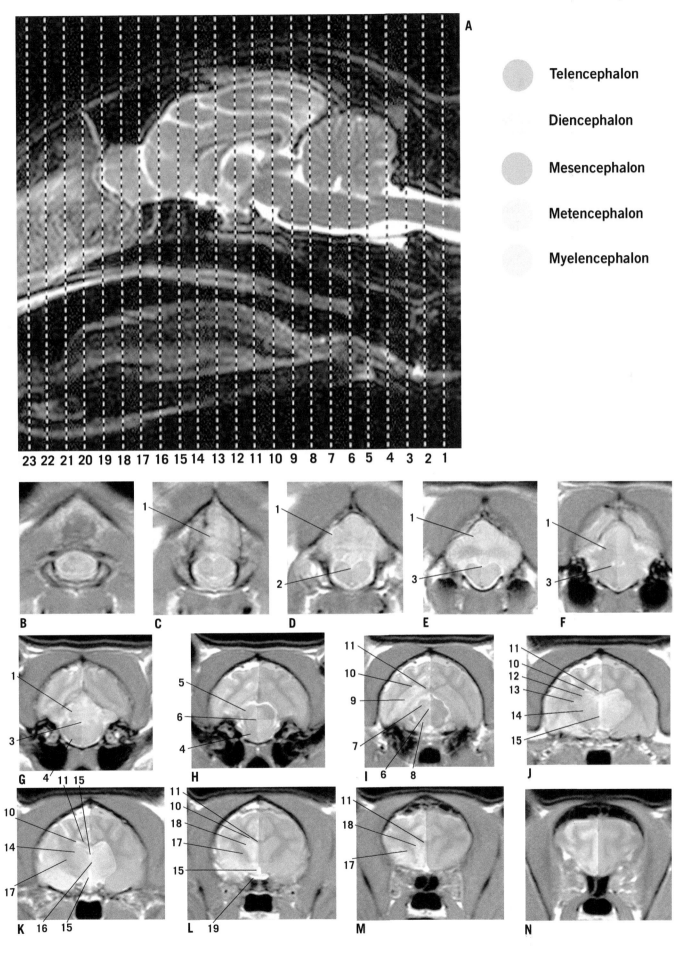

Plate 10-3

Figure A   Cervical and thoracic spinal cord in situ, with dorsal aspect of vertebrae and meninges removed, dorsal view. Cord segments and spinal nerves are denoted by C for cervical and T for thoracic plus an arabic number

Figure B   Schematic transverse section of spinal cord and associated spinal nerves with meninges and vessels at the level of an intervertebral foramen

Figure C   Transverse section of cervical (top) and thoracic spinal cord segments

a	Cervical vertebrae 1-7	**25**	Sympathetic ganglion
b	Thoracic vertebrae 1-11	**26**	Spinal a.
C1-8	Cervical spinal cord segments	**27**	Dorsal radicular branch
T1-11	Thoracic spinal cord segments	**28**	Ventral radicular branch
C1n	1st Cervical spinal nerve	**29**	Dorsal spinal a.
C8n	8th Cervical spinal nerve	**30**	Ventral spinal a.
T1n	1st Thoracic spinal nerve	**31**	Central a.
T6n	6th Thoracic spinal nerve	**32**	Vertebral venous sinus
T11n	11th Thoracic spinal nerve	**33**	Segments of cervical intumescence (C6-T2)
12	Spinal contribution to cn xi (accessory n.)	**34**	Dorsal median sulcus
13	Pia mater	**35**	Dorsolateral sulcus
14	Subarachnoid space	**36**	Dorsal intermediate sulcus
15	Arachnoid membrane (in green)	**37**	Ventral median fissure
16	Dura mater	**38**	Ventrolateral sulcus (indistinct)
17	Epidural fat in epidural space	**39-41**	White matter
18	Dorsal root of spinal n.	**39**	Dorsal funiculus
19	Spinal (dorsal root) ganglion	**40**	Lateral funiculus
20	Ventral root of spinal n.	**41**	Ventral funiculus
21	Spinal n.	**42-44**	Gray matter
22	Dorsal branch of spinal n.	**42**	Dorsal horn
23	Ventral branch of spinal n.	**43**	Zona intermedia
24	Ramus communicans of thoracolumbar spinal n.	**43'**	Lateral horn
		44	Ventral horn
		45	Central canal

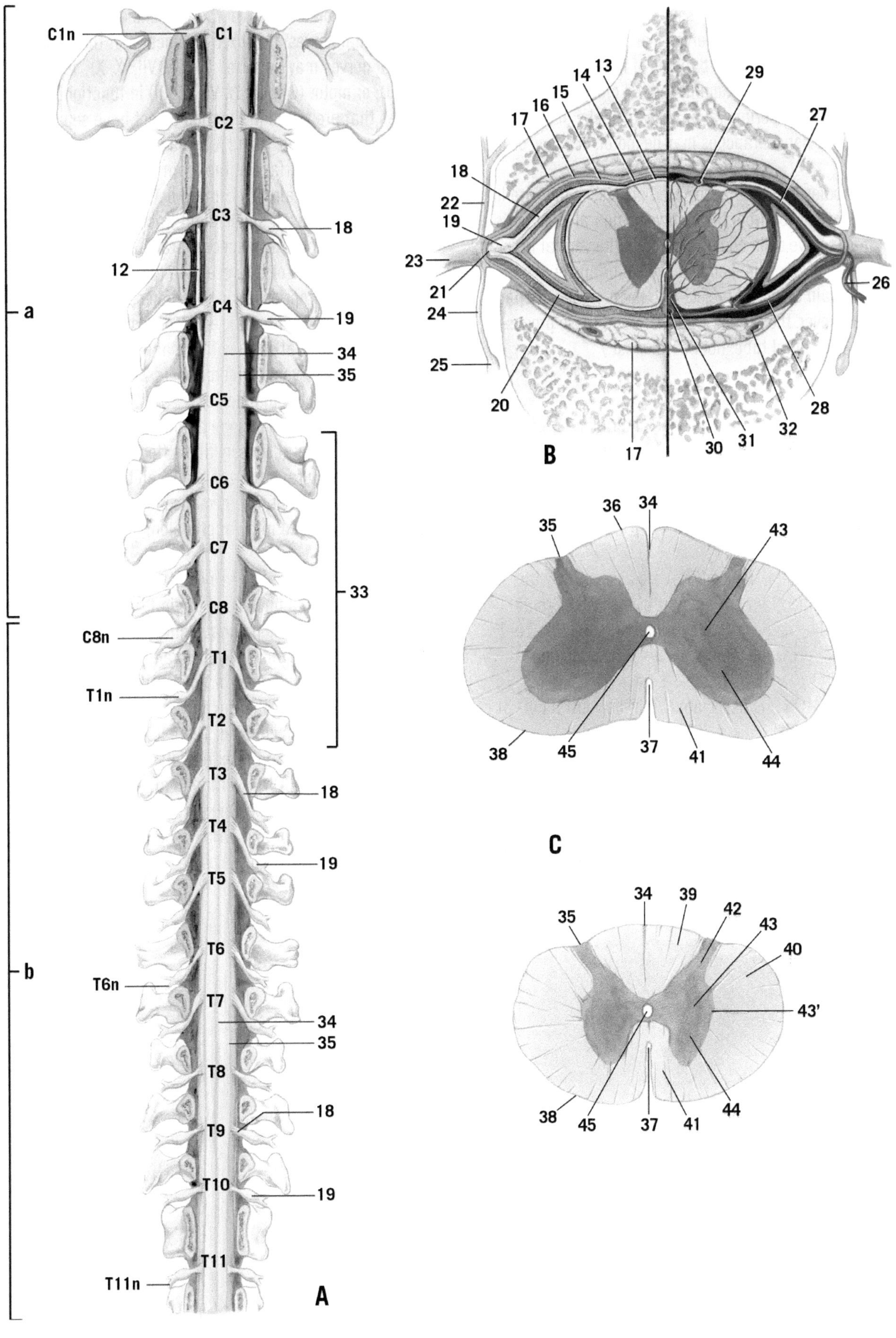
C1n
C1
C2
C3
18
12
a
C4
19
34
35
C5
C6
C7
33
C8
C8n
T1
T1n
T2
T3
18
T4
19
T5
T6
b
T6n
T7
34
35
T8
18
T9
T10
19
T11
T11n
A
13
14
15
16
17
29
27
18
22
19
23
21
24
26
25
20
17
30
31
32
28
B
36
34
35
43
38
45
37
41
44
C
34
39
35
42
43
40
43'
38
45
37
41
44

Peripheral Nervous System

The PNS is defined as nervous tissue other than the brain and spinal cord; this includes "nerves," and "ganglia" found throughout the body. Nerves are bundles of neuron processes in the PNS. A ganglion is a functionally related cluster of nerve cell bodies in the PNS (the peripheral analogy to nuclei of the CNS). Specific nerves or nerve branches may be motor, sensory, or mixed in function.

Nerve cell bodies and their associated processes that are located in the periphery develop from the embryonic neural crest cells. (Axons of many nerve cells bodies located in the ventral horn and zona intermedia of the spinal cord or the motor nuclei of cranial nerves in the brain stem will project into the periphery as part of the PNS. However, these cells and, therefore, these processes develop from the neural tube, not neural crest.)

Blood Supply

The PNS is supplied by spinal arteries and radicular branches in the immediate region of the vertebral column. Other parts of peripheral nerves are supplied by small branches, the vasa nervorum, of any nearby artery. Venous return is by satellite veins.

Cranial Nerves

The 12 pairs of cranial nerves (CNs) are associated with different areas of the brain but are part of the PNS.[d] Cranial nerves may be identified by name or Roman numeral (see Table 10-1). The general function of the cranial nerves is also included in Table 10-1.

The olfactory n. (CN I) is associated with the ventral part of the telencephalon while the optic n. (CN II) (see Chapter 11 also) is associated with the ventral diencephalon. The oculomotor n. (CN III) and trochlear n. (CN IV) (see Chapter 11 also) attach to the mesencephalon. CN IV is the only nerve that leaves the dorsal aspect of the brain. The trigeminal n. (CN V) leaves the lateral surface of the brain just caudal to the transverse pontine fibers.

The remaining cranial nerves (CN VI-XII) are associated with the lateral, ventrolateral, or ventral portions of the myelencephalon.

All spinal nerves are mixed in function at their origin, but the cranial nerves may be mixed (CNs V, VII, IX, X), sensory (CNs I, II, VIII), or motor (CNs III, IV, VI, XI, XII) in function. Also, cranial nerves that are mixed in function do not have separate dorsal and ventral "roots." CNs IX and X do have a series of rootlets emerging from the lateral surface of the brain that then merge into nerves, but these rootlets already contain both motor and sensory fibers. The special senses of smell, sight, taste, hearing, and equilibrium are associated only with specific cranial nerves, not any spinal nerves. The senses of exteroception (pain, touch, pressure, temperature), proprioception (position sense), and interoception (stretch, pressure) are also received from various structures of the head. These general sensory fibers are carried in CNs V, VII, IX, and X. Any cranial nerve with motor fibers will have LMN functions as do motor fibers in spinal nerves.

Cranial nerves that include autonomic motor fibers (CNs III, VII, IX, X) and/or general sensory fibers (for carrying modalities of pain, touch, temperature) have ganglia located somewhere along their length. Some, but not all, special sensory fibers have their nerve cell bodies gathered into ganglia along the appropriate nerve (see Table 10-1).

The cranial nerves that carry motor fibers and/or autonomic motor fibers have a nucleus of origin for those fibers within the brain stem. The location of each nucleus is within the division of the brain stem with which the cranial nerve is associated. For example, CN III (oculomotor n.) has both motor and autonomic motor fibers within it and the nerve is associated with separate nuclei in the mesencephalon. There is the oculomotor nucleus for innervation of some of the extraocular muscles, and the parasympathetic nucleus of CN III for innervation of the iris and ciliary muscles within the globe. The nerve cell bodies within these nuclei give rise to the motor and parasympathetic motor axons, respectively, that are carried in the oculomotor n.

---

[d]Cranial nerves I, II, and VIII are frequently considered extensions of the brain based on embryology. This is reflected by their meningeal coverings throughout their length unlike other cranial and spinal nerves. Nevertheless, they are referred to as "nerves" and are included in the PNS for that reason.

TABLE 10-1
General Function of Cranial Nerves

Number	Name	Exit from Skull	Associated Ganglia	Motor Function	Sensory Function
I	Olfactory n.	cribriform plate			smell
II	Optic n.	optic canal			sight
III	Oculomotor n.	orbital fissure	*ciliary g	dorsal, medial, ventral rectus mm., ventral oblique m., m. levator palpebrae superioris, *constrictor mm. of iris and ciliary body	
IV	Trochlear n.	orbital fissure		dorsal oblique m.	
V	Trigeminal n.		trigeminal g.	muscles of mastication	most structures of the head
	Ophthalmic	orbital fissure			orbit and eye, skin of dorsal nose, part of nasal cavity and sinuses
	Maxillary	round foramen			skin of cheek and lateral nose, mucous membrane of nasopharynx, soft and hard palate, superior teeth and gingivae
	Mandibular	oval foramen		Masseter, temporalis, medial and lateral pterygoid, digastricus, mylohyoid mm.	skin of jaw inferior teeth and gingivae, tongue
VI	Abducens n.	orbital fissure		lateral rectus and retractor bulbi mm.	
VII	Facial n.	stylomastoid foramen	geniculate g. *pterygopalatine, *mandibular, and *sublingual gg.	muscles of facial expression *salivary and lacrimal glands	taste, skin on concave surface of pinna
VIII	Vestibulo-cochlear n.	(does not leave skull proper)	spiral g. vestibular g.		hearing equilibrium
IX	Glosso-pharyngeal n.	tympano - occipital fissure	proximal and distal gg. *otic g.	muscles of the pharynx and soft palate, *salivary glands	taste, caudal 1/3 of tongue and pharyngeal mucosa
X	Vagus n.	tympano- occipital fissure	proximal and distal gg. *terminal gg.	muscles of pharynx, larynx, and esophagus *cervical, thoracic and abdominal viscera	pharyngeal and laryngeal mucosa cervical, thoracic, and abdominal viscera
XI	Accessory n.	tympano- occipital fissure		mm. trapezius, sternocephalicus, and omotransversarius	
XII	Hypoglossal n.	tympano- occipital fissure		muscles of tongue and some hyoid mm.	

*= autonomic motor innervation

Plate 10-4

Figure A   Lumbar, sacral and caudal spinal cord in situ with dorsal aspect of vertebrae and meninges removed. Cord segments and spinal nerves are denoted by T for thoracic, L for lumbar, S for sacral, and Ca for caudal plus an arabic number Enlargement of caudal region has dorsal roots removed on the right side.

Figure B   Transverse section of lumbar (left) and sacral spinal cord segments

a Thoracic vertebrae 12-13	**15** Dorsal median sulcus
b Lumbar vertebrae 1-7	**16** Dorsolateral sulcus
c Sacral vertebrae 1-3 (sacrum)	**17** Ventral median fissure
d Caudal vertebrae 1-3	**18** Ventrolateral sulcus (indistinct)
T12-13 Thoracic spinal cord segments	**19-21** White matter
L1-7 Lumbar spinal cord segments	**19** Dorsal funiculus
S Sacral spinal cord segments	**20** Lateral funiculus
Ca Caudal spinal cord segments	**21** Ventral funiculus
T13n 13th Thoracic spinal n.	**22-23** Gray matter
L1n 1st Lumbar spinal n.	**22** Dorsal horn
L7n 7th Lumbar spinal n.	**23** Zona intermedia
S1n 1st Sacral spinal n.	**24** Ventral horn
S3n 3rd Sacral spinal n.	**25** Central canal
Ca1n 1st Caudal spinal n.	**26** Dorsal root of spinal n.
14 Segments of lumbosacral intumescence (L4-S3)	**27** Spinal (dorsal root) ganglion
	28 Cauda equina

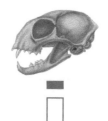

A

B

Plate 10-5

Figure A   Special areas of dura mater associated with the brain, median section with hindbrain removed, craniomedial view

Figure B   Position of spinal needle in subarachnoid space of cerebellomedullary cistern

Figure C   Position of spinal needle in subarachnoid space of more caudal spinal cord

Figure D   Cranial nerves exiting skull, cranial nerves (CN) I and VIII not visible; zygomatic arch and mandible removed, lateral view

1	Septum between frontal sinuses	17	Spinal subarachnoid space
2	Forebrain	18	Occipital condyle
3	Caudal cranial fossa	19	Tympanic bulla
4	Hypophyseal fossa	20	External acoustic meatus
5	Nasal septum	21	Zygomatic arch (cut and removed)
6-8	Double folds of dura mater	22	Infraorbital foramen
6	Falx cerebri	23	Optic n. (CN II)
7	Tentorium cerebelli	24	Oculomotor n. (CN III)
8	Diaphragma sellae	25	Trochlear n. (CN IV)
9	External occipital protuberance	26-28	Trigeminal n. (CN V)
10	Transverse process (wing) of atlas	26	Ophthalmic n.
11	Cerebellum	27	Maxillary n.
12	Caudal brain stem	28	Mandibular n.
13	Spinal cord	29	Abducens n. (CN VI)
14	Cerebellomedullary cistern (cisterna magna)	30	Facial n. (CN VII)
		31	Glossopharyngeal n. (CN IX)
15	L5 Vertebra	32	Vagus n. (CN X)
16	L6 Vertebra	33	Accessory n. (CN XI)
		34	Hypoglossal n. (CN XII)

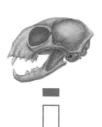

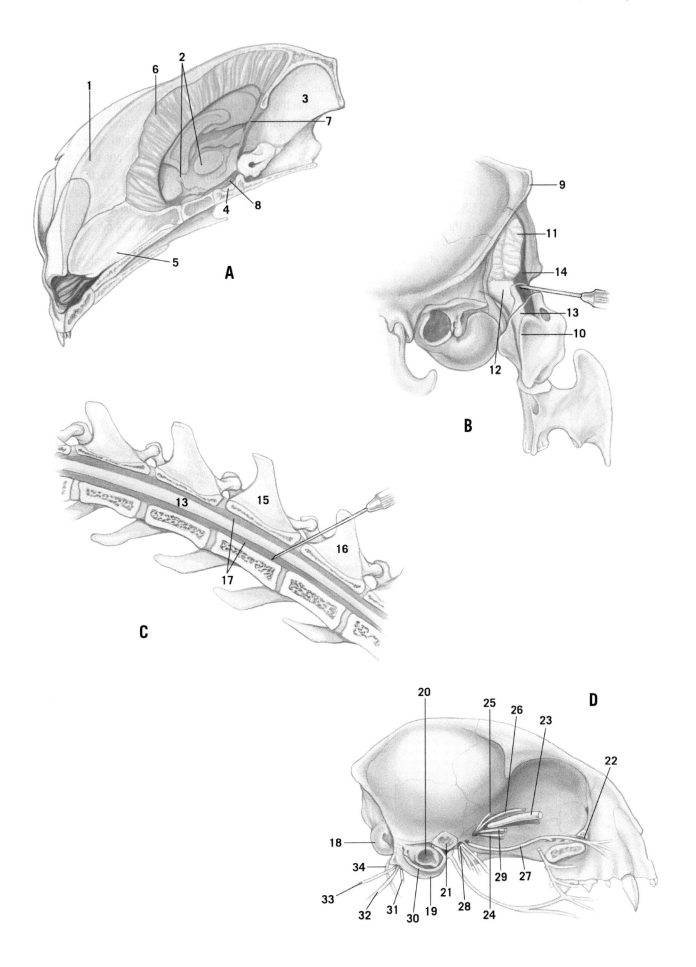

Spinal Nerves

Each segment of the spinal cord gives rise to a pair of spinal nerves, formed by a dorsal root and ventral root on each side. Each dorsal root has an enlargement along its length - the spinal (dorsal root) ganglion. The dorsal root has fibers associated with sensory functions and the spinal ganglion of a given dorsal root contains the nerve cell bodies of all of those sensory fibers. These sensory functions include exteroception associated especially with skin, proprioception associated especially with tendons, joints, and muscles, and interoception associated with viscera. The ventral roots have fibers associated with motor (LMN) function; but the nerve cell bodies of these fibers are found in the ventral or lateral horns of the spinal cord. The long roots of the caudal lumbar, sacral, and caudal nerves leave the tapering end of the spinal cord and travel to their exit foramina, forming the cauda equina.

The junction of dorsal and ventral roots generally lies at about the level of the appropriate intervertebral foramina. This junction marks the formation of the spinal nerve that is mixed (motor and sensory) in function and short in length. Whatever the location of the cord segment of origin within the vertebral canal, the spinal nerves have a very specific exit point. C_1 nerve leaves through the lateral vertebral foramen of C_1 vertebra. Spinal nerves C_2 through C_7 leave the intervertebral foramen just cranial to the vertebra of corresponding number, i.e., C_4 nerve leaves between C_3 and C_4 vertebra. Because there are 8 cervical spinal nerves but only 7 cervical vertebrae, there is a switch in the orientation of nerves and intervertebral foramina at the cervicothoracic junction. Nerve C_8 leaves through the space between C_7 and T_1 vertebrae. The remaining spinal nerves will leave the intervertebral foramina just caudal to the vertebra of corresponding number, i.e., T_{12} nerve leaves between vertebrae T_{12} and T_{13}.

Almost immediately upon leaving the vertebral canal, a spinal nerve divides into a dorsal branch, a ventral branch, and, in the thoracolumbar nerves, a ramus communicans. The dorsal branches innervate epaxial muscles and give rise to dorsal cutaneous nerves. The ventral branches innervate hypaxial muscles and give rise to lateral cutaneous and ventral cutaneous nerves. The ventral branches of spinal nerves C$_6$-T$_1$(T$_2$) and L$_4$-S$_3$ are of particular interest because these nerves form the brachial and lumbosacral plexi, respectively. The brachial and lumbosacral plexi in turn give rise to named nerves innervating the thoracic and pelvic limbs (see Table 10-2). Each ramus communicans of the thoracolumbar spinal nerves is associated with the autonomic nervous system and connects to a ganglion of the sympathetic trunk.

The radial n. of the brachial plexus innervating the forelimb has particular importance because it provides motor fibers to the m. triceps brachii, the major extensor of the elbow joint. Loss of this innervation (or of the muscle itself through injury or muscle disease) results in an animal unable to bear weight on the forelimb. In a similar fashion, the femoral n. is the key nerve of the hindlimb because it innervates the m. quadriceps femoris, the major extensor of the stifle joint. Loss of this innervation or muscle results in an animal unable to bear weight on the hindlimb.

In Manx cats, there is not only variable agenesis of caudal and sacral vertebrae, but these animals also have corresponding malformations of sacral and caudal nerves and, possibly, associated spinal cord segments. This can affect fecal and urinary continence because of compromise/loss of innervation to anal and urinary sphincters.

Cats that have had their tails caught by a moving car may have torn caudal nerves or even spinal cord damage because of the sudden traction and stretch of nerve roots. Depending on the exact level of damage, such animals may have limp tails, fecal incontinence, and difficulties in urination.

Cats with cardiomyopathy and subsequent thrombus in the caudal aorta or its large branches such as the external iliac a. or femoral a. can develop ischemic neuromyopathy within a short time. Demyelination and Wallerian-type degeneration can be seen particularly affecting the sciatic n. and its branches in the crus.

Plate 10-6

Figure A   Cranial nerves of the orbital region; deep dissection with periorbita and zygomatic arch removed, lateral view

Figure B   Deep branches of the trigeminal n with zygomatic arch and mandible removed, lateral view

Figure C   Superficial branches of the facial and trigeminal nerves with parotid, mandibular, and sublingual salivary glands removed, lateral view

Figure D   Initial path of facial and vestibulocochlear nerves in caudal skull with brain removed, median section, medial view

Figure E   Cranial nerves of the tympano-occipital region, median section, medial view

Figure F   Facial and hypoglossal nerves with parotid, mandibular, and sublingual glands removed, lateral view

1	Zygomatic arch, cut and removed in figs A, B, F
2	Lateral rectus m., cut and retracted
3	Dorsal rectus m.,
4	Lacrimal gland
5	Retractor bulbi m.
6	Bulbus oculi
7	Ventral oblique m.
8	Optic n. (CN II)
9	Oculomotor n. (CN III)
10	Ciliary ganglion
11	Short ciliary nn.
12	Trochlear n. (CN IV)
13	Lacrimal n.
14	Infratrochlear n.
15	Maxillary n.
16	Abducens n. (CN VI)
17	Periorbita
18	Mandible, ramus cut and removed
19	Medial pterygoid m.
20	Pterygopalatine n.
21	Pterygopalatine ganglion
22-26	Branches of mandibular n.
22	Buccal n.
23	Lingual n.
24	Inferior alveolar n.
25	Mylohyoid n.
26	Auriculotemporal n.
27	Auricular concha
28	M. masseter
29	Parotid duct
30	Facial n. (CN VII)
31	Caudal auricular n.
32	Parotid branch
33	Auriculopalpebral n.
34	Rostral auricular n.
35	Palpebral n.
36	Dorsal buccal branch
37	Ventral buccal branch
38	Branches of auriculotemporal n. (CN V)
39	Petrous temporal bone
40	Internal acoustic meatus
41	Tympanic bulla
42	Vestibulocochlear n. (CN VIII)
43	Pharynx
44	M. longus capitis, cut and removed
45	Glossopharyngeal n. (CN IX)
46	Vagus n. (CN X)
47	Distal vagal ganglion
48	Cranial laryngeal n.
49	Cranial cervical ganglion
50	Cervical sympathetic trunk
51	Vagosympathetic trunk
52	Accessory n. (CN XI)
53	C1 Spinal n.
54	External carotid a.
55	M. digastricus, cut and removed
56	M. sternocephalicus, cut and removed
57	External jugular v.
58	Hypoglossal n. (CN XII)

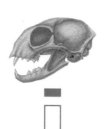

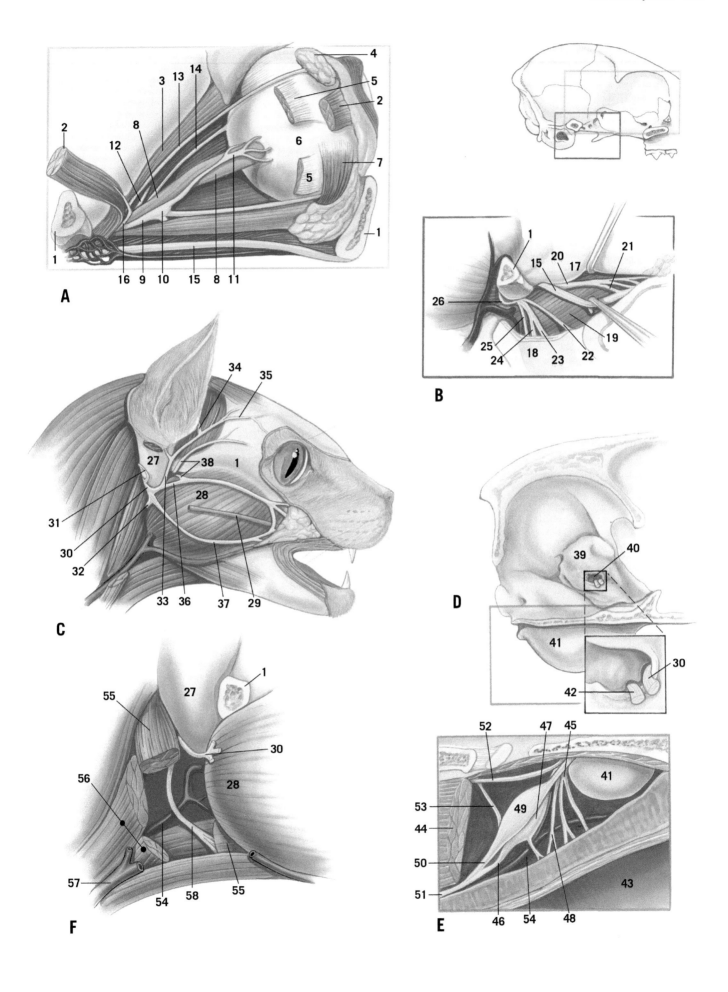

TABLE 10-2
Function of Nerves of the Brachial and Lumbosacral Plexi

Nerve	Motor Function	Sensory Function (Cutaneous Innervation as Autonomous Zones)
Brachial Plexus		
Cranial Pectoral nn.	superficial pectoral m.	
Caudal Pectoral nn.	deep pectoral m.	
Long Thoracic n.	m. serratus ventralis	
Thoracodorsal n.	m. latissimus dorsi	skin over lateral thorax
Suprascapular n.	m. supraspinatus, m. infraspinatus	glenohumeral joint skin over craniomedial brachium
Subscapular n.	m. subscapularis	
Axillary n.	m. teres major, m. teres minor, m. deltoideus, caudal margin of m. subscapularis	skin over lateral brachium and distal craniolateral brachium, skin over proximal cranial surface of antebrachium (via cranial cutaneous antebrachial n.)
Musculocutaneous n.		
proximal branch	m. coracobrachialis, m. biceps brachii	
distal branch	m. brachialis	cubital joint skin over medial surface of antebrachium (via medial cutaneous antebrachial n.)
Radial n.	m. triceps brachii, m. anconeus, m. tensor fasciae antebrachii, m. brachioradialis	
deep branch	m. extensor carpi radialis, m. common digital extensor, m. lateral digital extensor, m. extensor carpi ulnaris (ulnaris lateralis), m. supinator, m. abductor pollicis longus, m. extensor pollicis longus	
superficial branch		skin over lateral forearm (via lateral cutaneous antebrachial n.), skin over dorsum of digits II, III, and medial IV
Median n.	m. flexor carpi radialis, m. pronator teres, m. pronator quadratus, deep digital flexor m. (radial head), m. superficial digital flexor, m. superficial digital flexor, mm. interflexorii	cubital and carpal joints, skin over palmar digits II, III, and medial IV
Ulnar n.	m. flexor carpi ulnaris, deep digital flexor m. (ulnar and humeral heads)	cubital and carpal joints, skin over medial distal brachium and caudal antebrachium (via caudal cutaneous antebrachial n.)
dorsal branch		skin over lateral carpus and metacarpus, skin over dorsal digit V
palmar branch	mm. interossei, abductor and adductor muscles of digits I, II, and V	skin over palmar digit V and lateral palmar IV palmar digital joints

TABLE 10-2 (Continued)
Function of Nerves of the Brachial and Lumbosacral Plexi

Nerve	Motor Function	Sensory Function (Cutaneous Innervation as Autonomous Zones)
Lumbosacral Plexus		
Lateral Cutaneous Femoral n.	m. psoas minor	skin over craniolateral thigh and adjacent abdomen
Genitofemoral n.		scrotum and prepuce, or inguinal mammary gland, skin of medial proximal thigh
Femoral n.	m. iliopsoas (part), m. sartorius, m. quadriceps femoris	skin over medial thigh, crus, metatarsus (via saphenous n.), stifle joint (via saphenous n.)
Obturator n.	m. pectineus, m. gracilis, m. adductor longus, m. external obturator	
Cranial Gluteal n	middle gluteal m., deep gluteal m., m. tensor fasciae latae	
Caudal Gluteal n.	superficial gluteal m.,	
Caudal Gluteal n.	superficial gluteal m., m. gluteofemoris, cranial part of m. biceps femoris	
Caudal Cutaneous Femoral n.		skin over caudal thigh
Pudendal n.	m. ischiourethralis, urethral sphincter	skin over perineum (via perineal nn.), scrotum or labia, penis or clitoris
Caudal Rectal n.	external anal sphincter m., m. coccygeus, m. levator ani, m. bulbospongiosus or m. constrictor vulvae	
Sciatic n. (divides into common peroneal and tibial nn.)	m. gemelli, m. internal obturator, m. quadratus femoris, m. biceps femoris, m. semitendinosus, m. semimembranosus, caudal crural abductor m.	coxofemoral joint
Common Peroneal n.		
Common Peroneal n. (superficial and deep peroneal nn.)	cranial tibial m., long digital extensor m., lateral digital extensor m., m. peroneus longus, m. peroneus brevis, short digital extensor m.	stifle joint, skin over lateral crus, skin over dorsal tarsus, metatarsus, and digits
Tibial n.	m. gastrocnemius. m. soleus, m. popliteus, superficial digital flexor m., deep digital flexor m., m. caudal tibial, mm. interflexorii, short digital flexor m., m. quadratus plantae, mm. interossei, abductor and adductor muscles of digits II and V	stifle joint skin over caudal crus, skin over plantar tarsus, metatarsus, and digits

Plate 10-7

Figure A   Cervical nerves and formation of the brachial plexus, ventral view

Figure B   Caudal lumbar and sacral nerves, and formation of the lumbosacral plexus with muscles removed, ventral view

1	M. brachiocephalicus, cut	**23**	Fifth lumbar vertebra
2	M. pectoral profundus, cut	**24**	Sixth lumbar vertebra
3	M. latissimus dorsi	**25**	Seventh lumbar vertebra
4	First rib	**26**	Sacrum
5	Second cervical n.	**27**	Os coxae
6	Third cervical n.	**28**	Obturator foramen
7	Fourth cervical n.	**29**	Fourth lumbar n.
8	Fifth cervical n.	**30**	Fifth lumbar n.
9	Sixth cervical n.	**31**	Sixth lumbar n.
10	Seventh cervical n.	**32**	Seventh lumbar n.
11	Eighth cervical n.	**33**	Ventral branch of first sacral n.
12	First thoracic n.	**34**	Ventral branch of second sacral n.
13	Phrenic n.	**35**	Ventral branch of third sacral n.
14-21	Nerves of the brachial plexus	**36**	Contribution to pelvic n.
14	Suprascapular n.	**37-42**	Nerves of the lumbosacral plexus
15	Subscapular n.	**37**	Femoral n.
16	Axillary n.	**38**	Saphenous n.
17	Musculocutaneous n.	**39**	Obturator n.
18	Radial n.	**40**	Lumbosacral trunk (gives rise to cranial gluteal, caudal gluteal, sciatic, and caudal cutaneous femoral nn.)
19	Median n.		
20	Ulnar n.		
21	Thoracodorsal n.	**41**	Pudendal n.
22	Fourth lumbar vertebra	**42**	Caudal rectal n.

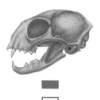

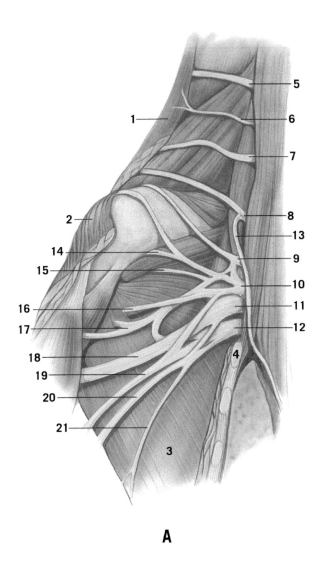

A

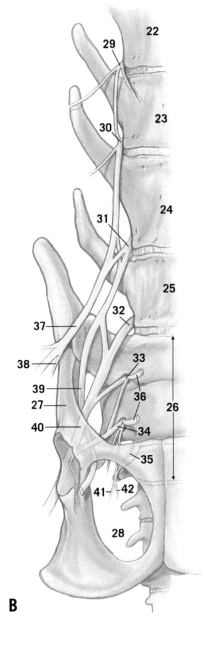

B

Plate 10-8

Figure A   Schematic illustration of brachial plexus nerves innervating intrinsic thoracic limb, medial view

Figure B   Superficial nerves of the forepaw, dorsal view

Figure C   Superficial (top) and deep nerves of the forepaw, palmar view

1	Subscapular n.	8	Medial cutaneous antebrachial n.
2	Suprascapular n.	9	Cranial cutaneous antebrachial n.
3	Musculocutaneous n.	10	Caudal cutaneous antebrachial n.
	3' Proximal branch	11	Dorsal common digital nn. I-IV
	3" Distal branch	12	Axial/abaxial dorsal proper digital nn. I-V
4	Axillary n.		
5	Radial n.	13	Superficial branch of palmar branch of ulnar n.
	5' Deep branch		
	5" Superficial branch	14	Deep branch of palmar branch of ulnar n.
6	Median n.		
7	Ulnar n.	15	Palmar common digital nn. I-IV
	7' Dorsal branch	16	Axial/abaxial palmar proper digital nn. I-V
	7" Palmar branch		
		17	Palmar metacarpal nn. I-IV

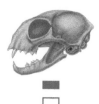

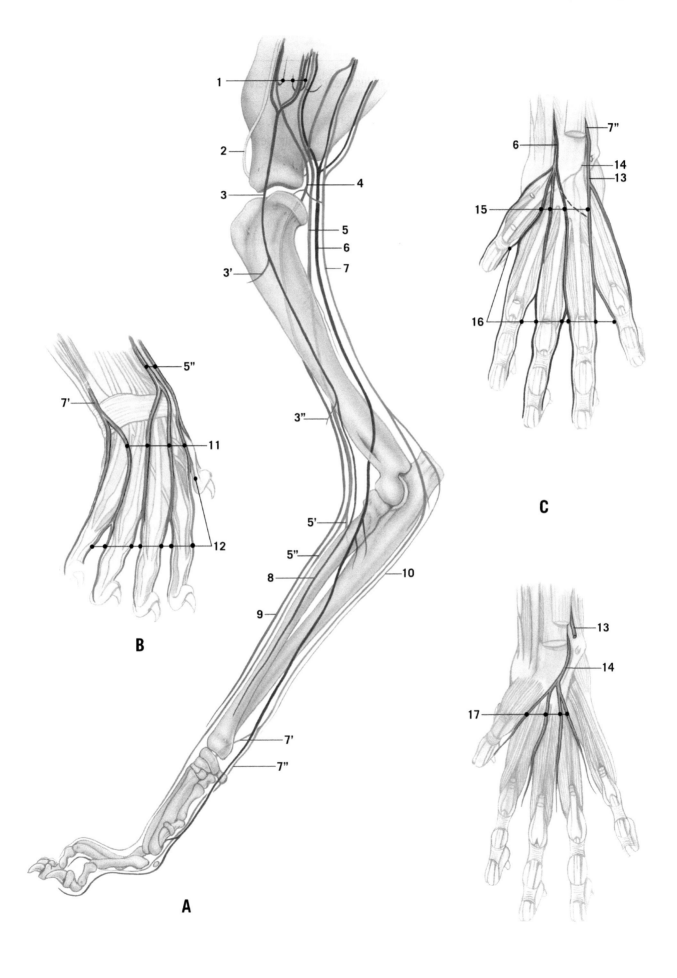

1

2

3

4

5

6

7

3'

3"

5'

5"

8

9

10

7'

7"

A

B

5"

7'

11

12

C

6

7"

14

13

15

16

13

14

17

Plate 10-9

Figure A   Schematic illustration of lumbosacral plexus nerves innervating the pelvic limb, lateral view

Figure B   Superficial and deep (inset) nerves of the pes, dorsal view

Figure C   Superficial (top) and deep innervation of the pes, plantar view

m   Medial
l   Lateral
1   Femoral n.
    1'   Saphenous n.
2   Obturator n.
3   Cranial gluteal n.
4   Caudal gluteal n.
5   Pudendal n.
6   Caudal cutaneous femoral n.
7   Sciatic n.
    7'   Caudal cutaneous sural n.
    7"   Lateral cutaneous sural n.
8   Tibial n.

9   Common peroneal (fibular) n.
    9'   Deep peroneal (fibular) n.
    9"   Superficial peroneal (fibular) n.
10   Dorsal common digital nn. II-IV
11   Axial/abaxial dorsal proper digital nn. II-V
12   Dorsal metatarsal nn. II, IV
13   Medial plantar n.
14   Lateral plantar n.
    14'   Superficial branch
    14"   Deep branch
15   Plantar common digital nn. II-IV
16   Axial/abaxial plantar proper digital nn. II-V
17   Plantar metatarsal nn. II-IV

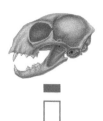

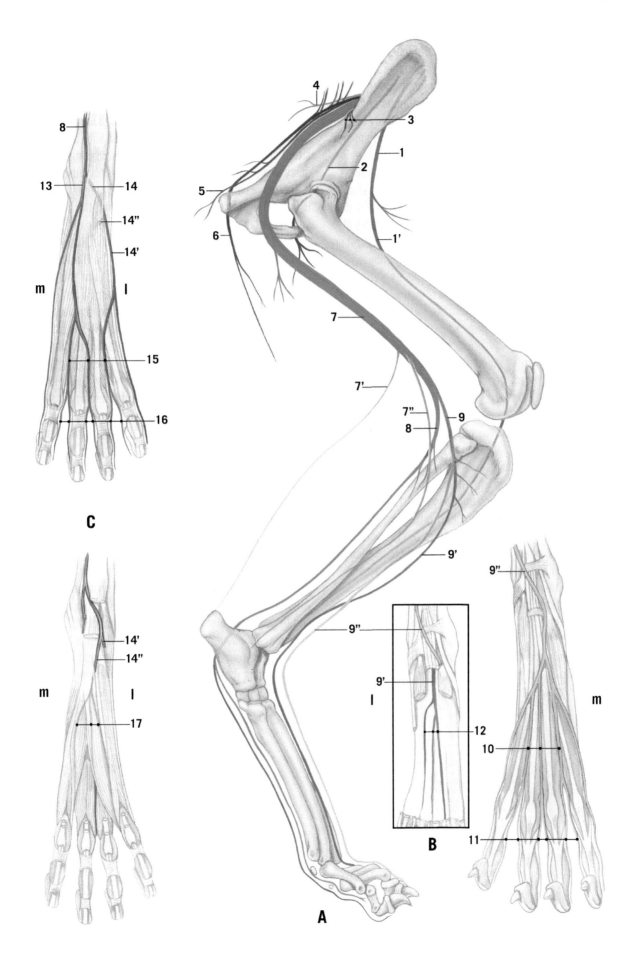

Autonomic Nervous System

The autonomic nervous system (ANS) is usually considered only in terms of its motor components, especially its peripheral motor neurons. However, the system includes sensory input and input from motor areas in the brain such as the hypothalamus and the reticular formation, i.e., vomiting center. The ANS is largely responsible for innervation of viscera, glands, blood vessels, and smooth muscle throughout the body. Appropriate responses to changes in the external and internal environments are mediated by the ANS. Autonomic motor impulses travel from a nerve cell body located in the parasympathetic nuclei of CNs III, VII, IX, or X of the brain stem or the zona intermedia of thoracolumbar and sacral segments of the spinal cord (preganglionic neuron), outwards into the periphery and through a synapse onto a second neuron (postganglionic neuron). The nerve cell bodies of the second neuron are gathered into ganglia, which contain one to thousands of neurons. The axon of the postganglionic neuron will innervate the target organ, such as smooth muscle or gland. One known exception to the rule of a 2-neuron connection in the ANS is the medulla of the adrenal gland, which receives only preganglionic fibers. However, the adrenal medulla cells are considered to be modified postganglionic neurons.

The autonomic nervous system is usually divided into sympathetic and parasympathetic divisions based on both anatomic and physiologic characteristics. In general, all tissue receiving autonomic innervation will receive fibers from both divisions, which, in turn, have basically opposite effects upon that tissue. As an example, sympathetic stimulation increases heart rate while parasympathetic stimulation decreases heart rate. Exceptions to this rule of both divisions innervating structures are the adrenal medulla, sweat glands, blood vessels, and mm. arrectores pilorum in the skin; these tissues receive only sympathetic innervation.

The two divisions have a constant basal rate of activity producing sympathetic or parasympathetic tone so that loss of one type results in a net effect of increased tone of the opposite type on the target tissue.

Feline dysautonomia is a disease of unknown etiology affecting the nerve cell bodies of the preganglionic and postganglionic neurons. Clinical signs relate to decreased function of lacrimal and salivary glands, decreased esophageal and intestinal motility, bradycardia and inability to increase heart rate, protrusion of the 3rd eyelid, and dilated pupils.

Sympathetic Division

This division is largely involved with body reactions in response to "flight or fight" situations. A cat faced with an emergency situation will react by dilating pupils, increasing heart rate, decreasing gut motility, vasodilation of limb muscles, etc.

The nerve cell body of the sympathetic preganglionic neuron is located in the zona intermedia, including the lateral horn, of spinal cord segments T_1-L_4. (The sympathetic division is sometimes referred to as the thoracolumbar division because of the location of the preganglionic nerve cell bodies in the thoracolumbar spinal cord.) The axon leaves in the ventral root, joins the spinal nerve and then leaves in the ramus communicans. Each ramus joins with a sympathetic (paravertebral) ganglion located ventrolateral to the thoracolumbar vertebral column. Additionally, these ganglia are interconnected with each other along the longitudinal axis forming bilateral, elongate sympathetic trunks. These ganglia positioned along the sympathetic trunks contain postganglionic sympathetic nerve cell bodies. At the cranial end of the thoracic sympathetic trunk is the cervicothoracic ganglion. This relatively large ganglion is formed by the fusion of the caudal cervical ganglion, and the T_1 and T_2 sympathetic trunk ganglia.

In the sympathetic division, the 2-neuron connection between CNS and target tissue must begin at the T_1-L_4 spinal cord initially, a relatively small area. But, the sympathetic division will target structures in the cat from the tip of the nose to the tip of the tail. Therefore, pathways for extending sympathetic fibers beyond the level of thoracolumbar vertebrae are present.

The sympathetic trunks, which are formed in the thoracolumbar region, are extended cranially by the (sympathetic part of the) vagosympathetic trunks in the neck. The vagosympathetic trunk and the cervicothoracic ganglion are connected by a loop of nerves, the ansa subclavia, which travels around the subclavian a. Each vagosympathetic trunk has the cranial cervical and middle cervical ganglia along its length where synapses of preganglionic and postganglionic sympathetic neurons can occur. Also in the neck region is the vertebral n. This is a bundle of postganglionic sympathetic fibers leaving the cervicothoracic ganglion and passing through successive transverse foramina of the cervical vertebrae.

There are nerves extending from the thoracic and lumbar sympathetic trunks into the abdominal cavity to sympathetic (prevertebral) ganglia. The major splanchnic n., minor splanchnic nn., and lumbar splanchnic nn. on each side of the body are examples of such nerves. The sympathetic ganglia in the abdominal cavity are most often located around large arteries and have the same name as the artery. These include the celiac ganglia, cranial mesenteric ganglion, and caudal mesenteric ganglion. The celiac and cranial mesenteric ganglia may be fused into a single mass called the celiacomesenteric ganglion. The tangle of fibers entering and leaving each ganglion forms a plexus - celiac, cranial mesenteric, and caudal mesenteric plexi. Generally, sympathetic fibers leaving these abdominal ganglia to viscera travel in unnamed rami along the surface of arteries supplying the various organs.

The hypogastric nn. extend the sympathetic division caudally. The hypogastric nn. leave the caudal mesenteric ganglion to travel into the pelvic cavity to pelvic organs. As a hypogastric n. enters the pelvis, the fibers mesh with the pelvic n. (parasympathetic division) and form a pelvic plexus on the lateral surface of the rectum before traveling to the target organs.

The neurotransmitter at the synapse of preganglionic and postganglionic neurons is most commonly acetylcholine. The neurotransmitter at the postganglionic neuron - target junction is most commonly norepinephrine in the sympathetic division. Development of different neurotransmitters (alpha, beta 1, beta 2, etc) allows different reactions in different tissues to the same neurotransmitters.

The diversity of possible routes for both the preganglionic and postganglionic sympathetic fibers within the sympathetic trunks and its branches has made it difficult to map the pathways to specific organs. However, the pathway to the dilator muscles of the pupil is known (see Chapter 11 also). Horner's syndrome is the clinical condition resulting from disruption of this pathway.

Parasympathetic Division

This division is involved with body responses of an animal in a relaxed state. Parasympathetic stimulation causes pupil constriction, increased gut motility after eating, decreased heart rate, increased salivation, etc.

The nerve cell bodies of the preganglionic neuron of the parasympathetic division are located in the parasympathetic nuclei of CNs III, VII, IX, and X, located in the mesencephalon and myelencephalon, and in the zona intermedia of the sacral spinal cord segments. (The parasympathetic division may be referred to as the craniosacral division because of the location of the preganglionic nerve cell bodies in the brain and sacral segments of the spinal cord.) Again, although there is a finite location of preganglionic neurons, the postganglionic neuron-target junctions are throughout the body.

The pathways beginning in CNs III, VII, and IX innervate certain structures of the head - the smooth muscles of the eye, lacrimal, nasal, and salivary glands. These cranial nerves have autonomic ganglia along their length (see Table 10-1). Parasympathetic fibers in CN X are distributed to cervical, thoracic, and abdominal viscera via the vagus portion of the vagosympathetic trunk and various branches of the vagus nerves. Upon reaching the abdomen, various unnamed rami travel along the large arteries (with sympathetic nerves) to reach the organs. The synapse of vagal preganglionic parasympathetic fibers with postganglionic parasympathetic neurons is usually within the wall of the target organ. This type of ganglia is collectively referred to as terminal ganglia.

Parasympathetic preganglionic fibers of the sacral spinal nerves initially travel in the pelvic n. The pelvic n. and hypogastric n. (sympathetic) meet and form a pelvic plexus on the lateral surface of the rectum. Imbedded within the pelvic plexus are pelvic ganglia. These ganglia are the location of some synapses of parasympathetic preganglionic fibers in the pelvic n. with parasympathetic postganglionic neurons. Parasympathetic pathways beginning in the sacral spinal cord segments are distributed to pelvic viscera and parts of the colon.

The neurotransmitter at the preganglionic and postganglionic neurons, and at the postganglionic neuron - target junction is usually acetylcholine.

Plate 10-10

Figure A　Location of cutaneous nerves and vessels of the trunk deep to the skin and superficial to most musculature

Figure B　Schematic illustration of the autonomic nervous system; distribution of parasympathetic division (orange) and sympathetic division (green) innervation. Solid lines indicate preganglionic nerves and dotted lines indicate postganglionic nerves.

1　Dorsal cutaneous branches of (dorsal branches of) cervical spinal nn.
2　Dorsal cutaneous branches of (dorsal branches of) thoracic spinal nn.
3　Dorsal cutaneous branches of (dorsal branches of) lumbar spinal nn.
4　Dorsal cutaneous branches of (dorsal branches of) sacral spinal nn.
5-6　Ventral branch of second cervical n.
5　Great auricular n.
6　Transverse cervical n.
7　Lateral cutaneous branches of (ventral branches of) cervical spinal nn.
8　Lateral cutaneous branches of intercostal (ventral branches of thoracic spinal) nn.
9　Lateral cutaneous branches of (ventral branches of) lumbar spinal nn.
10　Ventral cutaneous branches of intercostal (ventral branches of thoracic spinal) nn.
11　Thoracodorsal a.
12　Lateral thoracic n.
13a　Cranial superficial epigastric a.
13b　Caudal superficial epigastric a.

14　Lateral cutaneous femoral n.
15　Cranial abdominal a.
16　Caudal abdominal a.
17　Caudal cutaneous femoral n.
T_1　First thoracic spinal segment
T_{13}　Thirteenth thoracic spinal segment
L_1　First lumbar spinal segment
L_4　Fourth lumbar spinal segment
S_1　First sacral spinal segment
S_2　Second sacral spinal segment
18　Ciliary ganglion
19　Pterygopalatine ganglion
20　Submandibular ganglion
21　Mandibular ganglion
22　Otic ganglion
23　Cranial cervical ganglion
24　Middle cervical ganglion
25　Cervicothoracic ganglion
26　Sympathetic trunk
27　Sympathetic trunk ganglia
28　Celiacomesenteric ganglion (celiac ganglia and cranial mesenteric ganglion)

29　Caudal mesenteric ganglion
30　Pelvic ganglion
31　Cranial nerve III (oculomotor n)
32　Cranial nerve VII (facial n)
33　Cranial nerve IX (glossopharyngeal n)
34　Cranial nerve X (vagus n)
35　Ramus communicans of thoracolumbar spinal nn
36　Major splanchnic n
37　Minor splanchnic nn
38　Lumbar splanchnic nn
39　Hypogastric n
40　Pelvic n
41　Lacrimal gland
42　Nasal gland
43　Zygomatic salivary gland
44　Polystomatic sublingual salivary gland
45　Monostomatic sublingual salivary gland
46　Mandibular salivary gland
47　Parotid salivary gland

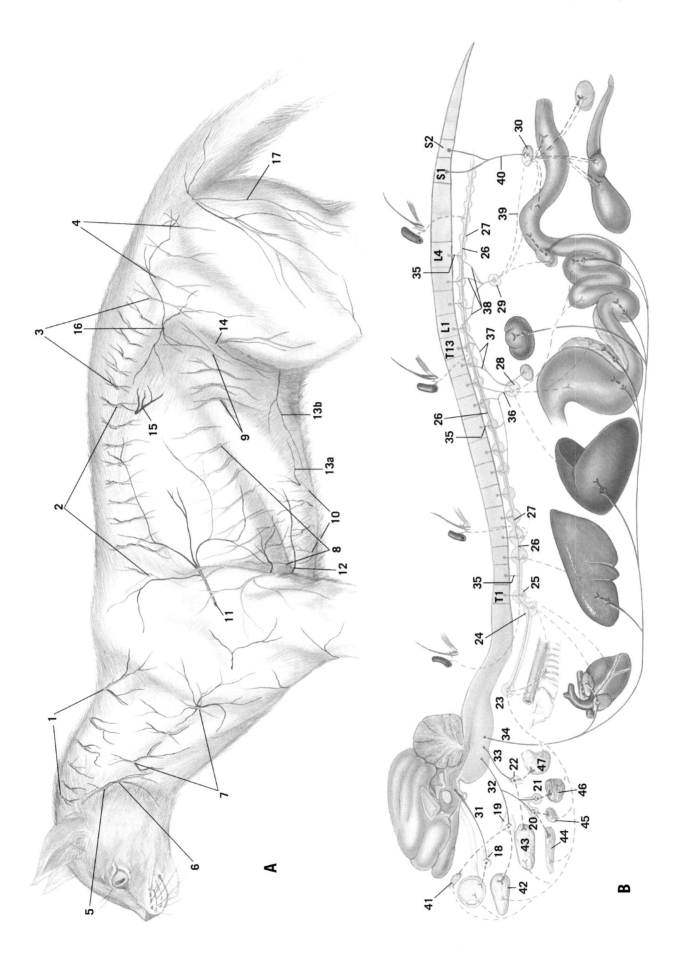

Plate 10-11

Figure A   Autonomic nervous system (ANS) of neck and thorax ribs and thoracic limb removed, lateral view.

Figure B   ANS of the abdomen and pelvis, left abdominal wall and os coxae removed and intestines retracted, lateral view

1   Trachea
2   Esophagus
3   Heart
4   Diaphragm
5   First rib
6   Eighth rib
7   Aorta
8   Phrenic n.
9   Distal vagal ganglion
10-16   Parasympathetic ANS
10   (Vagus part of) vagosympathetic trunk
11   Vagus n.
12a   Dorsal branch of vagus n.
12b   Ventral branch of vagus n.
13   Dorsal vagal trunk
14   Ventral vagal trunk
15   Pelvic n.
16   Pelvic plexus
17   Recurrent laryngeal n.
18-30   Sympathetic ANS
18   Cranial cervical ganglion
19   (Sympathetic part of) vagosympathetic trunk
20   Ansa subclavia
21   Vertebral n.

22   Cervicothoracic ganglion
23   Sympapastic trunk
24   Sympathetic trunk ganglia
25   Major splanchnic n.
26   Minor splanchnic nn.
27   Celiacomesenteric ganglion (fused celiac and cranial mesenteric ganglia)
28   Lumbar splanchnic nn.
29   Caudal mesenteric ganglion
30   Hypogastric n.
31   Adrenal gland
32   Rectum

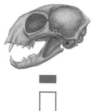

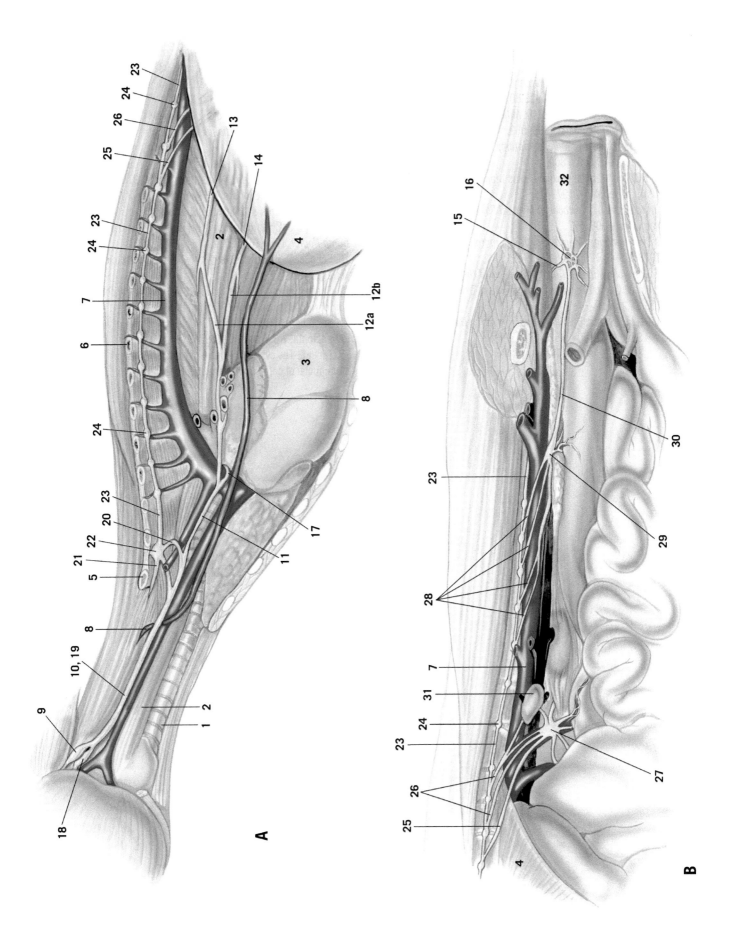

Selected References

1. Beitz AJ, Fletcher TF. In: Evans HE. *Miller's Anatomy of the Dog.* 3rd Ed. Philadelphia, WB Saunders, 1993; 894.

2. DeLahunta A. *Veterinary Neuroanatomy and Clinical Neurology.* 2nd Ed. Philadelphia, W.B. Saunders, Co., 1983;30, 95.

3. Evans HE, Kitchell, RL. In: Evans HE. *Miller's Anatomy of the Dog.* 3rd Ed. Philadelphia, WB Saunders, 1993; 953.

4. Fletcher, TF. In: Evans HE. *Miller's Anatomy of the Dog.* 3rd Ed. Philadelphia, WB Saunders, 1993; 800.

5. Ghoshal NG. The brachial plexus (plexus brachialis) of the cat (Felis domesticus). *Zbl Vet Med C* 1972;1:6.

6. Guyton A and Hall, JE. *Textbook of Medical Physiology,* 11th Ed. St Louis, Elsevier Saunders, 2006; 57.

7. Jenkins TW. *Functional Mammalian Neuroanatomy.* Philadelphia, Lea & Febiger, 1978;97,146,166,302.

8. King AS. *Physiological and Clinical Anatomy of the Domestic Mammals.* Vol 1. Central Nervous System. Oxford, Oxford University Press, 1987;1,8,13,24,255.

9. Kitchell RL. In: Evans HE. *Miller's Anatomy of the Dog.* 3rd Ed. Philadelphia, WB Saunders, 1993; 758.

10. Kitchell RL, et al. Electrophysiologic studies of cutaneous nerves of the forelimb of the cat. *J Comp Neurol* 1982;210:400.

11. Kitchell RL, Evans HE. In: Evans HE. *Miller's Anatomy of the Dog.* 3rd Ed. Philadelphia, WB Saunders, 1993;829.

12. Kornegay JN. Feline Neurology. In: Kay WJ and Brown NO (eds): *Problems in Veterinary Medicine.* Philadelphia, JB Lippincott, 1991:309,363,382,391

13. Nickel R, Schummer A, and Seiferle E. *Lehrbuch der Anatomie der Haustiere, Band IV. Berlin,* Verlag Paul Parey, 1975;30,60,174.

14. Noden D and DeLahunta A. *The Embryology of Domestic Animals.* Baltimore, Williams & Wilkins, 1985;92.

15. Rexed B. A Cytoarchitectonic atlas of the spinal cord in the cat. *J Comp Neurol,* 1954;100:297.

16. Schaller O. Illustrated Veterinary Nomina Anatomica. Stuttgart, Enke Verlag, 1992: 414.

17. Sharp NJH and Wheeler SJ. *Small Animal Spinal Disorders,* 2nd Ed. Edinburgh, Elsevier Mosby, 2005; 1, 261.

18. Stromberg MW. In: Evans HE. *Miller's Anatomy of the Dog.* 3rd Ed. Philadelphia, WB Saunders, 1993; 776.

19. Taber E. The cytoarchitecture of the brain stem of the cat. I. Brain stem nuclei of cat. *J Comp Neurol* 1961;116:27.

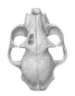

Chapter 11

Part 1: Ear

▌Lola C. Hudson

Modified from the original chapter by Randall Scagliotti

Ear

The ears, specifically the internal ear, house the receptors for the special senses of hearing and balance, which are extraordinary in the cat. Knowledge of the special anatomy of the ears of the cat is the basis for understanding the physiology of these special senses as manifested in health and disease.

The ear consists of three anatomically and functionally distinct parts: the external ear, the middle ear, and the internal ear. The entire middle and internal ear, and a small part of the external ear are located in the temporal bone of the skull.

Temporal Bone

The paired temporal bones are the most prominent bones in the ventrolateral walls of the skull. Separable into squamous, tympanic and petrous parts, the different areas house and protect delicate elements of the ear and also act as a conduit for the passage of nerves and vessels that are unrelated to the direct functions of the ear. Therefore, disease in certain areas of the ear within the petrous bone can affect more than one body system simply due to structures passing each other closely, if functionally distinct.

The External Ear

The external ear consists of a sound collecting part, the auricle (pinna) on the head surface and a short sound conducting tube, the external acoustic meatus (ear canal) that ends medially at the tympanic membrane located at the osseous external acoustic meatus of the skull.

Auricle

The auricle includes a number of ridges and prominences that give the ear base its distinct appearance. The ridge forming the lateral edge of the canal opening is the tragus and the margin of the ear flap is called the helix. Along the caudolateral edge is a marginal cutaneous pouch, which has no known function. The auricle is covered by integument on all surfaces and has a thin curved plate of auricular cartilage, sandwiched in between, to which numerous auricular muscles are attached. The integument on the convex surface is often injured when the cat scratches vigorously. Most cats have erect auricles, but an exception is the Scottish Fold, in which the most distal portion of the auricle is bent rostroventrally beginning at 3-4 weeks of age.

The auricular muscles move the auricle for optimal sound wave gathering and can alter the shape of cartilage at the entrance to the acoustic meatus. The inner surface of the initial part of the external ear canal has numerous prominent ridges with furrows between them. These ridges are due to folds in the cartilage, which correspond to projections to which intrinsic ear muscles attach.

External Auditory Meatus

The external auditory meatus extends more or less ventrally at its more superficial part, and then turns essentially medially to the tympanic membrane. The canal consists of two parts; a long, lateral cartilaginous meatus formed by the deeper parts of the auricular cartilage and the annular cartilage, and a more medial, short osseous external acoustic meatus. The external auditory meatus is lined by integument including the lateral surface of the tympanic membrane. The subcutaneous tissue of the canal contains ceruminous glands, which secrete the ear wax commonly seen during an otoscopic exam. *Otodectes cynotis*, a mite, lives on the surface of the canal and feeds on the epidermal debris. This causes intense irritation and causes the canal to fill with thick reddish brown crusts mixed with cerumen.

The rostral wall of the auricular cartilage is connected by muscle to the angular process of the mandible. Chronic otitis externa, especially with ossification of the cartilaginous portion of the canal, can lead to pain during jaw opening because of pressure on the canal by the mandible and rostral auricular muscles. The ventral and lateral canal wall is closely bound by the parotid gland.

Scutiform Cartilage

The long, narrow scutiform cartilage, although not forming part of the external ear, is closely connected with it. It lies in the temporal fossa between the integument and the m. temporalis, beneath the rostromedial portion of the auricle. It serves as the attachment for a number of rostral auricular muscles.

Muscles of the External Ear

One group of muscles connects the cartilages of the external ear with other parts of the head (extrinsic auricular muscles); while another group mostly interconnects the cartilages of the external ear or parts of these cartilages (intrinsic auricular muscles) (see Tables 11-1 and 11-2).

Innervation and Blood Supply

The general sensory nerves of the auricle are from branches of the auricular branch of the vagus (CN X) n., facial (CN VII) n. and second cervical (great auricular) n. All of the muscles of the external ear are innervated by the facial n. The arteries supplying the auricle are branches of the caudal auricular and superficial temporal aa., both of which are derived from the external carotid a. Venous drainage occurs from the caudal auricular and superficial temporal vv. into the maxillary v.

The Middle Ear

The middle ear includes the tympanic membrane, the tympanic cavity and its contents, and the auditory tube. It is located within the large, hollow, olive-shaped bone known as the tympanic bulla of the temporal bone. The bulla develops from two bones, the pars tympanica (lateral) and pars endotympanica (medial), that are well delineated in kittens and a little less so in adults. The pars tympanica makes up the lateral wall and surrounds the opening of the osseous external auditory meatus. In the cat, there is an incomplete bony septum bullae that subdivides the middle ear cavity into small dorsolateral and large ventromedial compartments. The septum bullae extends from the lateral (internal) wall of the tympanic bullae to the barrel-shaped promontory (petrous temporal

TABLE 11-1
Extrinsic Auricular Muscles

Muscle	Function
Rostral auricular muscles	Pull the ear rostrally
Scutuloauricularis superficialis	Draws the external ear rostrally
Scutuloauricularis profundus	Pulls the concha rostrodorsally
Frontoscutularis	Pulls the external ear rostrally
Zygomaticoscutularis	Pulls the external ear rostrally
Zygomaticoauricularis	Pulls the external ear rostrodorsally
Dorsal auricular muscles	Pull the ear dorsally
Interscutularis	Draws the ears dorsally toward the midline
Parietoscutularis	Pulls the external ear dorsally
Parietoauricularis	Pulls the external ear dorsally
Caudal auricular muscles	Pull the ear caudally
Cervicoscutularis	Pulls the external ear dorsocaudally
Cervicoauricularis superficialis	Pulls the external ear dorsocaudally
Cervicoauricularis medius	Pulls the external ear caudally
Cervicoauricularis profundus	Pulls the external ear caudally
Ventral auricular muscles	Pull the external ear ventrally
Parotidoauricularis	Draws the external ear ventrally
Styloauricularis	Pulls the ear ventrally and rotates it outward

bone). The two compartments communicate with each other by an opening at the caudodorsal margin of the septum bullae near the cochlear window.

Tympanic Membrane

As a thin, slightly opaque membranous partition, the tympanic membrane serves as the deep border of the external acoustic meatus and superficial border of the tympanic cavity. It is oval to elliptical in outline and much of its surface, especially the periphery, is not visualized during routine otoscopic exam. What often passes as an intact tympanic membrane is frequently perforated near its periphery, thus, explaining signs of acute otitis media present shortly following an ear cleansing. The lateral surface of the membrane is lined by a layer of skin that is continuous with the skin of the external auditory meatus; the medial surface is lined with the mucous membrane that also lines

TABLE 11-2
Intrinsic Auricular Muscles

Muscle	Function
Helicis	Draws rostral margin of auricle proximally
Helicis minor	
Tragicus	Flexes concha
Antitragicus	Constricts the external auditory opening
Caudoantitragicus	Constricts concha
Transversus auriculae	Flexes scapha medially on concha

the tympanic cavity. The manubrium of the malleus traverses the dorsal third of the membrane and is firmly attached to it. It draws the membrane medially, imparting a slight depression that can be seen with an otoscope.

Tympanic Cavity and Contents

The air-filled space of the tympanic cavity communicates via the auditory tube with the nasopharynx to maintain equal pressure on either side of the tympanic membrane. It is lined with mucous membrane. Removal of the thin, ventrolateral surface of the tympanic bullae reveals the septum bullae and the ventromedial compartment of the tympanic cavity of the middle ear. The dorsolateral compartment walls are marked by four apertures: the vestibular (oval) and cochlear (round) windows on the medial wall, the tympanic membrane on the lateral wall, and the tympanic ostium leading into the auditory tube on its rostral wall. There are additional openings associated with the tympanic cavity to allow passage of several nerves and small blood vessels. The dorsolateral compartment or true tympanic chamber contains the auditory ossicles that transmit vibrations from the tympanic membrane across the cavity to the labyrinth, and the muscles of the ossicles.

Auditory Ossicles

Within the tympanic cavity are three small, movable bones collectively called the auditory ossicles. They extend like a chain across the tympanic cavity and functionally connect the tympanic membrane with the vestibular window. The most lateral ossicle is the malleus, which is attached to the tympanic membrane. The most medial ossicle is the stapes that is in direct contact with the perilymph fluid through its footplate attachment in the vestibular window. Between and articulating with the other two ossicles, is the incus. In this way, vibrations of the tympanic membrane are transmitted through the chain of bones to the perilymph fluid within the vestibule.

Malleus

The malleus (hammer) consists of a head, a neck, a manubrium (handle) and rostral, muscular, and lateral processes. The head, which is smoothly rounded, articulates with the incus. The neck is a long, curved cylinder. The muscular process serves for attachment of the tendon of the m. tensor tympani. The feline manubrium is symmetrical and is the part of the malleus attached to the tympanic membrane.

Incus

The incus (anvil) shape is similar to a premolar tooth, with two roots forming a more or less right angle in between. The "tooth crown" corresponds to the body of the incus. The roots, represented by two processes of unequal length, correspond to crus breve and crus longum. The body articulates with the malleus. The crus breve is directed caudally and is attached at its tip by a strong ligament to the caudal wall of the middle ear. The crus longum extends ventrally and medially, nearly parallel to the neck of the malleus.

Plate 11-1

Figure A   Schematic illustration of structures of the right ear, transverse section through the external ear canal, cranial view

Figure B   Articulation of the left middle ear ossicles, caudal view

Figure C   Schematic illustration of sympathetic nerves through the middle ear cavity, ventral tympanic bulla and ventral septum bulla removed, ventral view

Figure D   Enlargement of structures of middle ear cavity, ventral bulla removed, ventral view; slight rostral rotation (above) to see additional middle ear structures

1	Skull	**11'**	Long crus
2	M. temporalis	**11"**	Short crus
3-6'	External ear	**12**	Stapes
	3-4 Auricular cartilage	**12'**	Base
	3 Scapha	**13**	Auditory tube
	4 Concha	**14**	Petrous temporal bone
	5 Annular cartilage	**15-17**	Osseous labyrinth
	6 External ear canal, vertical part	**15** Osseous semicircular canals
	6' External ear canal, horizontal part	**16** Osseous vestibule
		17 Osseous cochlea
7-12	Middle ear	**18**	External acoustic meatus
	7 Tympanic bulla	**19**	Tympano-occipital fissure
	8 Septum bullae	**20**	Cochlear window
	9 Tympanic membrane	**21**	Cervical sympathetic trunk
	10-12 Ear ossicles	**22**	Cranial cervical ganglion
	10 Malleus	**23**	Sympathetic rami
	10' Manubrium	**24**	Facial n.
	10" Head	**25**	M. tensor tympani
	11 Incus	**26**	M. stapedius

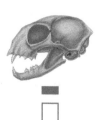

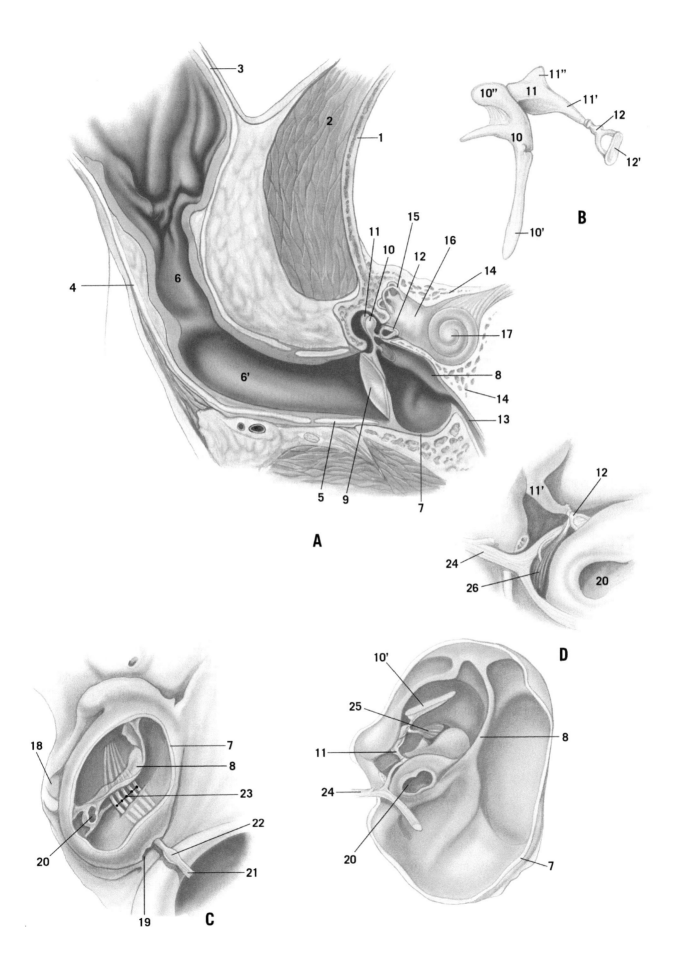

The extremity of the crus longum has a lenticular process, which articulates with the cupped head of the stapes. In the cat, this process is sometimes separate instead of joined, and is called the lenticular bone.

The ratio between the lengths of the manubrium of the malleus and the long process of the incus, is known as the lever ratio, varies in different species. The lever ratio in the cat (3.1 ± 0.6 Malleus: 1 Incus) is almost 3 times that of humans, and, in part, explains why sounds not heard by humans are easily detected by the cat. The long neck of the malleus in the cat increases the lever ratio, which in turn increases the magnification at the tip of the long process of the incus.

Stapes

The stapes is shaped like a stirrup. It consists of a head, which articulates with the incus; a neck; rostral and caudal legs, and a base (footplate). The rostral leg is shorter and straighter. The footplate corresponds to the shape of the vestibular window into which it fits and fills almost completely. The stapes is held in position by the m. stapedius, which is attached to a small process near the head of the stapes.

Auditory Muscles of the Middle Ear

In addition to ligaments that attach the auditory ossicles to the wall of the tympanic cavity, there are two striated muscles that move the articulations between ossicles and/or their borders. The m. tensor tympani is a short conical muscle that attaches on the neck of the malleus and a small fossa in the lateral surface of the petrous bone, near the vestibular window. This muscle serves to draw the manubrium medially and, thus, tighten the tympanic membrane. It is innervated by the tensor tympani n. (of the mandibular n.) of the trigeminal n. The m. stapedius, the smallest of all skeletal muscles, attaches to the head of the stapes and a narrow fossa on the lateral surface of the petrous bone. The muscle draws the cranial border of the base of the stapes laterally. It is innervated by the stapedial n. of the facial n.

Nerves of the Middle Ear

The nerves of the middle ear are of two types- those in transit through the middle ear destined for a distant location, and those that play a role in the normal function of the middle ear. All are susceptible to injury by disease in the middle ear.

Postganglionic Sympathetic Nerves

Sympathetic postganglionic neurons to the eye and orbit originate from nerve cell bodies located in the cranial cervical ganglion and pass through the middle ear cavity. The postganglionic fibers course through the tympano-occipital fissure with CNs IX, X, and XI and out from beneath the medial portion of the septum bullae at the margin of the promontory of the petrous temporal bone. They fan out as they pass over the promontory and disappear under the rostrolateral margin of the septum bullae. Occasionally a few fibers curve around the caudal portion of the promontory near the cochlear window. The fibers lie beneath the thin layer of mucous membrane lining the tympanic cavity and can be seen and manipulated easily with a fine probe during surgical ventral bulla osteotomy. The sympathetic fibers pass over the promontory of the petrous bone toward its apex to join the ventral surface of the trigeminal ganglion. They then pass with the ophthalmic n. of the trigeminal n. through the orbit to the eye and adnexa. Clinically, any otitis media or surgical manipulation of the bullae (such as resection of nasopharyngeal polyps that extend into the bullae from the auditory tube,) can lead to ocular signs associated with postganglionic sympathetic irritation or denervation (see Chapter 11, part 2 also).

Chorda Tympani Nerve

The chorda tympani n. arises from the facial n. within the petrous temporal bone. The chorda tympani n. then enters the cavity of the middle ear and passes medial to the malleus to ultimately join the lingual n. of the trigeminal n. The sensory fibers of the chorda tympani n. supply the taste buds of the rostral tongue and the autonomic motor fibers innervate the glands of the tongue to control secretion and vasodilation.

Tympanic Nerve and Tympanic Plexus

The tympanic n., a branch of the glossopharyngeal n., enters the tympanic cavity and then arborizes to form the tympanic plexus on the promontory of the petrous bone. In the cat, the tympanic plexus lies rostral and ventral to the fossa of the m. tensor tympani. The branches reunite forming the minor petrosal n. Some branches supply the mucous membrane lining the bony wall of the tympanic bulla.

Minor Petrosal Nerve

The minor petrosal n., a branch of the glossopharyngeal n., arises from the tympanic plexus on the promontory of the petrous temporal bone. It passes dorsal to the m. tensor tympani and through the medial aspect of the auditory tube to the otic ganglion. Its preganglionic parasympathetic fibers synapse with the postganglionic neurons in the otic ganglion, which are distributed to the parotid and zygomatic salivary glands. Cases of chronic otitis media may injure these nerves, which can lead to dry mouth.

Tensor Tympani Nerve

The tensor tympani n. issues from the mandibular n. of the trigeminal n. near the location of the otic ganglion. It enters the tympanic cavity below the auditory tube to innervate the m. tensor tympani.

Stapedius Nerves

Three to four stapedial nn. emerge from the facial n. near the point where the facial n. is crossed by the stapedial tendon. These nerves provide the motor supply to the m. stapedius.

Auditory Tube

The auditory tube is 1.5 to 2 cm long and extending rostromedially from the tympanic cavity to the nasopharynx. The pharyngeal opening is a small slit in the nasopharyngeal wall. The tube lumen is elliptical and has a thick cartilaginous medial wall and a thin connective tissue lateral wall. The lining of the auditory tube is mucous membrane continuous with that of the tympanic cavity. The auditory tube leaves the skull via the musculotubal canal near the rostromedial tympanic bulla.

The Internal Ear

The internal ear is located within the petrous temporal bone and consists of three primary parts: the membranous endolymphatic labyrinth, the osseous perilymphatic labyrinth, and the surrounding otic capsule. The internal ear contains the sensory organs of hearing and equilibrium for the cochlear and vestibular divisions of the vestibulocochlear (CN VIII) n. The petrous temporal bone consists of two parts, the dense, pyramidal-shaped portion and a flattened, triangular mastoid process, which is seen on the external surface of the skull. The pyramid has rostral, medial, ventral, and occipital faces and encloses the internal ear. The medial surface of the petrous bone bears the internal auditory meatus which is partitioned into a dorsal and ventral part. The dorsal portion is the beginning of the facial canal for the facial n.; the ventral portion presents several small foramina for the vestibulocochlear n.

Otic Capsule

The otic capsule is the innermost layer of bone bordering the series of cavities (osseous labyrinth) within the petrous bone. Acting like a protective shell, it is harder than the rest of the petrous bone and can be separated from the rest of the petrous bone in neonatal kittens. The internal surface of the otic capsule is lined with periosteum. Fundamentally it is a protective osseous box, which ossifies from numerous centers that ultimately fuse without leaving any sutural demarcation.

Osseous Labyrinth

The osseous labyrinth is incompletely subdivided into three regions: the bony vestibule, three osseous semicircular canals, and the cochlea. The osseous labyrinth houses the membranous labyrinth within it. Perilymph, which is similar to cerebrospinal fluid, is located internal to the osseous labyrinth and external to the membranous labyrinth.

Vestibule

The vestibule is the most spacious cavity of the osseous labyrinth and is pyramidal in shape situated medial to the caudal end of the cochlea. Rostroventrally the vestibule leads into the cochlea; caudodorsally it receives the ends of the osseous semicircular canals. The vestibule opens into the tympanic cavity through the vestibular window.

Semicircular Canals

There are three osseous semicircular canals, anterior, lateral, and posterior, imbedded in the petrous bone caudodorsal to the vestibule. Each describes two thirds of a circle and lies at approxi-

mately right angles to the other two. At one end each becomes dilated into an osseous ampulla, twice as large as the canal. Five apertures from the semicircular canals open into the vestibule, since the nonampullated ends of two canals fuse to form the crus commune.

The relationship of the canals' right angle planes is similar to the three adjoining sides about the corner of a cube. The anterior and posterior semicircular canals lie in nearly vertical planes with the right angle between them opening laterally. The rostrolateral end of the anterior canal and the ventral end of the posterior canal are ampullated while their nonampullated ends fuse to form the crus commune. The lateral semicircular canal is the shortest as it bows in the horizontal plane with its ampulla close to that of the anterior canal. The lateral semicircular canal occupies the same plane as its fellow canal in the opposite ear, although they can subtend as much as a 12 degree difference between each other in the cat. However, the anterior canal of one ear is essentially parallel to the posterior canal of the other, although here again the difference can subtend as much as 14 degrees. This relationship can best be viewed by bringing one corner of a cube against the corner of another while creating right angles without their sides touching each other.

Cochlea

The cochlea is situated in the promontory, the ventral, barrel-shaped elevation of the petrous bone and extends ventrorostrally from the cochlear window. The bony cochlea bears its name because it resembles a snail shell. Overall it is conical in shape with its base lying upon the internal acoustic meatus and its apex directed ventrorostrally and slightly laterally. It consists mainly of a spiral tube, the spiral cochlear canal that makes three turns (in the cat) about a central bony axis, or modiolus. Projecting part way out from the modiolus is a thin, bony plate, the osseous spiral lamina. It winds about the modiolus like the flange on a screw and ends in a hook-like hamulus at the apex of the modiolus. In this way, the osseous canal or tube is partly divided into an upper passage, the scala vestibuli, and a lower passage, the scala tympani, each containing perilymph. The two spaces join at the apex of the cochlea, the helicotrema, where the partitioning spiral lamina ends freely at the hamulus. The osseous labyrinth has three major openings: 1) the vestibular window, normally filled by the stapes, lies between the vestibule and tympanic cavity, 2) the cochlear window lies between the tympanic cavity and the scala tympani space, 3) the cochlear canaliculus, which carries a perilymphatic duct that in turn communicates with subarachnoid space and scala tympani.

Scala Vestibuli

The scala vestibuli is an extension of the space of the vestibule along one surface of the cochlea and contains perilymph. The epithelium lining the scala vestibuli fuses with epithelium of the membranous cochlear duct to form a partition of the two cavities called the vestibular membrane.

Scala Tympani

The scala tympani lies along the opposite side of the cochlea from the scala vestibule and contains perilymph. The epithelium lining the scala tympani fuses with the epithelium lining the cochlear duct to form a partition of the two cavities called the basilar membrane. The scalae tympani and vestibuli communicate at the apex of the cochlea. The scala tympani opens into the tympanic cavity by means of the cochlear window, which is closed by the secondary tympanic membrane.

Membranous Labyrinth

The membranous labyrinth is an interconnecting system of epithelial lined tubes and spaces filled with clear fluid called endolymph. It is contained within the osseous labyrinth. The cochlear duct and the semicircular ducts closely follow the configuration of the similarly named bone-lined channels, the cochlea and semicircular canals. The membranous components of the bony vestibule, rather than conform to their spacious cavity, form into two sacs, the utricle and saccule. Both sacs connect indirectly with each other and also with the cochlear and semicircular ducts.

Utricle

The utricle, occupies the caudodorsal region of the osseous vestibule. Internally, the macula acustica utriculi marks the location of sensory receptors which respond to movement of the surrounding endolymph and where the fibers of the vestibular n. leave. The caudal wall contains the openings of the semicircular ducts and on the rostral wall a slender utriculosaccular duct communicates with the saccule.

Saccule

The saccule is smaller than the utricle. It lies in the rostroventral part of the osseous vestibule. Internally, the macula sacculi is the location of sensory reception that responds to movement of the surrounding endolymph and where fibers of the vestibular n. leave. Ventrally, an opening connects the saccule with the cochlear duct. Caudally the saccule communicates with the utricle.

Semicircular Ducts

Within the bony semicircular canals, run three membranous tubes that open into the utricle and follow closely the configuration of the similarly named bony canals. Each semicircular duct is less than one third the diameter of the containing bony canal, from which it is separated by a large perilymphatic space. Each duct has a dilated end, the membranous ampulla. Each ampulla contains a crista ampullaris where sensory receptors that respond to movement of the fluid are located. Each crista has fibers from the vestibular n.

The semicircular ducts with their crista ampullaris and the utricle and saccule with their maculae constitute the organ for equilibrium. Disturbances of this system will lead to signs of vestibular disease, including vestibular ataxia, circling, head tilt, strabismus and nystagmus.

Cochlear Duct

The epithelial lined and endolymph filled cochlear duct lies within the bony cochlea and spirals within it as a coiled tube between the osseous spiral lamina and the outer bony wall. It lays between the perilymphatic space of the scala vestibuli and scala tympani in the cochlea. It winds through a basal, middle and incomplete apical turn, then ends blindly just beyond the hamulus of the spiral lamina in a blind pouch. It is somewhat triangular in shape on cross section and has a tympanic wall (roof), a vestibular wall (floor) and an outer wall.

The tympanic wall, towards the scala tympani, has a fibrous basilar membrane, reaching from the free border of the spiral lamina to the periosteum that lines the peripheral wall of the osseous cochlear canal. A specialized area of thickened epithelium in the basilar membrane constitutes the spiral organ (of Corti) in which the nerve endings of the cochlear n. terminate. This organ constitutes the peripheral sense organ of hearing. The spiral organ consists of inert supporting cells, shorter sensory hair cells and tectorial membrane.

Damage to these hair cells leads to hearing deficits or loss. Aminoglycoside therapy can lead to drug induced ototoxicity and is a leading cause of iatrogenic hearing loss. White cats with congenital deafness have numerous cochlear abnormalities, including damage in the spiral organ and spiral ganglion.

Nerve fibers from the cochlear division of the vestibulocochlear n. take a complex course, but their terminal branches finally innervate the sensory hair cells.

The vestibular wall, towards the scala vestibuli, consists of the vestibular membrane that passes unsupported from the outer wall of the osseous cochlea to the osseous spiral lamina near its free margin.

Nerve Supply of the Internal Ear

The vestibulocochlear n. (CN VIII) innervates the entire membranous labyrinth. It divides into two distinct nerves, the vestibular and cochlear nn., inside the internal acoustic meatus of the petrous temporal bone. The vestibular ganglion, located within the internal acoustic meatus, consists of bipolar cells whose peripheral fibers pass to the cristae ampullae of the semicircular ducts and to the maculae of the utricle and saccule. These neurons also have central projections (vestibular n.) that enter the brain stem and synapse in the vestibular nuclei and cerebellum. Within the cochlear modiolus, the bipolar cells of the spiral ganglion send dendrites through the spiral lamina to reach the sensory hair cells in the spiral organ, about which they arborize. Central (cochlear n.) projections synapse in the dorsal and ventral cochlear nuclei on the surface of the caudal brain stem.

Plate 11-2

Figure A Left membranous labyrinth, medial view

Figure B Schematic illustration of orientation of left and right semicircular ducts in 3 spatial planes, dorsocaudal view. Ducts in same color block are in the same plane.

Figure C Schematic illustration of cochlear duct, transverse section

Figure D Extraocular muscles, dorsal view

Figure E Anterior globe and adnexa, rostral view

r	Rostral	21	Frontal bone
c	Caudal	22	Zygomatic arch
l	Lateral	23	Bulbus oculi
1	Anterior semicircular duct	24	Lateral rectus m.
2	Lateral semicircular duct	25	M. retractor bulbi
3	Posterior semicircular duct	26	Dorsal rectus m.
4	Crus commune	27	M. levator palpebrae superioris
5	Ampullae of semicircular ducts containing cristae	28	Medial rectus m.
		29	Dorsal oblique m.
6	Utricle with macula	30	Trochlea
7	Endolymphatic duct	31	Zygomatic n.
	7' Endolymphatic sac	32	Infratrochlear n.
8	Utriculosaccular duct	33	Maxillary n.
9	Sacculus with macula	34	Inferior palpebra
10	Cecum vestibulare of cochlear duct	35	Superior palpebra
11	Osseous labyrinth	36	Lateral commissure
12	Scala vestibuli	37	Medial commissure
13	Scala tympani	38	Third eyelid (plica semilunaris) (nictatans)
14	Cochlear duct	39	Deep gland of the third eyelid
15	Vestibular membrane	40	Lacrimal gland
16	Stria vascularis	41	Excretory ducts
17	Spiral ligament	42	Puncta lacrimalis
18	Basilar membrane	43	Lacrimal canaliculi
19	Spiral organ (of Corti)	44	Lacrimal sac
20	Tectorial membrane	45	Nasolacrimal duct

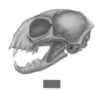

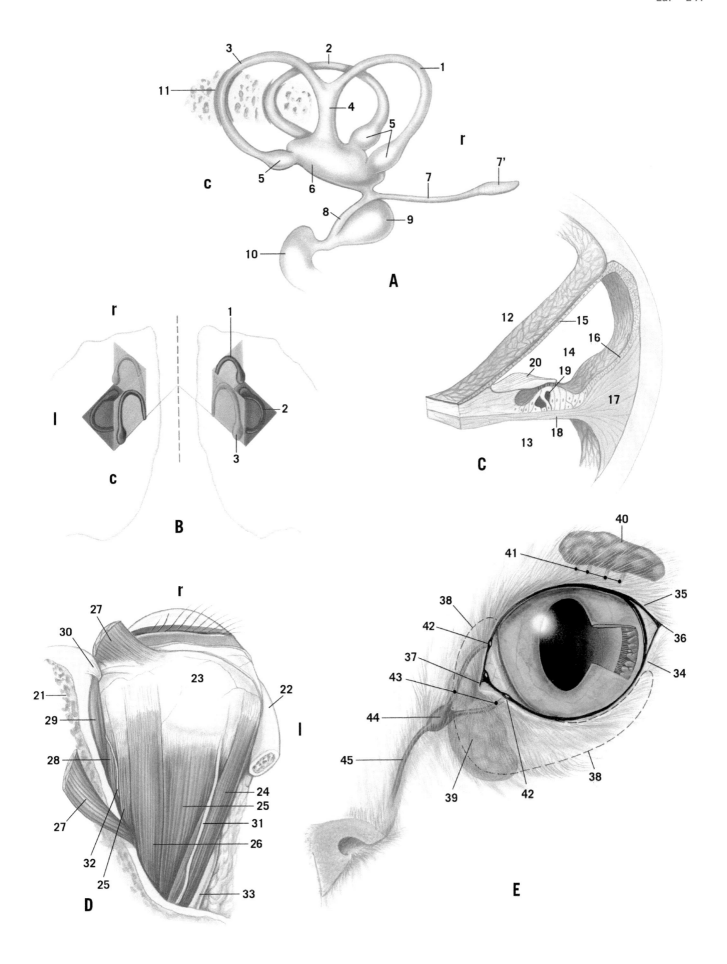

Selected References

1. Anson BJ and Donaldson JA. *Surgical Anatomy of the Temporal Bone.* 4th Ed. New York, Raven Press, 1992.

2. Barone R. *Anatomic Comparee des mammiferes domestiques.* Tome 2 Arthrologie et myologie. Paris, Editions Vogot, 1976.

3. Blevins CE. Studies on the innervation of the stapedia muscle of the cat. *Anat Rec* 149:157, 1964.

4. Durato S. *Submicroscopic Structure of the Inner Ear.* New York, Pergamon Press, 1967.

5. El-Mofty A and El-Serafy S. The ossicular chain in mammals. *Ann. OtoRhino Laryng* 76:903, 1967.

6. Reighard J and Jennings HS. *Anatomy of the Cat,* 3rd Ed. New York, Henry Holt and Company, 1935.

7. Schaller O. Illustrated Veterinary Nomina Anatomica. Stuttgart, Enke Verlag, 1992: 526.

8. Wilson VJ and Jones GM. *Mammalian Vestibular Physiology.* New York, Plenum Press, 1979.

Part 2: Eye

The eyes of the cat are the receptors for the special sense of sight. Each is a living optical instrument that partly mimics the properties of a camera, a hydroelectric plant, and a computer. The eye responds to light in its visual field by controlling the amount of its entry through a shutter-like iris diaphragm: then turbine-like photoreceptors in the retina convert these photons into electrochemical energy. Within the multiple retinal layers, complex processing then occurs similar to the integrated microchip circuits of a computer. This information is then sent to various areas of the brain for development of, and response to, the image.

Orbit

In the cat, the orbit is incomplete in the temporal or dorsotemporal region. This portion is bridged by the orbital ligament. The cat, as a predator, possesses large prominent eyeballs situated well forward in the head. They are positioned with a 10 to 15 degree angle between them resulting in a comparatively large binocular visual field and an extensive panoramic view that varies between 250 and 280 degrees.

Bony Orbit

The bony orbit is formed from six bones: lacrimal, palatine, sphenoid, maxillary, zygomatic, and frontal. Near the rostral border, the lacrimal bone contains the small lacrimal fossa and lacrimal canal. The dorsal limits are defined by the frontal and sphenoid bones. The lateral boundary is defined by the zygomatic and maxillary bones with the orbital ligament bridging the small gap between processes of these bones. The caudal extremity of the orbit is defined by the presphenoid and basisphenoid bones. In the suture between these bones, the large orbital fissure is located. The presphenoid bone contains the optic canal. The basisphenoid bone is pierced by the round and oval foramina. The ventral bony border of the orbit is defined by a thin shelf of maxilla located rostrally in the orbit, just dorsal to the premolar and molar teeth.

Soft Tissue Orbit

The non-bony portion of the orbit consists of two soft tissue regions, the intraperiorbital and extraperiorbital areas. Soft tissue orbit pathology can occur in either area, but rarely in both. The signs of soft tissue orbit disease will differ for each area.

The eyeball, extraocular muscles, lacrimal gland, nerves and most blood vessels of the eye are surrounded by a thin, tough, fascial sheath shaped like an ice cream cone called the periorbital sheath or periorbita. This "cone" is widest rostrally and tapers caudally in a ventromedial direction to surround the optic canal and orbital fissure. Fat is dispersed within the periorbital sheath and separates the extraocular muscles.

The extraperiorbital area is located between the bony orbit and the periorbita and is mainly occupied by muscle, except along the medial bony wall. It is the most common site of soft tissue orbital disease. The ventral extraperiorbital area (floor) is comprised of medial and lateral pterygoid mm. The most rostral extent of the dorsal extraperiorbital region (roof) is partly covered by the frontal bone, while the majority of the roof and the lateral extraperiorbital borders are formed by the m. temporalis. The zygomatic salivary gland lies in the rostrolateral extraperiorbital area.

Extraocular Muscles

The extraocular muscles consist of the mm. rectus dorsalis, rectus lateralis, rectus ventralis, rectus medialis, obliquus dorsalis, obliquus ventralis, and retractor bulbi (with four bellies). (Another muscle within the periorbita, the m. levator palpebrae superioris, is discussed with the muscles of the eyelid.) The function of these muscles is to move the globe within the orbit. The bellies of the m. retractor bulbi are of unequal size, with the ventral pair twice the size of the dorsal pair. Their origin is from the medial wall of the orbital fissure just dorsal to the origin of the ventral rectus m. An imaginary line connecting the insertion points of the m. retractor bulbi onto the eyeball forms a trapezoid. This shape results from one of the two ventral bellies of the m. retractor bulbi inserting ventral to the path of the medial rectus m. while the other is similarly positioned relative to the lateral rectus m. The two dorsal bellies of the m. retractor bulbi insert on either side of path of the dorsal rectus m.

The feline recti mm. make their insertions well posterior to the limbus. The dorsal, medial, and lateral recti mm. originate from the margin of the optic canal. The ventral rectus m. has its origin on the medial wall of the orbital fissure. The lateral rectus m. crosses dorsal to the origin of the ventral rectus m. and in so doing provides a space between the dorsal and lateral recti mm. through which the retractor bulbi m., and several nerves pass into the cone of muscles.

Vessels of the Orbit

The vascular network of arteries and veins which support the orbit and eyeball in the cat is generous, unusual and complicated.

The maxillary a., a terminal branch of the external carotid a., develops into a large vascular plexus called the maxillary rete which gives off most of the orbital arteries. This maxillary rete may be as much or more venous as arterial for a great number of small and large veins drain to it. The maxillary rete is partly extraperiorbital and intraperiorbital. Several arterial branches arise from the rete and the maxillary a. to serve the eye and orbit including the ciliary a., external ethmoidal, zygomatic, lacrimal, muscular, rami retis, and rostral deep temporal aa. The largest artery from the maxillary rete, the ciliary a, hugs the course of the optic n. Before reaching the globe, the ciliary a. divides into many short posterior ciliary aa. Several retinal arteries branch from the short posterior ciliary aa. before passing through the optic disc. Two long posterior ciliary aa. issue directly from the maxillary rete after which they travel rostrally on either side of the optic n. and then on opposite sides of the globe in the horizontal meridian, where they penetrate the sclera and enter the choroid just beyond the equator.

The remaining arteries support the eyelids and orbit as well as extraocular areas. The zygomatic a. arises from the maxillary rete and serves the skin at the lateral commissure. The lacrimal a. also arises from the maxillary rete and supplies the lacrimal gland and combines with branches of the superficial temporal and zygomatic aa. to form the lateral palpebral aa. serving the conjunctiva and eyelids. The external and internal ethmoidal aa. supply the frontal area of the eye. The muscular a., as the name implies, is the main supply to the extraocular muscles, while the rostral deep temporal a. supplies the temporalis m. The ophthalmic a. (corresponding to the internal ophthalmic a. in other animals), is missing in many cats. If present, it originates from the rostral region of the arterial circle, passing with the optic n. through the optic canal to join with the ciliary a. The maxillary a. gives rise to the artery that supplies the third eyelid and the infraorbital a. The large malar a., derived from the infraorbital a., divides into medial palpebral aa. that supply the medial part of the upper and lower eyelid and third eyelid as well as anastomosing with the lateral palpebral aa.

The maxillary rete is drained primarily by the ophthalmic plexus, which lies beside the maxillary a., and by small orbital veins that drain through the orbital fissure and optic canal. The maxillary rete has three main veins draining it from the orbit. The supraorbital v. enters the rete intraperiorbitally and drains the dorsal vortex v. that drains the anterior segment of the eyeball. The other two major veins draining into the rete are the two ventral orbital vv. that drain into the extraperiorbital portion of the rete after having passed through the periorbita first. The lateral ventral orbital vein drains the ventral vortex v. Each vortex vein leaves the globe only a few millimeters from the limbus. These can be easily injured during trauma or surgery to the anterior segment. The posterior ciliary vv. that enter directly into the maxillary rete drain the retinal veins of the globe.

Nerves of the Orbit

The optic n. enters the periorbital cone through the optic canal. The oculomotor (CN III), trochlear (CN IV), ophthalmic (of the trigeminal n. - CN V), and abducens (CN VI) nn. enter the intraperiorbita through the orbital fissure.

Optic Nerve (Cranial Nerve II)

The cat has approximately 193,000 optic nerve axons, which transmit the information gathered by the retina to the brain. The optic n., unlike the other nerves of the orbital region, is enclosed by meninges that are continuous with the meninges covering the brain. The long axons that form the optic n. originate in the ganglion cell layer of the retina and extend uninterrupted, through the optic chiasm and optic tracts to synapse on brain stem nuclei. Most fibers are vision fibers, some are pupillomotor fibers for the pupillary light reflex and others relay general muscle responses to light (e.g., the dazzle reflex). (For more information on these pathways, see the last section of this chapter.)

The segment from the optic disc to the optic chiasm is the optic n. Clinically it can be subdivided by location into ocular, orbital, intracanalicular, and intracranial portions which is useful for localizing the site of pathologic lesions. In the cat, there are three distinct classes of optic n. axons based on their axon diameters. These originate from the three functionally and morphologically distinct types of retinal ganglion cells: X-cells, Y-cells and W-cells. All axons of the ocular portion of the optic n. are non-myelinated as they converge to exit the eyeball at the optic disc. In the cat, all optic n. axons become myelinated posterior to the lamina cribrosa of the sclera. This myelination, along with the meningeal coverings, accounts for the marked increase in optic n. diameter after leaving the eye and entering the periorbita. The different sized fibers are evenly distributed in the optic n.

The orbital segment is excessively long with a mild flexure. The intracanalicular portion (within the optic canal) and intracranial segment are short.

Within the normal feline optic chiasm where the two optic nn. merge, a decussation of about 65% of fibers occurs, with the optic n. axons from the nasal region of the retina crossing to the opposite side, and those from the temporal region of the retina remaining uncrossed as they enter the optic tracts.

Oculomotor Nerve (Cranial Nerve III)

The oculomotor n. is involved in the pupillary light reflex, eyelid movement and ocular motility. The fibers of the oculomotor n. originate from the oculomotor nucleus and parasympathetic nucleus of CN III. The oculomotor n. divides into two rami soon after entering the intraperiorbital space. Injury to the oculomotor n. proximal to the rami can lead to external ophthalmoplegia (ptosis, lateral strabismus with an inability to rotate the globe dorsally, ventrally, or medially, and the presence or absence of a fixed dilated pupil). The dorsal ramus supplies the dorsal rectus and levator palpebrae superioris mm. The ventral ramus supplies the ventral oblique, ventral rectus, and medial rectus mm., and conducts preganglionic parasympathetic fibers to the ciliary ganglion. These parasympathetic fibers are small myelinated fibers concentrated around the periphery of the oculomotor n. making them particularly and preferentially vulnerable to injury. Occasionally a patient is found with normal vision and a fixed dilated pupil secondary to denervation of the oculomotor preganglionic parasympathetic fibers, but without concurrent damage to the oculomotor fibers innervating the extraocular muscles.

Preganglionic parasympathetic fibers of the oculomotor n. synapse on the postganglionic parasympathetic nerve cell bodies, which form the ciliary ganglion. The ciliary ganglion is a small, flattened, ovoid or triangular body located lateral to the optic n. and dorsal to the ventral ramus of the oculomotor n. Two myelinated short ciliary nn. emerge from the rostral ciliary ganglion and contain only postganglionic parasympathetic fibers. The larger, lateral short ciliary n. (malar n.) lies along the lateral surface of the optic n. and the smaller, medial short ciliary n. (nasal n.) lies ventrolaterally to the optic n. until it bifurcates into numerous branches before entering the globe. Both short ciliary nn. are joined by the long ciliary nn. from the nasociliary n. of the ophthalmic n. of CN V. The lateral and medial short ciliary nn. innervate the lateral and medial portions of the iris sphincter m, respectively.

Injury to the pre- or postganglionic parasympathetic axons or the ciliary ganglion leads to internal ophthalmoplegia (fixed dilated pupil).

Trochlear Nerve (Cranial Nerve IV)

The trochlear n. innervates the dorsal oblique m. Trochlear n. injury results in extorsion of the eye as the ventral oblique m. becomes unopposed. Clinically, the dorsal extent of the slit pupil will be rotated temporally as will the dorsal retinal vessels. Central lesions involving the trochlear nucleus produce this strabismus in the contralateral eye, since each trochlear n. crosses to the contralateral side.

Trigeminal Nerve (Cranial Nerve V)

The ophthalmic n. of the trigeminal n. is purely sensory and smaller than the other two branches of CN V. It supplies sensation to the entire eyeball, forehead, upper eyelids, lacrimal gland, and lacrimal drainage system. The sensory innervation of the periocular skin by the ophthalmic n. overlaps with the maxillary n. It enters the intraperiorbital area through the orbital fissure and has several branches.

The frontal n. branches from the ophthalmic n. before leaving the orbital fissure and is sensory to the upper eyelid and the forehead. Once the frontal n. branches, the remaining fibers of the ophthalmic n. become the nasociliary n. Postganglionic sympathetic fibers from the cranial cervical ganglion merge with the nasociliary n. to create a mixed (sensory and postganglionic sympathetic) nerve, which sends a sensory branch curiously through the belly of the lateral rectus m. that then passes near the ciliary ganglion. (In the cat, sympathetic fibers do not traverse the ciliary ganglion.) Further rostrally along the nasociliary n., a variable number of long ciliary nn. branch off and merge with the short ciliary nn. (from the oculomotor n.) before entering the globe. The long ciliary nn. are sensory to the eyeball and conduct the postganglionic sympathetic fibers to the ciliary body and iris dilator m. of the globe. Injury to these sympathetic fibers leads to Horner's syndrome. At its terminus, the nasociliary n. becomes the infratrochlear n. which is sensory to the medial commissure and part of the upper eyelid. Denervation of the nasociliary n. leads to a miotic pupil, upper lid ptosis, and protrusion of the third eyelid. Lesions occurring more distally along the infratrochlear n. lead to ptosis and protrusion of the third eyelid without miosis.

The maxillary n. of the trigeminal n. leaves the cranium via the round foramen and enters the area of the maxillary rete. Immediately after leaving this area, the nerve gives off the zygomatic and lacrimal nn. and continues toward the nose.

The zygomatic n. is sensory to the eyelids near the lateral commissure and the temporal region. Occasionally the lacrimal n. arises from the ophthalmic n. in the cat. The lacrimal n. innervates the lacrimal gland and branches from it continue rostrodorsally to the skin of the area. Abducens Nerve (Cranial Nerve VI). The abducens n. enters intraperiorbital space through the orbital fissure in close approximation with the ophthalmic n., oculomotor n., and trochlear n. The abducens n. sends fibers to the lateral rectus and retractor bulbi mm. Lesions of the abducens n. peripherally usually lead to paralysis of both muscles. With the normal eye fixating in the primary position of gaze, a convergent (medial) strabismus will be seen on the affected side.

Facial Nerve (Cranial Nerve VII)

The pathway for innervation of the lacrimal gland and presumably the gland of the 3rd eyelid originally comes from the parasympathetic nucleus of cranial nerve VII. The preganglionic fibers pass from the facial n. to the major petrosal n. and nerve of the pterygoid canal to synapse on postganglionic neurons in the pterygopalatine ganglion. From here, postganglionic fibers may join the maxillary or ophthalmic nn. to be distributed along with their branches.

Adnexa
Eyelids

The eyelids are covered externally with skin and hair, but lack appreciable cilia. Palpebral conjunctiva lines the inner surface. Along the lid margin, the orifices of the tarsal (Meibomian) gland ducts are in a shallow groove near the center of the lid margin. Each eyelid has one lacrimal puncta, which are openings into the nasolacrimal drainage system, located at the medial commissure posterior to the orifices of the tarsal gland ducts.

Muscles of the Eyelid

The eyelid proper has two muscles, the mm. orbicularis oculi and levator palpebrae superioris. The m. orbicularis oculi originates from the facial musculature while the m. levator palpebrae superioris takes origin from deep within the orbit.

The m. orbicularis oculi consists of two thin bands of muscle fibers, one in each eyelid, parallel to the lid margins and uniting at the commissures. The muscle is innervated by the auriculopalpebral n. of the facial n. (CN VII) and serves to close the eyelid.

The m. levator palpebrae superioris takes origin dorsal to the optic canal, passes dorsal to the medial surface of the dorsal rectus m. and ventral to the lacrimal gland to form a thin tendon of insertion into the margin of the upper eyelid. This muscle is innervated by the oculomotor n. and serves to elevate the upper eyelid. Denervation leads to a slight ptosis.

The m. frontalis is a broad, thin sheet of superficial head muscle that takes origin near the midline, passes laterally, then curves cranially to converge and insert into the upper eyelid, especially near the lateral commissure. It serves to raise the upper eyelid and is innervated by the facial n. The m. retractor anguli oculi lateralis arises from fibers of the m. frontalis and converges to form a narrow band that inserts at the lateral commissure where it unites with the m. orbicularis oculi. It serves to pull the lateral commissure caudally.

Third Eyelid

The third eyelid (plica semilunaris) arises from the periorbita at the medial angle of the orbit and when protruded is large enough to cover the entire anterior surface of the eyeball. Between its conjunctival-lined outer convex and inner concave surfaces lies a supporting, tilted "T" shaped strip of cartilage. The leading edge of the third eyelid is supported by the horizontal part of the "T," while the vertical part extends to the medial angle. The gland of the third eyelid extensively surrounds the base of the cartilage and produces a significant portion of the tear film. On the concave surface, a patch of lymphoid follicles is present.

Passive protrusion of the third eyelid is minimal because of the shallow orbit and weak m. retractor bulbi action. Active protrusion of the third eyelid occurs during different emotional or physical situations and is under the nervous control of the abducens n. This nerve innervates the lateral rectus m., which has a strip of fascia connecting the muscle to the third eyelid.

Retraction of the third eyelid results from medial and ventral smooth muscle sheets arising from the orbital fascia and that are innervated by postganglionic sympathetic nerves. The medial smooth muscle inserts into the upper eyelid and into the dorsal portion of the third eyelid and is supplied by sympathetic nerves that travel by way of the nasociliary n.

The ventral smooth muscle attaches to the lower eyelid and ventral half of the third eyelid and is supplied by postganglionic sympathetic nerves that run with the infraorbital and zygomatic nn. of the maxillary n. Denervation leads to elevation of the lower eyelid (reverse ptosis), and protrusion of the third eyelid without miosis.

Conjunctiva

The bulbar conjunctiva is a thin, vascularized, transparent layer that covers the anterior eyeball from the limbus to the fornix where it is continuous with the palpebral conjunctiva on the inner surface of the eyelids.

Lacrimal Apparatus

The lacrimal apparatus is responsible for tear production from the lacrimal gland, gland of the third eyelid, and accessory lacrimal glands. It is also responsible for tear drainage from the eye to the nasal cavity via the lacrimal puncta and canaliculi, lacrimal sac, nasolacrimal duct, and nasal puncta. The health of the ocular surfaces, the conjunctiva and cornea, are dependent upon a steady secretion of tears and their unimpeded removal by the nasolacrimal drainage apparatus.

The periorbital sheath divides to enclose the large reddish lacrimal gland located in the dorsolateral orbit. The gland is in contact with the zygomatic process of the frontal bone and its anterior edge lies very close to the limbus. It is a rather square, thin, and slightly lobulated and is the major source of tears. These tears enter the dorsal conjunctival sac by numerous microscopic ducts and are then distributed over the cornea by gravity flow and blinking action. The gland of the third eyelid, discussed previously, contributes to the tear production by a significant but lesser degree. Least contribution is made by the accessory lacrimal

glands, which are situated near the eyelid margin and include tarsal glands, ciliary (Moll) glands, and sebaceous (Zeis) glands.

The tears are moved medially toward the dorsal and ventral lacrimal puncta, which lie on the palpebral conjunctiva as slit-like openings near the medial limits of the tarsal gland openings. From the puncta, dorsal and ventral canaliculi lead to a poorly developed dilatation called the lacrimal sac. This sac lies in the lacrimal fossa of the lacrimal bone but in the cat, the most distal part of the sac has no osseous protection medially. From the sac, the nasolacrimal duct passes ventrally, then rostrally in a bony canal on the medial surface of the maxilla and then into a soft tissue canal in the nose to open into the ventral meatus of the nasal cavity.

Bulbus Oculi

The bulbus oculi (eyeball) of the cat extensively fills the rostral orbit and cannot be easily displaced to any direction by finger pressure. The anterior-posterior[a] axis is slightly longer than the vertical or horizontal axes. The eyeball is composed of three tissue layers, fibrous, vascular, and nervous, which enclose the internal chambers and the lens. The eyeball is internally partitioned by the iris into the anterior and posterior chambers. The posterior chamber is separated from the vitreous chamber by the lens and its zonular ligaments.

"Fundus" is a term often used in ophthalmology that refers to the various structures of the posterior hemisphere of the eyeball that can be viewed through the normal cornea, pupil, and lens. This would include the retina, retinal vessels, optic disc, tapetum lucidum, and non-tapetal choroid.

Fibrous Tunic

The fibrous tunic is the outermost, enclosing connective tissue layer of the three ocular layers. It consists of the clear, transparent cornea anteriorly and the white, opaque sclera posteriorly. The sclera meets the cornea in a transition zone (limbus) which can be identified by a whitish zone or band.

Cornea

Typical of nocturnal animals, the large feline cornea comprises about 30% of the fibrous tunic of the eyeball. The cornea is slightly conical and has the strongest refracting surface of the eye with a steeper curvature than the sclera. It is almost circular in shape but on average the vertical diameter is slightly less than the horizontal diameter. The periphery is slightly thicker than the corneal center.

The cornea of the cat consists of four histological layers: 1) anterior epithelium, 2) stroma, 3) posterior limiting membrane (Descemet's membrane), and 4) posterior epithelium (endothelium). The anterior epithelium consists of the basal lamina (basement membrane), and several layers of epithelial cells. The bulk of the cornea is the stroma that is composed of collagenous fibers arranged in lamellae, fibroblasts (keratocytes), and ground substance. The posterior limiting membrane is actually the exaggerated basement membrane of the posterior epithelium.

[a]On the eyeball and certain associated areas, the directional terms anterior, posterior, superior, and inferior are used.

Although clinically an ulcer down to the level of the posterior limiting membrane can behave with a degree of elasticity when it bulges anteriorly into the ulcerated defect, the membrane consists of only fine collagen fibrils. The posterior epithelium is comprised of a single layer of cells lining the inner cornea and its main function is to keep the cornea detergescenced (clear). Normally, there are no vessels contained within the cornea but it has a rich sensory innervation.

Sclera

The sclera is a viscoelastic tissue that helps maintain the shape of the eye, but its elasticity diminishes with age because of changes in its collagen. Its thickness varies considerably. The posterior segment is quite thin along with localized thin areas anteriorly where the extraocular muscles make their insertions. In general, the sclera is white in the thicker parts, but dark in the posterior and limbal region. Posteriorly, the dark color is due to the choroidal pigment showing through it, while pigment in the limbal region creates a dark perilimbal ring. These normal dark areas can be confused with pigmented tumors, especially in the enucleated eye.

A venous plexus is located within the sclera and it receives aqueous humor draining from the internal chambers of the globe. The plexus is also connected with veins draining the more internal layers of the eyeball. The scleral venous plexus consist of two to four large midscleral vessels that course the full circumference of the eyeball. They communicate anteriorly with the anterior ciliary veins and with the conjunctival veins via the limbal venular loops; they communicate freely posteriorly with the vortex veins draining the choroid. The scleral venous plexus receives afferent channels superficially from the superficial episcleral network at the limbus and deeply from channels draining the iridocorneal angle, namely the trabecular veins and collecting veins.

Posteriorly, the sclera is punctured by a cluster of small openings, the area cribrosa, that allow the optic n. fibers to exit the globe.

Vascular Tunic

The middle layer of the eye is known as the vascular tunic, uveal tract, or uvea. It consists of the iris anteriorly, the choroid posteriorly and between, the ciliary body. The vascular tunic contains the principal blood vessels and non-optical nerves of the eye. Its function is largely nutritive.

Iris

The iris is the most anterior structure of the vascular tunic. It forms a thin and movable diaphragm between the anterior and posterior chambers and functions to control the amount of light entering the eye and the degree of spherical aberration.

The iris surface is divided into two zones, the anulus iridis major (peripheral ciliary zone) and anulus iridis minor (central pupillary zone). Rudiments of the fetal pupillary membrane sometimes can be seen originating from the iris postnatally as thin pigmented

strands. The thinnest portion of the iris occurs at the extreme iris periphery that gives rise to the pectinate ligament structure. The anulus iridus minor also has a sinuous, circumferential artery known as the major arterial circle. This vessel is derived from branches of the long posterior ciliary aa. after they enter the eye at 9 and 3 o'clock positions. Each branches dorsally and ventrally and anastomoses to complete the circle. The central posterior aspect of the iris normally rests against the anterior lens surface.

The free, unattached border of the iris forms the pupil near the center of the iris. The pupil is lined posteriorly by a pigmented ruff that is the extension of the nervous layer.

The anterior surface of the iris of an adult cat is typically golden yellow or greenish yellow. Blue irides are common in kittens but often change later. The anterior surface of the iris is covered by a modified layer of stromal cells. Iris freckles are occasionally seen in the feline iris and should be critically differentiated from diffuse iris melanoma.

Along the ciliary zone of the posterior iris, radial folds (iridic plicae) extend to the ciliary body. The posterior surface of the iris is lined by two layers of heavily pigmented epithelium derived from the nervous layer. The epithelial layer closest to the iris has a basilar smooth muscle portion that forms the iris dilator m. extending radially from near the iris sphincter m. to near the ciliary margin. The dilator m. of the cat is poorly developed on the vertical meridian, but is well developed on the horizontal meridian. Contraction of the muscle creates a circular, dilated pupil and is antagonistic to the sphincter m. The dilator muscle is innervated by postganglionic sympathetic nerves from the cranial cervical ganglion.

The sphincter m. surrounds the pupil near the pupil margin and is oriented vertically. The sphincter m., which is the stronger, produces a vertical slit during contraction. This muscle is innervated by the short ciliary nn. (malar and nasal nn.), which are postganglionic parasympathetic fibers from the ciliary ganglion.

Pupillary dysfunction serves as a clinical indicator for the presence of neurologic or ophthalmic disease. Denervation of one short ciliary n. will lead to the pupillary abnormality known as D-shaped or reverse D-shaped pupil. Denervation of the iris dilator m. anywhere along the nerve impulse pathway, will lead to a miosis along with other signs of Horner's syndrome.

The sphincter and dilator mm. react pharmacologically to various substances in specific ways that are used in therapy, diagnosis and prognosis.

Ciliary Body

The ciliary body is the midportion of the vascular tunic lying between the iris and the choroid and is rather small in the cat. It is divided into anterior ciliary processes (pars plicata), and posterior ciliary ring or pars plana. In the cat there are about 76 major ciliary processes and an equal number of smaller minor processes in between. These processes produce most of the aqueous humor. The ciliary ring is the flat, posterior portion of the ciliary body extending from the posterior termination of the ciliary processes to the level of the peripheral termination of the optical retina (ora serrata). The smooth muscle that helps give shape to the ciliary body, the ciliary m., is weak in the cat and accounts for the poor accommodation ability in this species. Contraction of the ciliary m. causes relaxation of the lens zonules, which allows the lens to change shape. Ciliary m. contraction also opens the iridocorneal angle and thereby increases drainage of aqueous humor.

Choroid

The posterior portion of the vascular tunic is the choroid. The choroid is highly vascular and can be compared to erectile tissue as it changes in response to blood volume. The choroid, proceeding from internal to external layers, consists of: 1) the basal complex, 2) choriocapillaris, 3) tapetum lucidum, 4) stroma containing large vessels, and 5) the suprachoroid. The basal complex separates the retina from the choroid and is a poorly developed thin membrane in the cat.

The choriocapillaris, derived from the fine branching of the short posterior ciliary aa., is a single layer of capillaries between the tapetum lucidum and the pigmented retinal epithelium, or in the absence of a tapetum lucidum, between the pigmented retinal epithelium and the choroidal stroma.

The feline tapetum lucidum is located in the dorsal one-half of the fundus within the vascular layer and extends nearly twice as far nasally as temporally. It is this structure that enhances nocturnal vision by reflecting light that creates the eye shine. The tapetal-nontapetal junction is irregular and not well defined. In the peripheral nontapetal region, the fundus is a patchy dark red color. In both pigmented and non-pigmented animals, the tapetum lucidum is granular and yellow to green in color. Occasionally, the tapetum lucidum is focally or diffusely missing. In such instances, the underlying choroidal pigment is revealed or, if choroidal pigment is lacking, the radial pattern of the choroidal vasculature is seen against a background of the yellowish sclera. The feline tapetum lucidum is cellular, consisting of rectangular cells histologically, and is many cell layers deep. It is thickest in its central region, and gradually reduces towards the periphery, until it is replaced by regular choroidal stroma.

The stroma consists of large numbers of vessels with heavily pigmented strands of connective tissue separating the vessels. The arteries in the stroma are branches of the short posterior ciliary aa. that enter the globe around the optic n. and supply the optic n., retina, and the choroid. Anteriorly, branches of the short posterior ciliary aa. anastomose with branches of the long posterior ciliary aa. The veins of the stroma anastomose freely and communicate anteriorly with the vortex vv. and the anterior ciliary vv. via the scleral venous plexus.

The suprachoroid is the transition between the choroid and sclera. The long ciliary nn. (sensory and sympathetic fibers) course in the suprachoroidal space in the horizontal meridian.

Nervous Layer

The third and innermost layer of the eyeball is an extension of

the central nervous system. The embryonic optic cup is a double layer of neuroepithelium. These two layers are continuous with each other at the anterior edge of the cup and will ultimately line the posterior surface of the iris, and the internal surfaces of the ciliary body and choroid. The outer epithelium of the nervous layer becomes the stratum pigmentosum (one layer) and the inner epithelium becomes the stratum nervosum (up to 9 layers). "Retinal detachments" generally occur between these strata.

Stratum Pigmentosum

The stratum pigmentosum (pigmented retinal epithelium or PRE) develops from the outer portion of the optic cup; it therefore lies closest to the vascular layer. The PRE contains a large amount of melanin, which accounts for much of the dark color seen when viewing the nontapetal fundus. In the area of the tapetum lucidum, the PRE does not contain pigment (despite its name) and is optically clear to allow the fundic view of the tapetum lucidum (through all nervous layer thickness). The PRE will continue anteriorly over the internal surface of the ciliary body and posterior surface of the iris. The basilar part of the RPE on the posterior iris is modified to form the iris dilator m.

Stratum Nervosum

The stratum nervosum develops from the inner layer of the optic cup. Most of the stratum nervosum is the sensory or optical retina- the actual light receptors, and transmitting neurons. The optical retina increases in thickness from its thinnest point in the periphery at the ora serrata,[b] to its thickest portion near the optic disc. The nerve fibers from the ganglion cell layer of the optical retina are responsible for most of this increased thickening as the axons converge toward the optic disc to exit the eye. From the external portion of the optical retina, the rod and cone layer, photons of light are converted to electrochemical energy and then processed and relayed to the bipolar cells, and finally to the ganglion cell layer and the axon filled nerve fiber layer. The ganglion cells are the nerve cell bodies of the optic n. axons.

The area centralis is a part of the sensory retina where there are increased numbers of cones in the receptor layer. This is located slightly dorsolateral to the optic disc. (The density of rods throughout the retina is always greater than cones.)

As the pupil limits the amount of light that enters the eye, there is also a limit as to how far anteriorly optical retina is needed. At this point the multilayered optical retina will be reduced to a single layer of neuroepithelium. The circumferential line at this reduction in layers is called the ora serrata. Anterior to the ora serrata, the innermost epithelium of the nervous layer lines the pigmented retinal epithelium (also of the nervous layer).

The double layer of epithelium (from strata pigmentosum and nervosum) lining the internal surface of the ciliary body and the posterior surface of the iris can be referred to as the pars ciliaris retinae and pars iridica retinae, respectively.

As indicated earlier, the optic disc is the point where the fibers of the ganglion cell layer converge and leave the posterior globe.

[b]The term ora serrata is listed in the *Nomina Anatomica Veterinaria*, but in domestic mammals, this structure is not actually serrated as in human beings.

Fundoscopically, the cat's optic disc lies slightly temporal and ventral to the posterior pole of the eye and histologically is usually located completely within the tapetum lucidum of the choroid. The disc is round, small and unmyelinated, with a color range from grey to beige. The disc may be partially or completely encircled by a pigmented ring or less frequently, by a zone of hyperreflectivity.

The retinal vessels at or near the optic disc margin appear as a crown of ciliary arteries while leaving the central portion of the disc free of blood vessels. In a small number of cats, a vestigial central retinal artery may give rise to one or more of the major vessels from the center of the nerve head. Three major arterioles start from the disc margin and run dorsally, ventromedially and ventrolaterally. A larger, less tortuous venule accompanies each arteriole. The vein always lies over (internal to) the artery at the crossings (viewed fundoscopically). Lesser sized arterioles, radiating outward from the disc margin, complete the arteriolar crown. Although the area centralis is considered an avascular zone, a few thin blood vessels run to the area centralis. Within the retina, the retinal vessels are located in the superficial part of the nerve fiber layer.

Lens and Zonular Fibers

The lens is a transparent, biconvex structure, located posterior to the iris and suspended from the ciliary processes by zonular fibers. Anteriorly the lens is in contact with the pupillary portion of the iris. Posteriorly, it fits into a depression of the anterior vitreous surface, the patellar (hyaloid) fossa, and is firmly bound to the anterior vitreous face.

The lens consists of a capsule, epithelium, and lens fibers. The capsule is the exaggerated basal lamina of the epithelium and surrounds the lens. The capsule thickness varies, being thinnest at the posterior pole. The epithelium lies deep to the anterior and equatorial capsule. The posterior epithelium disappears as it is utilized to form the embryonic primary lens fibers.

The lens increases in size throughout life. Cells of the epithelium multiply around the equator, and as this occurs, those most recently formed become elongated. Elongation results from the anterior part of the cell extending anteriorly beneath the lens capsule and the posterior part extending posteriorly creating a U-shaped cell with its nucleus near the equator. The extensions of adjacent cells unite with each other at suture lines that have the form of a Y, the anterior Y being erect and the posterior one being inverted. These are seen clinically with transillumination of the lens and can be distinguished throughout life. In the postnatal kitten the anterior and posterior Y sutures lie beneath the capsule and on the surface of the fetal nucleus. The Y suture then become a good landmark in later life for slit-lamp determination of the time of onset of developmental lens opacities (cataracts). All newly formed cells are slightly longer than the preceding ones, accounting for the increase in the size of the lens up to adult life.

The zonules are the suspensory ligaments of the lens. They appear as fibers enclosed in a gel-like sheet which extend from the valleys between the ciliary processes to a narrow zone anterior and posterior to the lens equator. The zonules are separated from the anterior vitreous surface by a potential space (canal of Petit). It is through this space, that we clinically see an anterior prolapse of vitreous humor into the posterior chamber with subsequent passage through the pupil into the anterior chamber. This can be an early indication of an impending lens luxation.

Chambers of the Bulbus Oculi

The interior of the eye is partially divided by the iris and lens into three chambers-anterior, posterior, and vitreous. The anterior chamber is located between the cornea and iris and contains aqueous humor. The posterior chamber is between the iris and lens and also contains aqueous humor. These two chambers communicate via the pupil. The vitreous chamber is located between the lens and the posterior globe and is reduced to a potential space occupied by the vitreous body.

The aqueous humor of the anterior and posterior chambers is produced by the ciliary body and released into the posterior chamber. It then normally flows through the pupil to the anterior chamber. Absorption of the aqueous humor occurs at the iridocorneal angle.

The iridocorneal angle includes those structures associated with the base of the iris, anterior ciliary body, inner peripheral cornea, and inner anterior sclera. Therefore it can be seen to lie in the periphery of the anterior chamber under the opaque limbus and extending circumferentially. Impaired outflow of aqueous humor through this angle can lead to glaucoma.

The pectinate ligaments located at the angle in the cat consist of two rows of long thin strands that attach the base of the iris to the inner peripheral cornea (i.e., posterior limiting membrane) and have numerous lateral connections with adjacent fibers. Behind the second or accessory row lies a more complex network of fibers called the uveal or ciliary trabecular meshwork, which in the cat are more numerous and finer than the pectinate ligaments. These arise from the base of the ciliary body and insert posterior to the pectinate ligaments on the cribriform ligament (corneoscleral trabecular meshwork), which is the anterior extension of the longitudinal ciliary m. The ciliary cleft is the space formed by the cribriform ligament on the outer side and the base of the iris and ciliary body on the inner side. The pectinate ligaments and uveal trabecular meshwork are located within this cleft. Trabecular veins (i.e., capillaries) drain the cribriform ligament which than drain into the larger scleral venous plexus.

The vitreous chamber is normally occupied by a vitreous body, which in turn is mostly a gel-like structure. The vitreous is the largest single structure in the eye. Its anatomical position and large volume enables it to provide metabolic and structural support for the ocular tissues, especially the lens and retina, and to assist in the maintenance of the intraocular pressure.

The vitreous hydrogel contains 99% water with a specific gravity only slightly higher than that of water. It can be divided into three distinct components based on embryologic development. The primary vitreous develops first and consists of the hyaloid a. system that regresses with postnatal maturation. In the young eye remnants of it can be visualized. The neuroectodermally derived secondary vitreous forms around the primary vitreous and is the heavy, large volume gel of the mature eyeball. The tertiary vitreous is the zonular fibers of the lens. When referring to the vitreous as an anatomical structure, it includes the primary and secondary vitreous only.

The vitreous body is irregularly opposed to the lens and retina with separating spaces and areas of firm and weak attachments. The vitreous base is the firm attachment of the vitreous near the ora serrata. The other firm attachment, the ligamentum hyaloideo-capsulare, binds the anterior vitreous to the posterior lens capsule. Posteriorly, the vitreous firmly attaches to the edge of the optic n. The peripheral portion of the vitreous, the cortex, is mainly fluid in the cat and is weakly attached to the internal limiting membrane of the retina. The hyaloid canal represents the remnant of the primary vitreous with its vessel system and appears as an undulating tube that extends from the anterior vitreous face behind the lens to the optic disc. The anterior insertion of the hyaloid a. remnant within hyaloid canal can present as a dense, white, small dot often with a cork screw tail. It is clinically visible on the anterior vitreous face (anterior hyaloid membrane) just posterior to the lens and can be mistaken for a cataract. Congenital abnormalities of the vitreous can occur and usually involve the primary vitreous. The hyaloid a. may persist postnatally and contain blood, or it may appear as a cord or fine thread of vascular tissue accompanied by fibrous and glial elements.

Optic Nerve Pathways

All nerve impulses involved in visual perception, responses, or reflexes must travel in the optic n., optic chiasm, and optic tract initially. The medium size X cell axons within the optic n./tract have slower conduction velocities than the Y cells, and project to the pretectal nuclei. The thickest fibers arise from Y cells and have rapid conduction, and project to the dorsal nucleus of the lateral geniculate body and the rostral colliculus. The W ganglion cells have the thinnest fibers, very slow axonal conduction velocities, and project to the rostral colliculus. In contrast to the optic n., a striking segregation of fibers according to diameter occurs in the optic tract. The optic tracts of normal cats contain both crossed (nasal retina) and uncrossed (temporal retina) fibers, which become segregated on their way to synapse in brain stem nuclei. The deepest part of the tract is occupied by oldest X cells, while the youngest Y cells are in the most superficial part of the tract. The optic tract fibers that synapse in the lateral geniculate body have the same percentage of crossed and uncrossed fibers as in the optic chiasm.

Pupillary Light Reflex

The pupillary light reflex consists of a three neuron afferent pathway and a two neuron efferent pathway linked in a chain-like fashion. Those afferent optic n./tract axons that subserve pupillomotor function travel in the brachium of the rostral colliculus and enter the pretectal nuclei to synapse on the pretectal neurons. As majority of the optic n. axons for pupillomotor function that come from the nasal retina will cross at the optic chiasm, they synapse on contralateral pretectal nucleus. Axons from each pretectal nucleus carrying this impulse subsequently cross in the caudal commissure to the contralateral parasympathetic nucleus of the cranial nerve III (anteromedian nucleus, formerly thought to be Edinger-Westphal nucleus). A small number of nasal retinal axons in the optic n. will not cross at the chiasm but synapse on ipsilateral pretectal neurons that in turn project their axons to the to the ipsilateral parasympathetic nucleus of CN III.

The optic n. axons from the temporal retina do not cross at the optic chiasm but do project to the ipsilateral pretectal nucleus. However, most of these temporal retinal optic n. fibers synapse on pretectal neurons whose axons then cross in the caudal commissure to the contralateral parasympathetic nucleus of the cranial nerve III. The remaining few temporal retinal optic n. axons that do not cross at the optic chiasm synapse on pretectal neurons that project to the ipsilateral parasympathetic nucleus of the cranial nerve III.

The effect that a lesion has on the non-decussating efferent arm of the pupillary light reflex was discussed under the oculomotor n. previously. Clinically, the result of this neuroanatomic scheme for the entire light reflex can be demonstrated by applying a very strong focused light to one eye. The direct light reflex response will be more intense (greater miosis on the side receiving the light) than in the fellow eye, thereby creating a physiologic anisocoria. This neuroanatomic pathway also explains why a unilateral injury to the prechiasmal portion of the optic n. leads to pathologic anisocoria, a positive swinging flashlight test, and the more dilated pupil on the affected side.

Geniculocalcarine Pathway (Conscious Vision Pathway)

Optic n., chiasm, and tract axons destined for conscious vision enter the lateral geniculate body and synapse there. The geniculocalcarine tract extends from nerve cell bodies of the lateral geniculate body to the visual area in the occipital lobe. It contains all the visual fibers of that side and their axons form the optic radiation of the internal capsule.

Rostral Colliculus Pathway

A majority of the optic tract fibers of the cat originate from the contralateral eye and synapse on nuclei of the rostral colliculus. The rostral colliculus receives inputs from and generates outputs to various brain stem nuclei and cortical areas. These pathways serve to orient the body to visual stimuli.

Plate 11-3

Figure A   Schematic illustration showing 3 major tunics and internal structures of the globe, sagittal section

Figure B   Structures of the iridocorneal angle, sagittal section, anterolateral view

Figure C   Position and orientation of iris sphincter m. (right); dilated pupil (middle); "D-pupil" appearance (left) as a result of denervation to dilator mm. on one side of pupil

Figure D   Fundoscopic view of posterior globe

Figure E   Schematic illustration of neural pathways for pupillary light reflex, conscious vision pathway, and sympathetic pathway to the iris

1-2	Fibrous tunic
1	Cornea
2	Sclera
3-5	Vascular tunic
3	Iris
4	Ciliary body
5	Choroid
6-9	Nervous tunic
6a	Visual retina
6b	Pigmented retinal epithelium
7	Ora ciliaris retinae
8	Pars ciliaris retinae
9	Pars iridica retinae
10	Lens
11	Zonulary fibers
12	Anterior chamber
13	Posterior chamber
14	Vitreous chamber
15	Hyaloid canal
16	Limbus
17	Pectinate ligament
18	Scleral venous plexus
19	Pupillary margin
20	Major ciliary process
21	Ciliary mm.
22	Iris sphincter m. orientation
23	Tapetum lucidum
24	Nontapetal region
25	Retinal vessels
26	Optic disc

27-32	Conscious vision pathway
27	Optic n.
28	Optic chiasm
29	Optic tract
30	Lateral geniculate nucleus
31	Geniculocalcarine tract (within optic radiation of internal capsule)
32	Cortex of occipital lobe
27-29, 33-38	Pupillary light reflex
33	Pretectal nucleus
34	Parasympathetic nucleus of cranial nerve III
35	Oculomotor n. (contains preganglionic parasympathetic fibers)
36	Ciliary ganglion of cranial nerve III
37	Short ciliary n. (postganglionic parasympathetic fibers)
38	Iris constrictor mm.
39-46	Sympathetic pathway
39	Tectotegmentospinal tract
40	T1-T3 Spinal cord segments
41	Rami communicantes of T1-T3 spinal nn.
42	Thoracic sympathetic trunk
43	Vagosympathetic trunk
44	Cranial cervical ganglion
45	Postganglionic sympathetic fibers
46	Iris dilator mm.

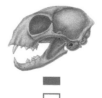

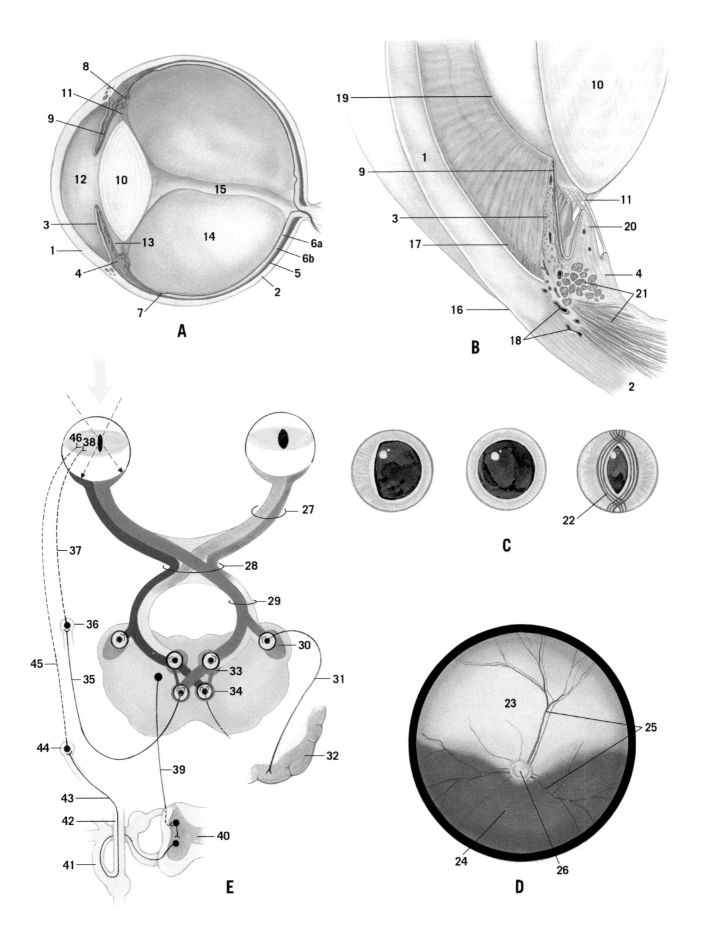

Selected References

1. Gelatt K. *Veterinary Ophthalmology,* 3rd Ed. Philadelphia, Lippincott, Willians & Wilkens, 1999.

2. Getty R. Sisson and Grossman's *The Anatomy of the Domestic Animals.* 5th Ed. Vol 2. Philadelphia, WB Saunders, 1975.

3. McClure RC, Dallman MJ and Ganett PG. *Cat Anatomy.* Philadelphia, Lea & Febiger, 1973.

4. *Noller C, Henninger W, Gronemeyer DH, Hirschberg RM, Budras KD.* Computed tomography-anatomy of the normal feline nasolacrimal drainage system. Vet Radiol Ultrasound. 2006 Jan-Feb;47(1):53-60.

5. Prince JH, Diesem CD, Eglitis I, Ruskell GL. *Anatomy and Histology of the Eye and Orbit in Domestic Animals.* Springfield, IL, Charles C. Thomas, 1960.

6. Schaller O. Illustrated Veterinary Nomina Anatomica. Stuttgart, Enke Verlag, 1992:510.

Index

anatomy of, 174-175
urinary functions of, 172-173

L

Labial granuloma, 154
Lacrimal apparatus, 246
Lacrimal gland, 243
    innervation of, 245
Lacrimal puncta, 245
Lacrimal sac, 246
Lactiferous ducts, 19
Langerhans cells, 13
Lanugo hair, 10
Laryngeal muscles, intrinsic, 48-49
Laryngeal nerve, 141
Laryngopharynx, 155
    in respiratory function, 139
Laryngospasm, 139-140
Larynx
    innervation of, 141
    lymphoid tissue in, 124
    musculature of, 140, 142-143
    in respiratory system, 138-141
Lateral cutaneous femoral nerve, 217
Lens, 249
Levator palpebrae superioris muscle, 245
Limbs
    lymph nodes of, 120
    pelvic, 35
        bones of, 38-39
        examination of, 3
        innervation of, 222-223
        muscle attachments sites of, 76-77
        muscles of, 74-75
            extrinsic, 66-67
            intrinsic, 72-73
            superficial and deep, 70-71, 74-75
        venous return of, 107
        vessels of, 106-109
    thoracic, 34-35
        bones of, 34-35, 36-37
        innervation of, 220-221
        muscle attachments sites of, 76-77
        muscles of, 60-61
            intrinsic, 60-61, 64-65
            superficial, 56-57
        vasculature of, 98-99
Lipids
    of skin surface, 12
    synthesis and mobilization of, 166
Lips, 154
    examination of, 3
    sebaceous glands of, 14
Liver
    anatomy of, 168-169
    blood vessels of, 100-101, 104-105
    digestive functions of, 166-167
    round ligament of, 166
Long thoracic nerve, 216
Longissimus muscles, 49
Lumbar nerves, caudal, 218-219
Lumbar vertebrae, 30
Lumbosacral plexus, 213, 222-223
    formation of, 218-219

functions of nerves of, 217
Lung fluke, 147
Lungs
    anatomy and function of, 145-151
    blood vessels of, 146-147
    examination of, 3
    innervation of, 146
    parasites of, 147
Lungworm, 145
Luteinizing hormone, 133
Luteotropin releasing factor, 133
Lymph nodes, 117
    abdominal, 118-119, 121
    function of, 117
    of head and neck, 120
    infection and, 117
    of limbs and trunk, 120
    location of, 126-127
    peripheral, 122-123
    splenic, 126-127
    thoracic, 118-119, 121
Lymphadenopathy, 117
Lymphatic vessels, 15, 116
    cisterna chyli, 117
    thoracic duct, 117
    tracheal trunks, 116
    visceral and lumbar trunks, 117
Lymphoid system
    functions of, 116
    primary organs of, 116
    secondary organs of, 116-127
Lymphoid tissue, aggregated, 124

M

Malleus, 233
Mammary glands, 18-19
    of non-lactating and lactating queen, 20-21
    tumors of, 19
    vascularization of, 19
Mandible, 25, 28-29
Mandibular nerve, 207
Manus, 36-37
    arterial supply to, 96-97
    muscles of, 64-65
    superficial musculature and tendons of, 68-69
Mast cells, 13
Mastication, muscles of, 48
Mastitis, 19
Maxillary artery, 243
Maxillary nerve, 207
Maxillary rete, 244
Mechanoreceptors, 15
Median nerve, 216
Megacolon, 163
Melanin, 11
Melanocytes, 13
Membranous labyrinth, 238-239
    anatomy of, 240-241
    innervation of, 239
Menace response, 2
Meninges, 194
Meningioma, 194
Meningitis, 93
Mesencephalon, 196

9781591610441